Public Communication in the Time of COVID-19

Public Communication in the Time of COVID-19

Perspectives from the Communication Discipline on the Pandemic

Edited by

Jim A. Kuypers

LEXINGTON BOOKS
Lanham • Boulder • New York • London

Published by Lexington Books
An imprint of The Rowman & Littlefield Publishing Group, Inc.
4501 Forbes Boulevard, Suite 200, Lanham, Maryland 20706
www.rowman.com
86-90 Paul Street, London EC2A 4NE, United Kingdom

Copyright © 2022 by The Rowman & Littlefield Publishing Group, Inc.

All rights reserved. No part of this book may be reproduced in any form or by any electronic or mechanical means, including information storage and retrieval systems, without written permission from the publisher, except by a reviewer who may quote passages in a review.

British Library Cataloguing in Publication Information Available

Library of Congress Cataloging-in-Publication Data

Names: Kuypers, Jim A., editor.
Title: Public communication in the time of COVID-19 : perspectives from the communication discipline on the pandemic / edited by Jim A. Kuypers.
Description: Lanham : Lexington Books, [2022] | Includes bibliographical references and index. | Summary: "This edited collection focuses on how public communication practices and the communication discipline were impacted by the 2020–2022 COVID-19 Pandemic. By discussing a wide range of issues from nine disciplinary positions, ultimately, they are able to reveal key insights about the relationship between the pandemic and public human communication"— Provided by publisher.
Identifiers: LCCN 2022029585 (print) | LCCN 2022029586 (ebook) | ISBN 9781793643667 (cloth) | ISBN 9781793643681 (paper) | ISBN 9781793643674 (epub)
Subjects: LCSH: COVID-19 Pandemic, 2020– , in mass media. | COVID-19 Pandemic, 2020—Influence. | Communication in public health.
Classification: LCC P96.C69 P83 2022 (print) | LCC P96.C69 (ebook) | DDC 302.209/052—dc23/eng/20220815
LC record available at https://lccn.loc.gov/2022029585
LC ebook record available at https://lccn.loc.gov/2022029586

To all the victims of COVID-19

Contents

Acknowledgments ix

Introduction xi
   Jim A. Kuypers

Chapter 1: Digital Rhetoric and the COVID-19 Pandemic 1
   Amber Davisson and Michelle Gibbons

Chapter 2: Journalism Framing in (Times of) Crisis: The Inevitability of Poor Reporting During the COVID-19 Pandemic 23
   Michael Horning and Jim A. Kuypers

Chapter 3: The Politicization of Protests and Protection: The Major Free Speech Issues during COVID-19 Pandemic 55
   Benjamin Medeiros, Ann E. Burnette, Rebekah L. Fox, and David R. Dewberry

Chapter 4: Confronting the Coronavirus: How Public Relations Can Foster Trust during Crisis 81
   Nneka Logan and Chelsea Woods

Chapter 5: This Just Got Real: Implications of the COVID-19 Pandemic on Sport Communication 111
   Brandi Watkins

Chapter 6: Public Address in a Time of Crisis 137
   Robert C. Rowland, Justin W. Kirk, and Michael Eisenstadt

Chapter 7: Health Communication Research and Social Implications during the COVID-19 Pandemic 167
   YoungJu Shin, Yu Lu, and Shristi Bhochhibhoya

Chapter 8: Religious Communication in the Age of COVID-19 189
  Dennis D. Cali

Chapter 9: "Saturday Nite Is Dead" at Least for a While: Changes in Popular Culture Theory during a Time of Crisis 213
  David Nelson and Kimberly Kulovitz

Index 225

About the Editor and Contributors 237

Acknowledgments

I thank my family for their unreserved and continual support of my writing. It is with gratitude that I mention Virginia Tech, which paid my salary and also funded library services such as interlibrary loan and EBSCOhost, all absolutely necessary to the completion of this project. The value Virginia Tech places on research allows projects such as this book to be undertaken and completed.

I also wish to acknowledge the encouragement and strong support of the chapter authors in this volume. Their hard work and positive attitude coming out of the pandemic was greatly appreciated. Additionally, thank you to Nicolette Amstutz, my editor at Lexington Books.

Introduction

Jim A. Kuypers

The ongoing COVID-19 pandemic, which as of this writing has moved beyond the two-year mark, has touched all of us in various ways. The impacts have been profound, encompassing the economic, social, personal, cultural, political, religious, and physical aspects of our human existence. All of these areas, however disparate at first glance, are united by the simple fact that they need effective communication to function well. This project was begun with this understanding in mind, that the discipline of communication is particularly well suited for exploring the effects—good and bad—the pandemic has had, and is having, on our communication with each other. The pandemic has not only influenced how humans communicate with each other, it has also greatly impacted the various subfields in the communication discipline; how they view, research, and teach about their area of communication. These impacts, positive and negative, are profound yet relatively unexplored; thus the writing of this book, to begin the process of exploration into this unknown area. In order to facilitate a wide range of understanding, authors from a variety of well-established communication sub-disciplines write from their area's point of view about the impact the pandemic has had on human communication, and also about how the pandemic has impacted their area of study. As such, these chapters are not about reporting the results of a specific empirical research project, but instead are about the application of general theoretical knowledge from an author's subject area to that author's observations about the pandemic and its impact on both human communication and the discipline of communication. This book focuses in particular on nine wide-ranging aspects of public communication,[1] each represented by a communication subdiscipline: digital rhetoric, journalism, free speech, public relations, sports communication, public address, health communication, spiritual communication, and popular culture.

Within these areas authors ask and answer wide-ranging and different questions, essentially focusing on how people communicate with each other: what aspects of communication have changed? How so? What has remained the same? How has the pandemic impacted scholarship in these areas? Or how has scholarship impacted our understanding of the pandemic? How has teaching, beyond the moving of courses online, been impacted? How has research in these areas been impacted, and what are some suggestions for future research in these areas when one considers the pandemic's impact? Collectively, then, these chapters offer a disciplinary response to the pandemic, a response that offers concrete ideas about the pandemic's impact and also about how to move forward while minimizing the negative consequences and maximizing our embrace of the positive. Of course, the above are general questions, and each chapter, as seen below, asks and answers questions specific to its own area of knowledge.

Certainly the pandemic would have been conceived of and responded to differently had it not been for the pervasive nature of the digital. The digital surrounds us, and in so many ways its expansive nature escapes our notice; yet many of us were forced to confront the digital when the pandemic thrust it upon us in ways we could not have imagined before. Amber Davisson and Michelle Gibbons look at the nature of digital rhetoric during the pandemic in their chapter, "Digital Rhetoric and the COVID-19 Pandemic," in which they specifically examine how the pandemic accelerated existing digital development trajectories that were being discussed in the communication discipline. In their chapter they discuss three such trajectories: ambient digital rhetoric, digital publics and privacy, and digital realities. In terms of the ambient, the authors argue that to fully understand digital rhetoric, public understanding must expand to embrace digital rhetoric's increasingly ambient nature. The pandemic, they argue, "amplifies calls to move digital rhetoric beyond 'the screenic surface,' or a 'screen-centric' focus on what appears on our screens and how we interact with them." Instead, it served as an impetus to move beyond such narrow confines and looks to how the digital is actually embodied and infiltrates our environments. In terms of the public/private dichotomy, the authors note that the internet has always participated in that debate, yet the pandemic acted to exacerbate this tension, and it was especially noted in our engagement with multiple publics online simultaneously, the holding of classroom sessions often from our homes, and the notion of hyperpublicity, in which we are constantly aware of how our digital private communication can become public. In terms of digital realities, Davisson and Gibbons point to the ways in which contemporary digital technology complicates our sense of reality, or gives rise to so-called "digital realities." For the authors, "The phenomenological experience of engaging with the digital texts that comprise the internet, as suggested by the very phrase 'being online,' is that it involves inhabiting a different terrain, an ontological plain apart from the flesh and blood one." They conclude their chapter with suggestions for future research and teaching in this area.

When people wanted knowledge of the COVID-19 pandemic, they would regularly turn to the news, not just for information about lockdowns and new rules, but also for information about the very nature of the virus and potential treatments, or for the scientific aspects of the pandemic. Michael Horning and Jim A. Kuypers explore the problematic nature of looking at the mainstream news for quality science reporting in "Journalism Framing in (Times of) Crisis: The Inevitability of Poor Reporting during the COVID-19 Pandemic." These authors first provide a brief overview of the area of study known as journalism and mass communication, and following this, they relay observations about the educational preparation of journalists and how framing theory can help explain their reportorial practice during the pandemic. Putting the two together, they then look at an extended case study examining a specific instance of the reporting on hydroxychloroquine as a treatment for COVID-19 in which they find that educational preparation and journalistic political culture combined to produce both biased and poor reporting. They conclude with observations about how this knowledge impacts future teaching in this area, followed by suggestions for future research.

One public concern the news media highlighted throughout the pandemic was associated with free speech, particularly the perceived clash between public safety and the exercise of free speech. In "The Politicization of Protests and Protection: The Major Free Speech Issues during COVID-19 Pandemic," Benjamin Medeiros, Ann E. Burnette, Rebekah L. Fox, and David R. Dewberry examine the major conflicts around freedom of expression that have emerged during the COVID-19 pandemic. Focusing in particular on gathering restrictions to different kinds of expressive activity, the authors look intently at the tension between the government's ability to restrict activity in the name of public health and the Constitutional guarantees the First Amendment provides for freedom of speech, religion, and assembly. Noting that government imposed restrictions "on physical gathering have been among the central tools in the fight against the coronavirus pandemic," the authors also address their enormous public backlash; however, a central consideration for them are the questions about "where the government's ability to restrict activity in the name of public health ends and the First Amendment guarantees of freedom of speech, religion, and assembly begin." In examining these tensions Medeiros, Dewberry, Burnette, and Fox look specifically on the gathering restriction impacts on religious institutions, the protests in response to the death of George Floyd in spring of 2020, and mask mandates. They conclude with suggestions for teaching and future research.

In "Confronting the Coronavirus: How Public Relations Can Foster Trust during Crisis," Nneka Logan and Chelsea Woods note that the work of public relations is seen in a variety of strategies and tactics, and does consist primarily "of creating and disseminating strategic communication campaigns, news releases, press conferences, statements, social media posts, and other communication messages and materials" as well as "protecting an organization's reputation and contributing to its economic prosperity." Importantly, Logan and Woods note that relationships are a vital centering point to public relations practice and scholarship, and that this relationship-centric mission is not limited to organizations only, but applies to obtaining benefits to the larger society in which public relations exists. When an organization enters a time of crisis, when anxieties and uncertainties rise, as with the COVID-19 pandemic, public relations, they contend, "becomes even more important in helping stakeholders such as employees, customers, and communities make sense of what is happening, why it is happening, how it will affect them, and when they will emerge from troubling times." It is with this understanding that Logan and Woods use corporate social responsibility theory and relationship management theory to explore the pandemic's impact on corporations and society, noting how corporations acted and communicated in ways that fostered or diminished trust. Additionally, they use the theories to explore how organizations could better manage the complexities of doing business during the pandemic. Using corporate social responsibility theory and relationship management theory in this manner allowed them to provide a "novel theoretical framework to explore how American businesses experienced the pandemic and communicated to foster trust in their organizations among internal and external stakeholders, such as employees, customers and communities." In order to do this, Woods and Logan use their framework to examine the three stages of crises: precrisis, crisis, and postcrisis. Using numerous examples from various corporations they demonstrate how uniting a notion of corporate social responsibility with a relationship management approach to public relations allows organizations to better foster public trust through their crisis communications. They conclude by making suggestions for using corporate social responsibility theory and relationship management theory in communication teaching, research, and practice.

Sports have been a growing part of the lives of Americans since the dawn of the 20th century. So it is unsurprising that when the pandemic hit many turned to sports for comfort. Yet the sports viewing of Americans grew complicated not only due to pandemic dynamics, but also through the insertion of racialized politics into the mix. In "This Just Got Real: Implications of the COVID-19 Pandemic on Sport Communication," Brandi Watkins explores the intersections of sport communication, pandemic influences, and race. For Watkins, sport communication is an area of study that "encompasses the study of sport media, sport organizations, sport production, sport fandom, and the cultural and social structures that surround sport." Watkins takes the stance that sports are a powerful force in our society, one that should be taught so that the social dynamics are better understood. In this sense, her chapter invites us to more robustly appreciate how to consume and to understand sports, and importantly, how to communicate about sports. One has, after reading this chapter, a better sense of how sports may be used as a lens "to view and interpret world events and to critically analyze the systems" in which sports operate. In her chapter, Watkins specifically addresses the impact of the COVID-19 pandemic on sports in America, as well as its impact on the sports communication discipline. Additionally, she looks at the relationship between the George Floyd protests in conjunction with the COVID-19 pandemic within the context of sports communication. In doing so she analyzes the sports industry's reaction to the COVID-19 pandemic, and then recounts the events of the summer of 2020 after the death of George Floyd. She concludes with suggestions for future research in this area, and also suggestions for improving the teaching of sports communication.

In "Public Address in a Time of Crisis," Robin C. Rowland, Justin Kirk, and Michael Eisenstadt make the point that our various forms of democratic governance at all levels is "defined by the principle that citizen stakeholders talk first and then the public, often through their representatives in legislative bodies, decides." Those who study public address explore and explain such public talk, often identifying different genres, styles of discourse, ideological influences, cultural influences, political ramifications, often evaluating what works or does not work well. As Rowland, Kirk, and Eisenstadt put it, if "rhetoric is the lifeblood of democratic societies of all kinds, public address scholars are the rhetorical hematologists who study how effectively rhetoric circulates in the body politic." Certainly during times of national crisis the importance of understanding and analyzing public address is readily apparent. Starting from the premise that the COVID-19 pandemic eventuated with three interanimated crises—public health, economic crisis, and American policing. Rowland, Kirk, and Eisenstadt set aside the economic concerns to better highlight the centrality of public address scholarship when they focus on the public health and policing issues. They conduct case studies of a key moment in each of these areas: "a briefing on the pandemic conducted by President Donald Trump and his COVID Taskforce on April 23, 2020 and the contrasting rhetoric of protesters and President Trump prior to and following the action of the police to clear Lafayette Square and Lafayette Park of protesters before a photo op by President Trump at St. John's Church." In examining these public address examples the authors first provide a theoretical approach for examining rhetoric operating in a public sphere undergirded by Anglo-American liberal ideals followed by a detailed analysis of the two case studies. This is followed by comments concerning future research in this area and also how the insights generated could be applied to teaching public address.

Health was, obviously, a major concern during the pandemic, driving hard various discussions of public policy, and influencing all areas of our lives. However, what was not so much discussed was *how* issues of health were actually communicated. In "Health Communication Research and Social Implications during the COVID-19 Pandemic," YoungJu Shin, Yu Lu, and Shristi Bhochhibhoya first address health communication research concerning the COVID-19 pandemic as well as its social implications (detailing in particular the social, physical, and mental impacts). Following this, the authors look at the relationship between anti-Asian discrimination and health, focusing on America, where they argue that Americans of Asian descent were at even higher risk than others for adverse health effects "due to the surge of discrimination toward Asians since the outbreak." Following this they discuss the role of health communication in family and interpersonal relationships during the pandemic, and detail how a new perspective in family communication is necessary to account for the pandemic influences, in particular, the "uncertainty due to the adjustment to and threat caused by the COVID-19 and health related information." Interpersonal relationships were, of course, also impacted, and Shin, Lu, and Bhochhibhoya relay well how the pandemic "triggered a turning point for re-negotiation and re-formation of interpersonal relationships, including romantic relationships." This is followed by a short section on the practical implications for public health interventions in which they suggest that "health interventions should be designed to highlight the benefits of desirable health practices." In particular, they stress that health communication researchers must attempt to "reduce the spread of misinformation" by taking account of "the different usage of communication channels in interpersonal relationships," followed with a commitment to developing "intervention messages based on the target audience." They conclude with suggestions for future research and also practical applications for teaching.

Much in the hearts of Americans and also in the news was how pandemic lockdowns and restrictions impacted our religious lives. During the height of the pandemic we heard constantly about protests over intrusive government mandates concerning religious observances; considerably less was heard, however, about the overall impact of the pandemic on religious communication in general. In "Religious Communication in the Age of Covid-19," Dennis D. Cali addresses this lack. In his chapter Cali points out that, although rising concomitantly with the growth in popular culture studies, the transdisciplinary field of religious communication has emerged in some ways from the imbrications among established areas of scholarship, particularly since the advent of the digital age, and in so doing has advanced new lines of both inquiry and ways of teaching about how religious communication operates. Of note here, with the onset of the pandemic, is that religious communication took on especial importance, particularly since in so many countries, and in numerous states in America, lock downs prohibited or severely limited traditional forms of religious gatherings. Yet religious expressions also changed in other ways; for instance, with the rise of online use during the pandemic, or with the advent of parking lot religious services. Cali explores these areas and others, offering insight into the nuances of religious communication during the pandemic. In particular, he explores both religion in popular culture *and* popular culture in religion before commenting upon the dialectical tension between the two, notably looking at religion and popular culture in dialog. To achieve this he begins with an overview of the field's rather unique development. Once establishing this and the dimensions of the religion and popular culture dialectical tension he then identifies four key themes in the field: communitas, liminality, hierophany, and myth. He then applies these key themes to examine from a religious communication perspective the pandemic-induced social conditions upon religious practices. He concludes with suggestions for future research and teaching.

The pandemic also made its way into popular culture. In "'Saturday Nite Is Dead' at Least for a While: Changes in Popular Culture Theory during a Time of Crisis," David Nelson and Kimberly Kulovitz begin with the acknowledgment that the field of popular culture is difficult to define "because it crosses various academic disciplines, cultures, quantitative and qualitative values, influences, and experiences scholars have." They move to look instead at the various elements that inform attempts at defining popular culture, noting that the area is by its very nature transdisciplinary, and that numerous disciplines—math, geology, communication, sociology, anthropology, economics, for instance—have initiated work in this general area. Taking into consideration that as society changes so too does the manner of theorizing and teaching about popular culture, Nelson and Kulovitz argue that such changes, or alterations, "will have short and long-term effects to the lenses used in examining popular culture." Looking at popular culture during the pandemic, they share insight in five areas. First, they share theoretical views of popular culture, exploring the main contributors to current thinking on popular culture studies. Second, they define what they call the COVID Bubble, "that window of time that has created a disruption and restrictions for such things as the workplace, economic actives, communication between people, and entertainment for society and individuals during the COVID-19 pandemic." Additionally they look at how this bubble "shifted how technology was used and its effects on people's actions." They then look at the interanimation of pop culture, COVID, and research followed by exploring the interanimation of pop culture, COVID, and the classroom. They conclude with predictions for the future of popular culture research and teaching.

As can be seen, each of these chapters address an important area of communication within the context of the pandemic, and each offers insights into our collective public communication practices. Together they present a wide lens snapshot of public communication during the pandemic. As such they open the doors to insights that not only enhance our understanding of the pandemic's impact, but also provide ways of exploring new research and teaching opportunities. Collectively they argue for a positive and strong response from the communication discipline; for confidently acting with the knowledge that the insights and suggestions shared will allow us to emerge from the pandemic stronger than ever.

NOTE

1. If one is interested in the personal, as opposed to public, aspects of the pandemic's impact on human communication, see Kuypers, Jim A. ed. *Personal and Administrative Perspectives from the Communication Discipline during COVID-19* (Lanham, MD: Lexington Books, 2022).

Chapter 1

Digital Rhetoric and the COVID-19 Pandemic

Amber Davisson and Michelle Gibbons

In the early days of the COVID-19 pandemic, during the very first lockdown, an old newspaper ad circulated on Twitter. From the *St. Louis Post-Dispatch*, it showed a woman at home, talking on the telephone. Just behind her, a man with a blanket on his legs sits on a chair beside a bed reading a book. The text of the ad reads, in part, "People who are in quarantine are not isolated if they have a Bell Telephone."[1] Though social media posts mistakenly identified it as stemming from the 1918 pandemic, the ad was actually from 1910.[2] It referenced not the quarantine efforts around the well-known, misnamed Spanish flu, but the household quarantines many endured for other communicable diseases in the early 20th century, including smallpox, diphtheria, meningitis, and others. Its resonance in March 2020 not only spoke to the ways in which technology can enable connection, but to the ways in which pandemics can motivate technological adoption. At least that is what Bell hoped for the then fairly-new home telephone.

An early fall 2020 survey by the McKinsey Group found that "responses to COVID-19 have speeded the adoption of digital technologies by several years—and that many of these changes could be here for the long haul," noting that "digital adoption has taken a quantum leap."[3] McKinsey's survey focuses specifically on business contexts, but its findings apply more broadly. For digital rhetoric, that means that the pandemic has accelerated existing trajectories such that a number of the focal themes and topics that had already been part of the disciplinary conversation are even more pointedly salient. In this chapter, we discuss three such themes/topics: (1) ambient digital rhetoric, (2) digital publics and digital privacy, and (3) digital realities. For each one, we recap the ongoing disciplinary conversation and then address how COVID-19 has underscored its importance. In doing so, we also introduce some research questions and consider implications for pedagogy in digital rhetoric.

AMBIENT DIGITAL RHETORIC

The term "digital rhetoric" dates back to Richard Lanham's use of it in a 1992 essay entitled "Digital Rhetoric: Theory, Practice, and Property."[4] At the year of that piece's publication, the first photograph was just published to the web (a picture of the band, Les Horribles Cernettes), and the first website was just two years old.[5] Even a full three years later, on an episode of the *Today Show*, as Katie Couric, Bryant Gumbel, and Elizabeth Vargas discussed how to pronounce the @ in an email address, Couric quizzically asked, "What is Internet anyway?"[6] She meant the question in the most ordinary, literal of ways. In other words, when Lanham first referenced "digital rhetoric," the internet, our engagements with it, and our conceptualizations of it were vastly different than they are today. In its moment of birth as terminological designation, "digital rhetoric" referred to something more limited in scope than its current iteration. In fact, it challenges the imagination a bit to conjure up that very specific context, in which much digital writing occurred on offline computers, and while online spaces existed, only a tiny percentage of the population was using the internet, less than 5% by some measures, and were generally doing so for more occasional, limited purposes.[7]

Fast forward 30 years or so and today's scholars of digital rhetoric (and digital studies more broadly) contend with the digital's bigness, its unwieldiness, the fact that it is so utterly, almost incomprehensibly, encompassing. In 2017, Aaron Hess referred to digital technology as "less like a *technology* and more like a common feature of modern existence."[8] In the opening lines of *Ambient Rhetoric*, Thomas Rickert remarks on how "digital technologies are increasingly enmeshed with our everyday environment . . . not only converging but also permeating the carpentry of the world."[9] This observation constitutes one impetus for his argument that rhetoric orient toward the ambient, that is "what is lying around, surrounding, encircling, encompassing, or environing."[10] In 2018, Casey Boyle, James J. Brown, Jr., and Steph Ceraso similarly described digital rhetoric as an "ambient condition," noting that "rhetoricians first saw 'the digital' flickering on screens but now feel its effects transducing our most fundamental of social practices."[11] Or, as someone commented on the YouTube *Today Show* clip referenced earlier, "90's Internet was a harmless and fun guest you would occasionally invite into your home. Now it's a stalker that won't leave. And it follows you everywhere you go."[12]

All that said, although the digital may have felt like our lived environment prior to COVID-19's emergence as pandemic, in retrospect, there was clearly yet so much more room for it to expand, to even more fully encompass our experience. For one, the sheer hours that people spent in the typical digital spaces increased dramatically. Videogame usage increased by almost 50% during the pandemic.[13] Netflix added 26 million subscribers in the first half of 2020, and other streaming services saw unprecedented gains in new users.[14] Across the board, home bandwidth usage increased; broadband traffic in the early months of the pandemic was 20%–30% higher than pre-pandemic[15] So just in terms of temporal quantity, the sheer numbers of hours logged, the digital swelled.

But perhaps even more notable is the way the pandemic spurred the colonization of facets of social life that had previously been largely, or at least primarily operative, via the physical body, in shared material space with others. Social gatherings migrated into digital spaces. Take for example, the milestone life event, the 50th birthday, the 25th wedding anniversary, funerals, meeting the new baby, and so on. Such events are traditionally marked by large in-person gatherings. Or consider happy hours and public lectures. Although these were often organized (digital invites), recorded (iPhone photos), and replayed (social media posts) in digital space in prepandemic life, they now often *occur* in those digital spaces, begetting a whole industry of online party facilitators, services newly transitioned into online formats (Zoom birthday clown anyone?), and a litany of how-to guides. Other arenas now swept up in and encompassed by the digital include domains in which the one-on-one face-to-face encounter once felt almost sacrosanct, such as healthcare and psychotherapy. But perhaps no single example of the transition of otherwise in-person activity into online spaces has gotten more attention than the $1.5 trillion education industry.[16] From preschool to graduate school to tutoring and enrichment programs, education moved online.[17]

If we want to understand digital rhetoric, we must orient toward its ambience. The pandemic, therefore, amplifies calls to move digital rhetoric beyond "the screenic surface" and a "screen-centric" focus on what appears on our screens and how we interact with them.[18] It serves as impetus to attend to embodiment and environment; or, as Byron Hawk argues "situating bodies within ecological contexts."[19] Douglas Eyman similarly suggests attending to "the roles our bodies play in the production and reception of digital rhetoric."[20] For example, in prepandemic work that does just this, Catherine Gouge and John Jones introduce the concept of "diffractive wearing" to capture how people creatively, and materially, engage wearable technologies, as in the artist who walked through the streets of Tokyo to generate a hazard sign via GPS map, with its radius spanning the same area as the Fukushima nuclear fallout.[21]

The pandemic itself shaped embodiments around digital technologies. For example, for many, it involved contraction, perhaps even contortion, into small spaces, with so many ad hoc offices in cramped spare bedrooms, even closets, leading to the rise of the "cloffice," together with articles such as "A Cloffice is the Ultimate Work-From-Home Setup" and all manner of Pinterest inspiration boards.[22] News outlets reported on waves of back and neck pain complaints due to shifts in work patterns as more people worked remotely from home, many hunched over their devices.[23] If we theorize an expansive, creative "diffractive wearing," how might we theorize these hyperconfined embodiments into which so many were unceremoniously thrust? Similarly, interruption, by kids, pets, spouses, and so on, became part of the background against which so much digital engagement occurred. Teachers and students alike complained about parents who, suddenly in a position to watch their children's daily education, interrupted classes from kindergarten to college.[24] Such contexts of interruption—mitigated, in some part by the sensorial interventions of headsets and the like—are sites for rhetorical scholarship around attention, one with ambient, environmental concerns.

Contact tracing apps are perhaps an archetypal case study in pandemic digital rhetoric. Installed on a mobile device, contact tracing apps can use a device's Bluetooth signal to determine when app users are in close proximity to each other for a certain amount of time. If someone tests positive, the app then notifies those contacts of their potential exposure.[25] And while we could certainly adopt a screenic orientation to investigating them, looking at the details of app interface, for example, they also invite us to see just how much lies beyond that type of conceptual lens. Here, what appears on the screen is just one aspect of how the app serves as constellation point for the imbrication of bodies, digital signals, and virus in digital/material space, arguably distributing agency among a constellation of human and nonhuman actors.[26]

Another mode of attending to the digital's encompassing ambience is to focus on infrastructure. Ambient does not equal ephemeral, and ambience, in part, takes shape by various "surround systems." In the context of digital rhetoric, infrastructure refers to the underlying systems that enable, organize, and connect digital technologies, both on a large-scale, such as the web itself, or smaller one, such as the circuitry of a smartphone; it includes both hardware and software, such as code and algorithms.[27] As Samer Faraj, Wadih Renno, and Anand Bhardwaj argue, the pandemic acted as something of a "natural breaching experiment that has challenged taken-for-granted expectations about digitalization," one of which concerns access to digital infrastructures.[28] As illustrated by the viral photo of two children sitting on the sidewalk outside a Taco Bell to get wifi access, or the stories about school buses redeployed as mobile wifi hotspots, access is neither a given, not equally distributed.[29] In response, during the pandemic the FCC instituted an Emergency

Broadband Benefit program to provide low-income households with significantly discounted broadband access.[30] Therefore, underlying infrastructures both grew and bred modifications (i.e. new ad hoc mobile hotspots) during the pandemic, while also reminding us that the digital divide has not disappeared and may impact ambience, such that it is far from a uniform condition of contemporary life, but a much more variegated one.

The postpandemic landscape of digital rhetoric research also invites attention to those underlying systems that became newly essential and central to our efforts at connecting when in-person connection was ill-advised or even forbidden. For example, although tools that enable online collaboration and event hosting (e.g. Microsoft Teams, Zoom, and Facebook Live), learning management systems (e.g. Canvas and Blackboard), and online shopping tools had already existed prepandemic, they became even more a core technological infrastructure of our pandemic lives. As rhetorical scholars, we should consider how the underlying systems themselves, in terms of code, protocol, and interface, for example, exert rhetorical agency, shaping human exchange and action.[31] Just as grocery store layout fosters certain paths through the aisles and motivates certain purchases, how does a grocery store app foster certain behaviors with respect to food? How has the expansion of course management software, and our more robust use of it, made us different teachers, for better and/or worse?

Finally, given the time-sensitive nature of crisis, the pandemic highlights not only synchronic dimensions, but also diachronic trajectories of infrastructure. We tend to think of infrastructure as large, unwieldy, and slow-changing—and it often is. The prototypical example of traditional infrastructure, highway systems, clearly are. Yet the pandemic serves as a case study in infrastructural agility, one that may animate new ways of understanding digital infrastructures.

At the end of their essay, "The Digital: Rhetoric Beyond and Behind the Screen," Boyle et al. make the point that "the digital portends to be a momentary specialization that falls away and becomes eventually known as the conditions through which rhetorical studies finds itself endlessly transducing."[32] Has the COVID-19 pandemic hastened that future in which digital rhetoric's moment as specialization ends? In doing so, does it hasten some sort of disciplinary reconfiguration? Digital rhetoric has always felt a little like digital technology itself—constantly emerging, changing, and shifting—such that it seemed too slippery to grasp before the pandemic. So it is not surprising that in a global pandemic we are left to consider how the field might transform—whether its concerns have grown so big that we need to reconfigure how we understand our work. For example, what does it mean for digital rhetoric if being an expert in contemporary political discourse, popular culture, free speech, and so on, now demands expertise in digital rhetoric? For one, we might think of this in terms of pedagogy and what the future will bring for Digital Rhetoric courses. Will the singular, standalone Digital Rhetoric course, now standard in many Communication Departments, persist or will it, perhaps, splinter into multiple, more specialized iterations? In short, what does it mean to study digital rhetoric if so much of rhetoric is now digital?

DIGITAL PUBLICS AND DIGITAL PRIVACY

In the middle of April 2020, a month after President Donald J. Trump declared COVID-19 a national emergency, *Inside Higher Ed* published an editorial titled "Instructors, Please Wash Your Hair." The author lamented that after a month of teaching from home in the midst of a nationwide lockdown, professors were getting a little too casual. The article admonished educators for sloppiness and advised them to remember that when they log on to teach, they are entering a professional space: "Your piles of unattended laundry are not trophies for the amount of time you are putting into your coursework. They are distractions, signs of disorganization and, quite frankly, unsightly and off-putting."[33] As one might expect, the comments section included many heated responses to the essay, highlighting specifically the ways the criticisms in the essay reinforce expectations surrounding class and gender in the academy. One comment in particular pointed out that logging in does not transform one's home into a professional space. If anything, the professor said that when students log in to Zoom, she is visiting them, and they are visiting her, in the privacy of their homes. Whereas before the pandemic, one might conveniently label the homes of professors their personal space and the classroom a professional space (with a professor's office occupying a sort of in-between), Zoom rooms are disconcertingly liminal.

The liminal sense of the Zoom classroom—stuck somewhere between personal and professional or public and private—is a feeling common for those used to navigating digital technology. In his original conception of the public sphere, Jürgen Habermas intimated that it was distinct from the private sphere, calling it "a realm of our social life in which something approaching public opinion can be formed. Access is guaranteed to all citizens. A portion of the public sphere comes into being in every conversation in which private individuals assemble to form a public body."[34] The idea that individuals move from being private to public points to a dividing line between the two. Nancy Fraser took issue with the divisions between public and private in Habermas's conception of the public sphere;[35] mainly in that it assumed that the concerns of the private, intimate domestic sphere were separate from public life. The separation ignored the fact that much of women's participation in public life is tied to what takes place within the spaces that Habermas understood to be private and separate. The *Inside Higher Ed* editorial presumes, much like Habermas, that individuals cross over from being private to public when they join a public body in spaces like Zoom rooms, whereas Fraser, much like the professor in the comments, asks us to consider how much of intimate life is really left behind when we engage the public.

The internet has always occupied an uncomfortable space in the debate over the public/private dichotomy. On the one hand, the personalness of online media platforms—they are accessed often from one's phone, users are encouraged to develop personal profiles, and while we know that many people see the same things that we do, our viewing experiences often take place in isolation—works to make digital communication feel intimate. At the same time, there are constant reminders that our activities online are seldom if ever private. Many have had the experience of sharing something online with a small audience in mind, only to have that communication engaged by an unintended audience. Digital technology may feel intimate, but it is more accurately characterized as hyperpublic. Damien Pfister points to hyperpublicity as part of public life in a digital world: "The term 'hyperpublicity' captures a condition of public culture marked by ubiquitous recording technologies and networked circulation patterns. It signals an expansion in the capacity of personal media to record, archive, make searchable, and circulate opinions, events, and interactions in publicly accessible databases."[36] Even before the pandemic, the sense that every person you encountered had a camera in his or her pocket made public life fraught with the possibility that everyday embarrassing moments had the potential to become viral media events. That potential has, to varying degrees, introduced new cautiousness and increasingly guarded behavior. Pfister points out that "hyperpublicity constrains rhetorical experimentation"[37] because speakers are aware of the possible dangers of a misstep. In short, our constant awareness of the potential for our digital communication to be public makes it difficult to engage in digital rhetoric.

In America, privacy is generally considered both a right and a value, and thus the term is automatically provided with copious normative meaning. Normative definitions tend to err on the side of privacy as a matter of liberty, or privacy as a matter of secrecy.[38] To talk about how one's personal ability to choose what to keep private aids in the creation of digital rhetoric, it helps to begin with a more neutral definition of the concept of privacy. Rather than starting with the common understanding of privacy in terms of rights and privileges, one can conceive of it as a tool that individuals use to produce their rhetorical personas. Ruth Gavison, for instance, defines privacy as a matter of accessibility; our privacy consists of "the extent to which we are known to others, the extent to which others have physical access to us, and the extent to which we are the subject of others' attention."[39] Individuals make contextual choices about what to keep private and when to reveal private information for public consumption. It is this element of choosing and contextualizing that makes privacy a rhetorical tool. Helen Nissenbaum points out that public debates about privacy tend to flatten that concept of contextualization, and instead discuss all losses of privacy as if they are the same and as if they are all normatively bad. She suggests it may be more useful to think of it, not in terms of losses, but in terms of "constraints on access" and "control."[40] Herman Tavani explains control as relating to choice, consent, and correction. Meaning, control is the ability individuals have to make choices about access and distribution of private information, the right to consciously and actively consent to losses of privacy, and the ability to make corrections to private information once it is released.[41] Whether or not it is good or bad to constrain access to or control use of our private information, is largely contextual. In some contexts losing control of private information has a positive impact, and in some cases the inability to constrain access is dangerous. The operative issue when balancing privacy with other factors is control.

Online communication complicates our ability to constrain or control access to private information because individuals often engage in multiple publics online simultaneously. In day-to-day life, individuals travel through many distinct public bodies: work, school, parties, HOA meetings, and so on. The ability to decide what is private and what is public in each of the scenarios is important for developing an identity in these spaces.[42] For example, what one chooses to reveal at a party, or the way privacy is exercised at a party or on a date, is likely not the same as the choices they might make at school or work. From the outside these separate identities could potentially appear fragmented or even duplicitous. Facebook founder Mark Zuckerberg once told reporter David Kirkpatrick that "Having two identities for yourself is an example of a lack of integrity."[43] However, what Zuckerberg failed to grasp is that choices about identity are not about lying, they are about selecting what is private in any given setting. To some extent digital technology can aid individuals in carving out spaces to withhold information as private as a means to explore identity. Drag queens report creating multiple social media profiles as a means of separating out their participation in the drag community from their day-to-day life.[44] Many teenagers create what are called finsta (fake Instagram) accounts to share parts of their life with their friends and keep those things private from the watchful eyes of parents.[45] The internet can be a place to use privacy to control access and carve out distinct identities, but it can also force a type of hyperpublicity in which all elements of life are accessible somewhere online.

HYPERPUBLICITY

Life online during the pandemic brought the problem of hyperpublicity to a head. In March of 2020, as citizens across the United States entered lockdown, personal control over daily life was something that seemed to be in short supply. On the one hand, the answer to the coronavirus pandemic seemed simple: everyone stay at home! However, for most it was not possible to simply stay at home and binge Netflix. People still needed to "go" to work and school. Zoom videoconferencing became invaluable to daily life during the pandemic, and more than any other technology, it has pointed to the tenuousness of the public/private dichotomy. Using Zoom, college students suddenly found themselves attending college classes in their childhood bedrooms, while working in the family business to make ends meet, or taking care of siblings while parents worked. Professors signed on to office hours to find themselves in a bedroom with a student lying in bed. On a college campus, students might decide how much of their home or family life to keep private. Now, their classmates had a window into those private spaces.

Zoom was founded in 2011 by Eric Yuan, and went live in January of 2013. By May of that year, it had more than a million customers.[46] In 2014, that number had increased to more than 10 million participants, and a year later that number had quadrupled.[47] Zoom's IPO launched in 2019, and the founder quickly became a billionaire.[48] While food, transportation, and retail outlets were taking a financial hit from the coronavirus, Zoom saw the company's value soar to over $29 billion.[49] In the early days of the pandemic, on one day alone, Sunday, March 15, nearly 600,000 people downloaded the app.[50] Yuan faced a lot of stress as a result, telling a reporter: "I tell myself, every morning when I wake up, two things . . . Don't let the world down. Don't let our users down."[51] Shira Ovide explains that what made Zoom so popular in the days after the coronavirus was that it was incredibly easy for people to login by just clicking on a link.[52] The software did not require every user to download the same program or have compatible technology. It was simple and user friendly for people to adopt. Zoom began planning for its surge in popularity when the virus started spreading in China in January, and it eliminated a lot of its fees and limits in preparation for quarantines in the US.[53] During the lockdown phase of the pandemic, Zoom became a place to try to maintain the rituals of everyday life. However, as one columnist pointed out: "trying to translate your old social habits to Zoom or FaceTime is like going vegetarian and proceeding to glumly eat a diet of just tofurkey, rather than cooking varied, creative, and flavorful meals with fruits and vegetables."[54] As the pandemic stretched on, Zoom went from a primary meeting place for work and education to a technology to maintain connections with friends, see family from a distance, and even date.

For many people, home is a private place where work and school are public spaces. During the pandemic, Zoom allowed people to bridge the gap by logging into the publicness of work and school from the privateness of home. As rhetoricians, we are interested in the extreme publicness or hyperpublicity of platforms such as Zoom. Consider the classroom. Even though students might recognize themselves as being in a public place when they are in a classroom, they likely do not think of themselves as constantly addressing the public while they are in that space. Often the audience attention is on the teacher or whichever student is speaking, and that allows the majority of students to be in the space passively. When active, the video function of Zoom makes that passivity difficult. The Zoom classroom compounds personal awareness. Users can see themselves on the screen at all times, and there is a persistent reminder that they are being seen. There is no fading into the audience and no forgetting that their bodies are public.[55] Barbara Couture points out that, long before COVID-19, the mediation of private, intimate lives into the public sphere was normalized by talk radio, reality tv, and talk shows in the late 1900s.[56] Writing as early as 2004, she pointed to online teaching as a space where the seemingly private rhetoric of the classroom was made public through publication on the internet. Couture argues that one of the dangers of private lives made public is that the publicity can be used rhetorically to persuade people of changing social norms.[57] The speaker establishes that all private intimacies should be made public, and they attempt to persuade the audience that they must reciprocate. One sees this in the Zoom classroom as teachers struggled over establishing the normative practice of students keeping cameras on, while students argued they should not be forced to reveal their private spaces.[58] Couture expressed concern over the impact establishing norms and expectations of public intimacy has on the ability to form intimate relationships separate from relationships to the public and the impact it has on a person's ability to negotiate the different identities they occupy.

In the 90s, the term "meatspace" was coined to describe the physical experience of a body while interacting online.[59] The idea being that there is cyberspace where one's identity exists online, and there is meatspace where one's body physically exists. Though, Kazys Varnelis and Anne Friedberg push back on that delineation, arguing that physical space and bodies do not go away in favor of a digital world. The two worlds are extensions of each other, and individuals do not go back and forth between them. They are inhabited simultaneously.[60] Zooming during the pandemic has pushed awareness of the body in online interactions. Norm Friesen points out that seeing ourselves on screen both reminds us of the unblinking eye of the camera and makes us persistently aware of how we look to others.[61] As Madeleine Aggeler explains it:

"Though we may pretend to be looking at another person when we FaceTime or Zoom, really we're just looking at ourselves—fussing with our hair, subtly adjusting our facial expressions, trying to find the most flattering angle at which to hold our phones. Seeing someone else do this feels voyeuristic."[62] Take, for instance, fitness classes, which have always been a weirdly intimate space. Coronavirus brought those classes into our home and increased their intimacy. Leah Prinzivalli pointed out that when doing yoga over Zoom, she could not help but be captivated by the homes of other participants on the screen.[63] It was not the same as watching a premade fitness video of a group of people doing yoga in a well-lit studio. Instead, you were watching amateur bodies struggle to hold the poses in the privacy of their home while cats, partners, and children wandered through the screen. One nudist blogged about the difficulty of meeting up over the web.[64] Members of the community had all been nude together before, and live nudity on the internet is not exactly groundbreaking. There was a difference between simply being nude together and being mediated nude together. The meeting had the slight feeling of voyeurism and raised questions about the line between nudism and pornography.

When Zoom makes so many activities feel more public—simply sitting in class, group fitness, going to a meeting—it also makes these activities feel more rhetorical. Participants are aware of being watched, and this generates the feeling that one needs to perform a self that is likable, attractive, and persuasive to others. The hyperpublicity of Zoom constrains our ability to fully engage in digital rhetoric by not just depriving individuals of the private intimate space of home, but also making the participants constantly aware of their publicness. Sonia Livingstone wrote about the dangers of treating the digital as a place that transcends all boundaries. She argues that the seemingly artificial boundaries that we have carved out in society function to regulate and reinforce norms and values, which can be problematic. At the same time, when those boundaries are renegotiated, it is most often not in the interests of fighting norms. It is in the interests of creating new restrictions and norms: "transformations are effectively exploited by powerful commercial interests, ruthlessly undermining any surviving spaces for the exercise of freedom by either the traditional elite or the masses."[65] In the pandemic, for many people, home stopped being a place to potentially be free of the watchful eye of the public. Home became a classroom. Home became an office. Home became one more public space. The distinction between publicity and privacy is artificial, and the reinforcement of it is often about communicating social norms that maintain power structures. With that said, an individual's ability to use their privacy and control access is critical to the development of a rhetorical self that is capable of pushing back against those structures.

DIGITAL REALITIES

In an episode of the NBC sitcom *The Office*, paper salesman Michael Scott and his assistant Dwight drive to a sales call in an unfamiliar location, using their car's GPS as a guide. They head down a clearly incorrect path, off the main road, straight toward a lake. Dwight suggests that Michael is misinterpreting the GPS's instructions, as Michael desperately insists, "the machine knows" just as the car enters into the lake and begins to float. The joke here is that Michael trusts the technology over his own perceptions, even as it becomes increasingly impossible to imagine any way they could be headed in the right direction.[66] Behind that joke lies the real unease many feel about the role technology plays in shaping perceptions, maybe even overruling them, constructing realities. Indeed, the joke is reminiscent of the real life moment when a group of Japanese tourists visiting Australia followed their GPS directions and drove into the Pacific Ocean.[67] Driving into the ocean may be the rare extreme, but how many of us have had the experience of glancing at the phone's weather app showing crystal clear skies and then feeling unsettled and somewhat confused as we walk out the door and feel a light rain.

From its inception as a discipline, rhetoric's role in shaping reality has generated some of the most fundamental and enduring questions. From Protagoras's constructivist assertion about "man as the measure of all things," to the 1970s debates about rhetoric as epistemic, to Lloyd Bitzer's situation claims and subsequent discussions, rhetoricians have debated, in conversation with philosophy, the extent to which reality exists apart from our discursively mediated conception of it? We will not recap those arguments here except to say that they are often inflected by new technologies. And new technologies often lend new salience to them. Indeed, we see this concern starting in 1920 with some in the Cornell School wanting to broaden rhetorical studies' scope, calling for broader research applications, followed by new ways of looking at rhetoric, such as the works of Kenneth Burke, and Edwin Black's calls for expansion.[68] By 1972, as rhetoric was in the midst of a dramatic broadening, with a disciplinary awning expanding to encompass not just speeches as analytic site, but symbolic activity more generally, David Berg wrote an essay on mass media, reflecting on a "media produced reality."[69] Today, our discipline is turning a good deal of attention to the ways in which contemporary digital technology complicates our realities, or gives rise to "digital realities." The phenomenological experience of engaging with the digital texts that comprise the internet, as suggested by the very phrase "being online," is that it involves inhabiting a different terrain, an ontological plain apart from the flesh and blood one. Virtual reality purposefully highlights this immersive quality.[70] Now, of course, the two are thoroughly enmeshed, with server farms, with their blunt materiality, serving as one on-the-ground reminder of the fact that neither can be unfettered from the other. Even though we objectively realize it is not true in a literal sense, our screens still feel like portals to another realm.

In "Pushing Back on the Rhetoric of 'Real' Life," Jordan Frith challenges the continuing characterization of digital life as separate from "physical," or "real" life.[71] He argues that although scholarly literature has challenged this false dichotomy, it nonetheless persists, both in academic writing (especially outside of fields that take technology as central focus) and in the vernacular. Moreover, it comes with it a corollary that "real life" is more important than anything that happens online. This is not without repercussions. That distinction between the real and the digital allows people to ignore the environmental costs of digital technologies and deflects from the very real consequences of what happens in online spaces. Take, for example, crypto currency, which is traded entirely digitally and may feel to some like a really high stakes video game. Carbon emissions from cryptocurrency bitcoin demonstrate the entanglement between the digital and the real: "to put this into perspective, one Bitcoin transaction is the 'equivalent to the carbon footprint of 735,121 Visa transactions or 55,280 hours of watching YouTube.'"[72] Frith advocates Adria de Souza e Silva's vision of "hybrid space . . . [which] moves away from unrealistic dichotomies that ignore bodies, the vast physical infrastructure that enables the digital, and the ways experiences of the physical are influenced by what people see online (or vice versa)."[73] Awareness of the physical reality of the digital makes users more aware of the realness of digital life.

The both quick and seismic shift in living habits wrought by the pandemic, brought about a distinct change in the balance of time online/offline for many people. As already referenced in this chapter, we need no reminding of the hours logged on Zoom, ordering groceries online, binging TV shows, and endlessly "doomscrolling." Thus, while hybridity remains, the balance of the digital demonstrably tilted. What are the implications for digital rhetoric, especially around the issue of the relationship between "real life" and "digital life," and the realities they entail?

First of all, Frith published his piece in July of 2020, but one assumes he drafted it earlier than that. As we write this chapter a full year of pandemic later, one wonders whether the attitudes he described have changed (or not)? How has that metaphor fared in the face of the pandemic? Did hours of work hours logged on Zoom, with the neck aches and eye strain, finally dismantle the illusion that digital life is lived separately and apart from our physical bodies? What happens when the digital is no longer a place of escape? In the real life vs. digital life metaphor, there is sometimes an unspoken corollary that the digital is the space of freedom, an escape from the demands of real life. Anxieties around screen time, perhaps, reflect this sense that digital engagement is an indulgence to be moderated. But when baking sourdough bread becomes a form of escapism from all those Zoom meetings, when material engagements are now an escape from the oppressive screen, does the metaphor that digital life is not real life finally fall apart?

We can put aside questions about how digital realities exist in, through, and alongside other realities, focusing instead on the nature of those realities, the "truths" they craft. During the pandemic, as our immersion in digital spaces and contexts, and their imbrication in our lived environments, became even more extensive, the realities shaped therein and thereby became all the more enveloping. Media studies scholars have introduced the term "deep mediatization" to capture the way we live in an age "when the very *elements and building-blocks* from which a sense of the social is constructed become *themselves* based in technologically based processes of mediation."[74] There is a lot in that claim, which evokes a need to study such processes, the urgency of which has been heightened by the pandemic-related accelerations in technological trajectories, as noted at the beginning of this chapter. Here we focus on just a few points regarding digital realities, as underscored in the pandemic.

The pandemic has highlighted the very real, life-and-death stakes of those realities, ones that are not just individual, but collective. Given how both viruses and public health systems operate, someone's decision not to wear a mask or not to get a vaccine does not just affect that person, but potentially affects all of us. We need to better understand the mediatization of stories about the virus as a hoax or government plot, about masks as useless, and vaccines as dangerous, etc. . . . ,[75] the prevalence of which is so widespread that some characterize it as an infodemic.[76] There is an urgent social need to better understand how false claims and false realities both germinate and are sustained in and through the digital.

For rhetoric scholars, this serves as a call for, among other things, more research into the rhetorical ecologies in which discourse operates.[77] As Dana Cloud argues, "strategies of mediation," that is, those having to do with the presentation of information, often overshadow facts.[78] We should attend to those, including, as Cloud describes, myth, spectacle, and affect. This call also echoes the chapter's earlier argument regarding the importance of digital infrastructures and looking beyond the screenic surface. Within rhetoric, circulation studies remains, as Laurie Gries wrote in 2013, "an emergent area of study ripe for theoretical and methodological attention."[79]

LOOKING FORWARD TO THE RESEARCH AND TEACHING OF DIGITAL RHETORIC POSTPANDEMIC

The pandemic did not fundamentally alter the course of digital rhetoric so much as it worked to speed our way forward in many of the directions we were already headed. Well before a nationwide lockdown was even a possibility, researchers in the field were attending to questions about the increasing ambience of digital technology, the blurring of private and public communication online, and the uncanny way that digital technology could create realities and worlds. So, if the pandemic has caused these issues to take a quantum leap forward, how should scholars in digital rhetoric race to catch up? First, on the question of ambient digital rhetoric, the increasingly ambient nature of digital technology requires scholars of digital rhetoric to think about where they fit in the discipline. The digital now seemingly forms part of most rhetoric, which begs the question: are we our own community? Or do we more accurately belong in popular culture studies, political communication, media studies? If all rhetoric is now digital, is the study of digital rhetoric really just the study of rhetoric? And what might this criticism of digital rhetoric look like?[80] Conversely, scholars in other fields must begin to contend with the ways that digital technology shape all public conversations. Second, on the question of public and private, as ambient technology makes all rhetoric seem potentially public, we must be mindful of the impact of hyperpublicity on agency. Researchers should consider the way hyperpublicity shifts rhetorical agency from speaker to audience, as individuals lose the ability to make choices about privacy in a world where the audience can always see them. Finally, digital rhetoric scholars have an obligation to attend to Dana Cloud's warning that mediations are so persuasive that we often believe what digital technology is telling us regardless of the persuasiveness of the facts it is transmitting.

In the classroom, professors in digital rhetoric can use the kairotic moment of life shifting back to normal to highlight the increase in ambient rhetoric. In particular, conversations about ambient rhetoric and privacy during the pandemic intersect in the form of conversations about inequality and education. Previously, the infrastructure that supported digital technology may have felt like something far away, but as students have struggled to log in to classes and participate online, many have become painfully aware of infrastructure. This is a critical moment for professors to engage with students in conversations about infrastructure and technology. Those conversations transition well into the question of privacy and the requirement to turn on one's camera during a Zoom class. Many students are ready to talk about the ways that Zoom cameras became an uncomfortable window for classmates to see the financial difficulties they were experiencing. Education is often touted as a great equalizer, and when everyone is living in the same dorm and eating at the same dining hall it can feel like the playing field is level. Zooming in from home complicates that narrative of equality. Digital rhetoric classes, both in conversations about ambience and privacy, offer spaces to explore the precarity of discourses of equality in education. Finally, the pedagogical stakes of our inability to reconcile the digital and the real are clear. How do we best both teach students to be more critically aware of the ways in which digital life is real life and the ways in which realities are conditioned in and through the digital? As recent research has shown, just merely saying so is not always enough.[81]

Digital rhetoric, as rhetorical subfield, was borne out of technological development, taking shape alongside personal and mobile computing. And though we might trace its origins back to 1992, when Richard Lanham wrote of "digital rhetoric," many years later we can still find descriptions of it as "a new" or "emergent" field.[82] In some ways, perhaps digital rhetoric will always be somewhat emergent, perhaps always be somewhat inevitably new. It takes shape in response to technological change, considers that change as its focal subject matter, and finds, in new technologies, not only fresh sites for analysis, but new ways of understanding itself. It is, by nature, responsive.

The transformations to the technological landscape wrought by the COVID-19 pandemic, not just in new technologies, but in new habits of use, will inevitably shape what digital rhetoric is, does, and becomes. That said, the extent to which the field may reconfigure remains to be seen. This chapter ultimately suggests that the pandemic highlighted some already-existing disciplinary conversations, potentially accelerating (or serving as impetus to accelerate) research trajectories that were already in progress, particularly those around ambient digital rhetoric, digital publics and digital privacy, and digital realities.

NOTES

1. Bell Telephone, "When in Quarantine," print advertisement, *St. Louis Post-Dispatch* (St. Louis, Missouri), November 17, 1910, 16.

2. E.g., Ian Boudreau (@iboudreau), "More than a century ago, during the Spanish flu outbreak," Tweet, March 30, 2020, https://twitter.com/iboudreau/status/1244584907113930758/photo/1; see Dan Evon, "Is This a 1918 Quarantine Ad for the Bell Telephone?" *Snopes*, May 15, 2020, https://www.snopes.com/fact-check/1918-quarantine-ad-for-phone/; Harry McCracken, "How the Telephone Failed Its Big Test During the 1918's Spanish Flu Pandemic," *FastCompany*, April 3, 2020,

https://www.fastcompany.com/90484820/how-1918s-spanish-flu-outbreak-crushed-the-u-s-telephone-system.

3. "How COVID-19 has Pushed Companies Over the Technology Tipping Point—And Transformed Business Forever," McKinsey, October 5, 2020, https://www.mckinsey.com/business-functions/strategy-and-corporate-finance/our-insights/how-covid-19-has-pushed-companies-over-the-technology-tipping-point-and-transformed-business-forever#.

4. On Lanham's introduction of the term, see Elizabeth Losh, *Virtualpolitik: An Electronic History of Government Media-Making in a Time of War, Scandal, Disaster, Miscommunication, and Mistakes* (MIT Press, 2009), 82.

5. "World Wide Web Timeline," Pew Research Center, March 11, 2014, https://www.pewresearch.org/internet/2014/03/11/world-wide-web-timeline/#1992.

6. "1994: 'Today Show': 'What is the Internet, Anyway?'," video, January 28, 2015, https://www.youtube.com/watch/UlJku_CSyNg.

7. Max Roser, "The Internet's History has Just Begun," Our World in Data, October 3, 2018, https://ourworldindata.org/internet-history-just-begun.

8. Aaron Hess, "Introduction: Theorizing Digital Rhetoric," *Theorizing Digital Rhetoric*, ed. Aaron Hess and Amber Davisson (Routledge, 2018), 6.

9. Thomas Rickert, *Ambient Rhetoric: The Attunements of Rhetorical Being* (University of Pittsburgh Press, 2013), 1.

10. Rickert, *Ambient Rhetoric*, 5–6.

11. Casey Boyle, James J. Brown, Jr., and Steph Ceraso, "The Digital: Rhetoric Behind and Beyond the Screen," *Rhetoric Society Quarterly* 48, no. 3 (2018): 251.

12. Ryan Doyle, nd, comment on "1994: 'Today Show': 'What is the Internet, Anyway?'"

13. Drew Szala, "Gaming Sees an Increase During COVID-19 Pandemic," Fox43, February 8, 2021, https://www.fox43.com/article/tech/gaming/video-gaming-games-covid19-pandemic/521-4606d7d4-6989-4082-a601-7966a8ef7f6d; Adam Epstein, "The Pandemic Has Turned Everyone into Gamers," *Quartz*, September 16, 2020, https://qz.com/1904276/everyone-is-playing-video-games-during-the-pandemic/.

14. Jonathan Ponciano, "5 Big Numbers that Show Netflix's Massive Growth Continues During the Coronavirus Pandemic," *Forbes*, October 19, 2020, https://www.forbes.com/sites/jonathanponciano/2020/10/19/netflix-earnings-5-numbers-growth-continues-during-the-coronavirus-pandemic/?sh=7d5539fc225e; see also Daisuke Wakabayashi, Jack Nicas, Steve Lohr, and Mike Isaac, "Big Tech Could Emerge from Coronavirus Crisis Stronger than Ever," *The New York Times*, March 23, 2020, https://www.nytimes.com/2020/03/23/technology/coronavirus-facebook-amazon-youtube.html.

15. Doug Brake, "Lessons From the Pandemic: Broadband Policy after COVID-19," Information Technology & Innovation Foundation, July 13, 2020, https://itif.org/publications/2020/07/13/lessons-pandemic-broadband-policy-after-covid-19.

16. "Educational Services in the US - Market Size 2005–2027," IBIS World, May 26, 2021, https://www.ibisworld.com/industry-statistics/market-size/educational-services-united-states/.

17. For a discussion of that shift, with a focus on the Communication Studies, see Roy Schwartzman, "The (Post-)Pandemic Academic: Re-Forming Communication Studies," *Carolinas Communication Annual* 36 (2020):1–8.

18. Boyle et al., "The Digital," 252, 253

19. Byron Hawk. *A Counter-History of Composition: Toward Methodologies of Complexity* (Pittsburgh: University of Pittsburgh Press, 2007), 206. See also Brett Lunceford, "Where is the Body in Digital Rhetoric?" in *Theorizing Digital Rhetoric*, ed. Aaron Hess and Amber Davisson (Routledge, 2018), 140–152.

20. Douglas Eyman, "Looking Back and Looking Forward: Digital Rhetoric as Evolving Field," *enculturation*, November 22, 2016, http://enculturation.net/looking-back-and-looking-forward.

21. Catherine Gouge and John Jones, "Wearable Technologies and Invention," *Rhetoric Review* 37, no. 4 (2018): 421–433.

22. Jessica Bennett, "A Cloffice is the Ultimate Work-From-Home Setup If You're Short on Space," *Better Homes & Gardens*, January 11, 2021, https://www.bhg.com/rooms/home-office/makeovers/cloffice-ideas/; Jura Koncius, "Tiny Cloffices—Workspaces in Closets—Are Big, Thanks to the Pandemic," *The Washington Post*, May 27, 2021, https://www.washingtonpost.com/lifestyle/home/cloffice-ideas-home-office-closet/2021/05/25/2cb652f2-8d9e-11eb-a6bd-0eb91c03305a_story.html.

23. Cory Stieg, "Working from Home During Covid is Causing More Back and Neck Pain—Here's How to Find Relief," *CNBC*, March 3, 2021, https://www.cnbc.com/2021/03/03/back-and-neck-pain-working-from-home-amid-covid-exercises-for-relief.html.

24. Julie Jargon, "Parents are the New Remote-School Zoom Bombers," *The Wall Street Journal*, October 27, 2020, https://www.wsj.com/articles/parents-are-the-new-remote-school-zoom-bombers-11603800001.

25. Dyani Lewis, "Contact-Tracing Apps Help Reduce COVID Infections, Data Suggest," *Nature* February 22, 2021, https://www.nature.com/articles/d41586-021-00451-y.

26. See Anne Teresa Demo, "Hacking Agency: Apps, Autism, and Neurodiversity," *Quarterly Journal of Speech* 103, no. 3 (2017): 277–300.

27. See Nathan R. Johnson, "Information Infrastructure as Rhetoric: Tools For Analysis," *POROI* 8, no. 1 (2012).

28. Samer Faraj, Wadih Renno, and Anand Bhardwaj, "Unto the Breach: What the COVID-19 Pandemic Exposes about Digitalization," *Information and Organization* 31, no. 1 (2021).

29. Alisha Ebrahimji, "School Sends California Family a Hotspot after Students went to Taco Bell to use their Free WiFi," *CNN*, August 31, 2020, https://www.cnn.com/2020/08/31/us/taco-bell-california-students-wifi-trnd/index.html; Taylor Hannon, "School Bus Wi-Fi Hotspots Aide Student Learning During COVID-19 Closures," *School Transportation News*, April 8, 2020, https://stnonline.com/special-reports/school-bus-wi-fi-hotspots-aide-student-learning-during-covid-19-closures/.

30. "Emergency Broadband Benefit," Federal Communications Commission, https://www.fcc.gov/broadbandbenefit.

31. We might also approach this in terms of affordances, see Amber Davisson and Angela C. Leone, "From Coercion to Community Building: Technological Affordances as Rhetorical Forms," in *Theorizing Digital Rhetoric*, ed. Aaron Hess and Amber Davisson (Routledge, 2018), 85–97.

32. Boyle et al., "The Digital," 258.

33. Kristie Kiser, "Instructors, Please Wash Your Hair," *Inside Higher Ed*, April 16, 2020, https://www.insidehighered.com/advice/2020/04/16/teaching-online-should-not-mean-presenting-yourself-less-professionally-or.

34. Jürgen Habermas, "The Public Sphere: An Encyclopedia Article," *New German Critique* 3 (1974): 49.

35. Nancy Fraser, "Rethinking the Public Sphere: A Contribution to the Critique of Actually Existing Democracy." *Social Text* 25/26 (1990): 71.

36. Damien Smith Pfister, *Networked Media, Networked Rhetorics: Attention and Deliberation in the Early Blogosphere* (Penn State University Press, 2014), 176. Emphasis original.

37. Pfister, *Networked Media, Networked Rhetorics*, 181.

38. Herman T. Tavani, "Philosophical Theories of Privacy: Implications for An Adequate Online Privacy Policy," *Metaphilosophy* 38.1 (2007): 1–22.

39. Ruth Gavison, "Privacy and the Limits of the Law," *The Yale Law Journal* 89, no. 3 (1980): 423.

40. Helen Nissenbaum, *Privacy in Context: Technology, Policy, and the Integrity of Social Life* (Stanford University Press, 2010), 70.

41. Tavani, "Philosophical Theories of Privacy." On control over personal information in digital contexts, see also Nora A. Draper, *The Identity Trade: Selling Privacy and Reputation Online* (New York University Press, 2019).

42. danah boyd, *It's Complicated: The Social Lives of Networked Teens* (Yale University Press, 2014), 54.

43. David Kirkpatrick. *The Facebook Effect: The Inside Story of the Company that is Connecting the World* (Simon and Schuster, 2011), 199.

44. See Maggie MacAulay and Marcos Daniel Moldes, "Queen Don't Compute: Reading and Casting Shade on Facebook's Real Names Policy." *Critical Studies in Media Communication* 33, no. 1 (2016): 6–22; Alexander Cho, "Default Publicness: Queer Youth of Color, Social Media, and Being Outed by the Machine," *New Media & Society* 20, no. 9 (2018): 3183–3200. See also Amber Davisson, "The Politics of Authenticity in Facebook's Name Policy," in *Social Media and Politics: A New Way to Participate in the Political Process*, vol. 2, ed. Glen Richardson (New York: Praeger, 2016).

45. Brett Molina, "Does your Kid have a 'Finsta' Account? Why it's a Big Deal." *USA Today*. October 20, 2017, https://www.usatoday.com/story/tech/talkingtech/2017/10/20/does-your-kid-have-finsta-account-why-its-big-deal/783424001/.

46. Robbie Pleasant, "Zoom Video Communications Reaches 1 Million Participants," *TMCnet*, May 23, 2013, https://www.tmcnet.com/topics/articles/2013/05/23/339279-zoom-video-communications-reaches-1-million-participants.htm.

47. "How We Zoomed Past 10 Million Participants," Zoom [blog], July 22, 2014, https://blog.zoom.us/wordpress/2014/07/22/how-10-million/; "Zoom Raises

$30M in Series C Funding Led by Emergence Capital," Press Release, February 4, 2015, https://www.globenewswire.com/news-release/2015/02/04/1130354/0/en/Zoom-Raises-30M-in-Series-C-Funding-Led-by-Emergence-Capital.html.

48. Pranav Dixit, "Google Told Its Workers that They Can't use Zoom on their Laptops Anymore," *Buzzfeed*, April 8, 2020, https://www.buzzfeednews.com/article/pranavdixit/google-bans-zoom.

49. Taylor Lorenz, Erin Griffith, and Mike Isaac, "We Live in Zoom Now," *New York Times*, March 17, 2020, https://www.nytimes.com/2020/03/17/style/zoom-parties-coronavirus-memes.html.

50. Lorenz et al., "We Live in Zoom."

51. Drake Bennett and Nico Grant, "Zoom Goes from Conferencing App to the Pandemic's Social Network," *Bloomberg Businessweek*, April 9, 2020, https://www.bloomberg.com/news/features/2020-04-09/zoom-goes-from-conferencing-app-to-the-pandemic-s-social-network.

52. Shira Ovide, "Zoom is Easy. That's Why It's Dangerous," *New York Times*, April 9, 2020, https://www.nytimes.com/2020/04/09/technology/zoom-security.html.

53. Lorenz et al., "We Live in Zoom."

54. Ashley Fetters, "We Need to Stop Trying to Replicate the Life We Had," *The Atlantic*, April 10, 2020, https://www.theatlantic.com/family/archive/2020/04/why-your-zoom-happy-hour-unsatisfying/609823/.

55. Jeremy Bailenson, "Nonverbal Overload: A Theoretical Argument for the Causes of Zoom Fatigue," *Technology, Mind, and Behavior* 2 no. 1 (2021).

56. Barbara Couture, "Reconciling Private Lives and Public Rhetoric: What's at Stake?" in *The Private, the Public, and the Published: Reconciling Private Lives and Public Rhetoric*, ed. Barbara Couture and Thomas Kent (Utah State University Press, 2004), 2.

57. Couture, "Reconciling Private Lives," 4.

58. Tabitha Moses, "5 Reasons to let Students Keep their Cameras off During Zoom Classes," *The Conversation*, August 17, 2020, https://theconversation.com/5-reasons-to-let-students-keep-their-cameras-off-during-zoom-classes-144111.

59. "What is 'Meatspace'?" *Merriam-Webster*, https://www.merriam-webster.com/words-at-play/what-is-meatspace.

60. Kazys Varnelis and Anne Friedberg, "Place: The Networking of Public Space," in *Networked Publics,* ed. Kazys Varnelis (MIT Press, 2008), 25–27.

61. Norm Friesen, "The Bizarre Intimacy of Zoom Meetings," *Mic*, April 2, 2020, https://www.mic.com/p/the-bizarre-intimacy-of-zoom-meetings-22684781.

62. Madeleine Aggeler, "The Bizarre Intimacy of Video Chat," *The Cut*, March 20, 2020, https://www.thecut.com/2020/03/video-chat-intimacy-coronavirus.html.

63. Leah Prinzivalli, "The Bizarre Intimacy of Group Fitness on Zoom," *Outside*, April 15, 2020, https://www.outsideonline.com/2411585/zoom-fitness-classes-coronavirus.

64. "Social Nudity in the Age of Isolation: Naked on ZOOM!" *The Meandering Naturalist*, April 5, 2020, https://meanderingnaturist.com/2020/04/05/social-nudity-in-the-age-of-isolation-naked-on-zoom.

65. Sonia Livingstone, "In Defence of Privacy: Mediating the Public/Private Boundary at Home," in *Audiences and Publics: When Cultural Engagement Matters for the Public Sphere*, ed. Sonia Livingstone (Bristol, UK: Intellect Books, 2005), 163.

66. *The Office*, "Michael Drives into a Lake—The Office US," *YouTube*, August 8, 2017, https://www.youtube.com/watch?v=DOW_kPzY_JY.

67. Akiko Fujita, "GPS Tracking Disaster: Japanese Tourists Drive Straight into the Pacific," *ABC News*, March 16, 2012, https://abcnews.go.com/blogs/headlines/2012/03/gps-tracking-disaster-japanese-tourists-drive-straight-into-the-pacific.

68. Andrew King and Jim A. Kuypers, "Our Roots are Strong and Deep," in *Twentieth-Century Roots of Rhetorical Studies*, ed. Jim A. Kuypers and Andrew King (Westport, CT: Praeger, 2001), ix-xx.

69. David M. Berg, "Rhetoric, Reality, and Mass Media," *The Quarterly Journal of Speech* 58, no. 3 (1972): 255–263.

70. See Lisa Messeri "Realities of Illusion: Tracing an Anthropology of the Unreal from Torres Strait to Virtual Reality," *Journal of the Royal Anthropological Institute* 27 (2021): 340–359.

71. Jordan Frith, "Pushing Back on the Rhetoric of 'Real' Life," *Present Tense* 8, no. 2 (2020), http://www.presenttensejournal.org/volume-8/pushing-back-on-the-rhetoric-of-real-life/.

72. Andrew Ross Sorkin, "Bitcoin's Climate Problem," *New York Times*, March 9, 2021, https://www.nytimes.com/2021/03/09/business/dealbook/bitcoin-climate-change.html.

73. See Frith, "Pushing Back"; see also Nonny de la Peña, "Embodied Digital Rhetoric: Soft Selves, Plastic Presence, and the Nonfiction Narrative," in *Digital Rhetoric and Global Literacies; Communication Modes and Digital Practices in the Networked World*, ed. Gustav Verhulsdonck and Marohang Limbu (IGI Global, 2014), 312–327.

74. Nick Couldry and Andreas Hepp, *The Mediated Construction of Reality* (Polity, 2016), 7.

75. For a few of many news stories on pandemic misinformation, see Miles Parks, "Few Facts, Millions of Clicks: Fearmongering Vaccine Stories Go Viral Online," *NPR*, March 25, 2021, https://www.npr.org/2021/03/25/980035707/lying-through-truth-misleading-facts-fuel-vaccine-misinformation; Joseph Choi, "Russia Trying to Undermine Confidence in COVID-19 Vaccines: Report," *The Hill*, March 8, 2021, https://thehill.com/policy/international/russia/542092-russia-trying-to-undermine-confidence-in-covid-19-vaccines-report; Kat Eschner, "Get Wise to Covid Rumors," *New York Times*, February 12, 2021, https://www.nytimes.com/2021/02/12/well/covid-vaccine-misinformation.html; Geoff Brumfiel, "The Life Cycle of a COVID-19 Vaccine Lie," *NPR*, July 20, 2021, https://www.npr.org/sections/health-shots/2021/07/20/1016912079/the-life-cycle-of-a-covid-19-vaccine-lie?fbclid=IwAR0yeKXDxpq_lurG5bO_dtUKffRsjcCCGcWjGx3DfStlau5Mam21ZJuGRWo.

76. Riccardo Gallotti, Francesco Valle, Nicola Castaldo, Pierluigi Sacco, and Manilo DeDomenico, "Assessing the Risks of 'Infodemics' in Response to COVID-19 Epidemics," *Nature Human Behavior* 4, no. 12 (December 2020): 1285–1293.

77. See Jenny Edbauer, "Unframing Models of Public Distribution: From Rhetorical Situation to Rhetorical Ecologies," *Rhetoric Society Quarterly* 35, no. 4 (2005): 5–24.

78. See Dana L. Cloud, *Reality Bites: Rhetoric and the Circulation of Truth Claims in U.S. Political Culture* (Ohio State University Press, 2018), 9.

79. Laurie E. Gries, "Iconographic Tracking: A Digital Research Method for Visual Rhetoric and Circulation Studies," *Computers and Composition* 30 (2013): 346; see also Kelly A. Clancy and Benjamin Clancy, "Growing Monstrous Organisms: The Construction of Anti-GMO Visual Rhetoric Through Digital Media," *Critical Studies in Media Communication* 33, no. 3 (2016): 279–292.

80. For a primer on criticism of digital rhetoric, see, Michelle G. Gibbons, "Criticism of Digital Rhetoric," in *Rhetorical Criticism: Perspectives in Action*, 3rd edition, ed. Jim Kuypers (Rowman & Littlefield, 2021), 299–320.

81. Kathleen Hall Jamieson, "How to Debunk Misinformation about COVID, Vaccines, and Masks," *Scientific American*, April 1, 2021, https://www.scientificamerican.com/article/how-to-debunk-misinformation-about-covid-vaccines-and-masks/.

82. Douglas Eyman, *Digital Rhetoric: Theory, Method, Practice* (Ann Arbor: University of Michigan Press, 2015), 9.

Chapter 2

Journalism Framing in (Times of) Crisis

The Inevitability of Poor Reporting During the COVID-19 Pandemic

Michael Horning and Jim A. Kuypers

Reporting during any crisis is a challenging endeavor. The COVID-19 pandemic is particularly notable due to both the length of time it persisted and for the complex reportorial context that prevailed. COVID related news moved at an unprecedented rate of speed, often with new scientific discoveries becoming outdated or retracted as quickly as they were published or even prepublished. Within this environment the COVID crisis unfolded, and journalists were faced with the task of quickly interpreting complex, often changing, and imperfect data. Adding to this complicated context is the very nature of journalists themselves, who have historically been ill equipped to report on scientific matters because they so often lack the depth of knowledge to ask the right questions about studies, reports, etc.[1] During the pandemic we see a constantly changing narrative: wear masks, do not wear masks; this drug works, this one does not; the disease is virulent, the disease is difficult to contract; and so on. In some instances this changing narrative is reflective of the constant stream of changing information that comes from "experts"; yet, on the other hand, it also comes from the inability of journalists to communicate scientific data effectively, both in terms of background training and educational preparation. In fact, as the news media attempted to cover a number of constantly shifting narratives about everything from "flattening the curve" to the (in)effectiveness of wearing masks, the effect of changing narratives and new information seemed to be that members of the public became increasingly divided on what to believe,[2] even as the mainstream news media (MSM) increasingly pushed a preferred narrative, eventually limiting information that did not fit (for example, lockdowns are beneficial, or that the virus did not originate in the Wuhan lab).[3] Such outcomes suggest perhaps a significant deficiency in the way that the MSM covered the pandemic and indicate that journalists still have much to learn about how to report on scientific matters.[4]

In the pages that follow we explore these issues in six sections. First, we provide a brief overview of the area of study known as Journalism & Mass Communication which leads into our second area, observations about the educational preparation of journalists and how framing theory can help explain their reportorial practice during the pandemic. Following this we look at an extended case study examining a specific instance of the reporting on hydroxychloroquine as a treatment for COVID-19. We then look at how this knowledge impacts future teaching in this area, followed by suggestions for future research, and our final thoughts.

OVERVIEW OF JOURNALISM AND MASS COMMUNICATION AS AN AREA OF STUDY

The idea of the professional, formally trained journalist is a relatively young area of study in the university, tracing its origins to the end of the 19th century; prior to that, newspapers relied on public officials, printers, and volunteers to produce the news events of the day.[5] By the time America entered the 20th century, however, the newspaper business was booming, and the idea of journalists as paid professionals was becoming mainstream. This was the era known as Yellow Journalism when newspaper barons such as Joseph Pulitzer and William Randolph Hearst hired journalists to fill their pages with sensational and scandalous stories that appealed to mass audiences.[6] At this time, with no formal training, journalists learned their craft on the job.

In 1912, the University of Wisconsin formed the first journalism department. Although offering journalism classes as early as 1904, with the formalization of a degree it quickly became the key institution for journalist training. The journalism curriculum at that time was heavily influenced by the humanities with a strong emphasis on writing, and although journalists took classes in sociology, history, and politics, the focus even in those courses emphasized humanistic methods of inquiry. A similar program in journalism was established at the University of Iowa in the early 1900s, and by 1924 Iowa had also established a School of Journalism which offered a strongly applied journalism curriculum with courses in news editing, copyreading, advertising, and magazine writing—all of which were skills in high demand during the heyday of newspaper publishing.[7] This kind of program growth only continued during the ensuing decades across America.

Today journalism is often taught in Mass Communications schools and offers majors that focus on areas such as television, radio, and online news, with courses at the undergraduate level still largely emphasizing an applied approach to journalism education. There remains minimal opportunities for aspiring journalists to hone their scientific skills, however. For example, the Accrediting Council on Education in Journalism and Mass Communication, which is the largest accrediting body for journalism schools, does prescribe a specific curriculum for journalism education that requires certified journalism programs to focus on such areas as press law, history of media institutions, issues of diversity, ethics, writing style, and reporting accuracy. And yet, even though the standards for certification suggest that students of journalism be able to apply *basic* numerical and statistical concepts, the curriculum on the whole is still almost exclusively applied, and leaves it up to the individual student or the university to require any meaningful science education as a part of the journalism degree.[8]

EDUCATIONAL PREPARATION OF JOURNALISTS AND FRAMING THEORY

We turn now to exploring some of the critical issues faced by the MSM during the pandemic; specifically, we seek to better understand how matters of a scientific nature were covered by the news media. To do so we use both the idea of educational preparation (or lack thereof) and framing theory as critical lenses as we consider how journalists covered the reporting on the efficaciousness of hydroxychloroquine. We look specifically at how the MSM's reporting on this issue induces particular audience understandings (both epistemic and political) of the issues, and also relates to reportorial ability and ethics.

Journalist Educational Preparation

At the turn of the 20th century in the United States, journalism was relatively subjective, mired in low credibility, and often privileged sensational stories. However, a number of factors began to shift journalism to take a more objective style in its reporting. Although the lines of objective, fact-based reporting can be traced back to the use of the telegraph during the War Between the States, we see an especially strong embrace of it with the rise of public relations and advertising. Michael Schudson, for example, argued that as public relations used various propaganda techniques in advertising, and as it became increasingly difficult to assess truth from lies, publics began to crave a reporting style that relied on objective, more dispassionate reporting.[9] This, along with an increasingly complex, quickly industrializing world, eventually lead Adolph Ochs, the owner and publisher of the *New York Times* to famously state: "It will be my earnest aim that THE NEW YORK TIMES give the news, all the news, in concise and attractive form . . . to give the news impartially, without fear or favor, regardless of any party, sect or interest involved."[10] This marked a new era in journalism, with objectivity becoming a bedrock principle, although not always practice, for the remainder of the 20th century. Most journalistic codes of ethics today continue to stress such a view, even in the face of a growing practice of "advocacy journalism." For instance, The Society of Professional Journalists states that "public enlightenment is the forerunner of justice and the foundation of democracy. The duty of the journalist is to further those ends by seeking truth and providing a fair and comprehensive account of events and issues."[11] The Associated Press Managing Editors Code of Ethics states in part that, the "good newspaper is fair, accurate, honest, responsible, independent and decent" and that "Truth is its guiding principle."[12] The American Society of Newspaper Editors statement of principles, under the heading of "truth and accuracy," states: "Every effort must be made to assure that the news content is accurate, free from bias and in context, and that all sides are presented fairly. Significant errors of fact, as well as errors of omission, should be corrected promptly and prominently." Additionally, the "primary purpose of gathering and distributing news and opinion is to serve the general welfare by informing the people and enabling them to make judgments on the issues of the time."[13] Clearly "America's mainstream news media voluntarily pledge to follow ethical reporting practices by providing the public with complete, accurate details, within an unbiased context, so that the people may make informed political judgments."[14]

On the matter of truth, Thomas E. Patterson wrote that there is "no reason to question reporters' determination to deliver . . . 'the best obtainable version of truth.'"[15] Yet even he admits that reporters are often wrong, as did James Curran, who stated that, concerning forecasting outcomes in particular, they get it, "'repeatedly, wildly wrong.'"[16] Along these lines David Broder wrote his own "experience suggests that we [journalists] often have a hard time finding our way through the maze of facts—visible and concealed—in any story. And even when the facts seem most evident to our senses, we go astray by our misunderstanding and misjudgment of the context in which they belong."[17] Yet reporters speak with such certainty, often arrogantly so,[18] even as in the next breath they append qualifiers to facts to the point of meaninglessness, as in this sentence: "*Most* people who recover from COVID-19 *could have* immunity that lasts at least a year or even longer—and *may not need* a booster shot after being vaccinated."[19] And although they may well strive to provide "the truth," so often this "truth" is not the objective reality in front of them, but their presuppositions and *a priori* truths that guide both their observations and evaluations. These journalistic "shared values" are often the cause of going astray from the truth.[20]

Certainly reporting on science-oriented topics should be especially fact based, but when confronted with ideologically influenced observations, the challenges of comprehending complex scientific data, and a trend toward ever more opinion-filled hard news, this becomes problematic.[21] Much of reporting is simply conjectural, especially where discussion of policy and science is concerned, as during the pandemic. As Walter Lippmann wrote, "where the issue is complex, as for example in the matter of the success of a policy, or the social conditions among a foreign people,—that is to say, where the real answer is neither yes or no, but subtle, and a matter of balanced evidence . . . the report causes no end of derangement, misunderstanding, and even misrepresentation."[22] Given that scientists devote years of schooling and spend entire careers attempting to master their trade, how can we expect journalists, with little to no scientific training, to be able to report comprehensively on it, especially when we add into the mix considerations of public policy? As Patterson points out, "Almost alone among the professions, journalism is . . . not grounded in a systemic body of substantive knowledge that would protect its practitioners' autonomy and inform their judgment. Medicine, law, and the sciences . . . have disciplinary knowledge that guides practitioners' decision, narrowing the choices and reducing the chances of error."[23] So from where do these decisions flow? As will be seen below, from the shared world views, values, and ideology through which the scientific content is filtered. Most journalists today have a journalism degree, which essentially instills the skills of obtaining and writing a story, all while not being an expert upon that which they report.

This lack of knowledge has consequences impacting the quality of reporting, as concluded by C.W. Anderson, Emily Bell, and Clay Shirky: "most journalists . . . do not spend most of their time conducting anything like empirically robust forms of evidence gathering. . . . [T]he belief in the value of original reporting often exceeds the volume at which it is actually produced."[24] Journalism "students are instructed in the skills of the craft and taught how to construct a broadcast, print or online story. Few journalism schools systematically train student how to access, gain command of and apply subject matter knowledge."[25] Thus context suffers. According to one journalist researcher, science

> journalists are increasingly confronted with covering complicated technical information as well as the potential social, legal, religious, and political consequences of scientific research. Avian flu, embryonic stem cell research, genetic

engineering, global warming, teaching of evolution, and bioterrorism are just a few of the topics on journalists' plates today.[26]

Of course, even in this age of instant and unlimited information, such access has not guaranteed quality reporting or truth. As pointed out by Patterson, unless "the reporter knows something about the subject at hand, the odds of making a mistake are uncomfortably high."[27] Part of this is so since the training of journalists is essentially skills based, focused on "getting" and "presenting" a story. Important elements such as basic knowledge of statistics, the ability to analyze large sets of data and data distributions, are something of which the overwhelming majority of journalists are ignorant. Although there are some rare exceptions, in a large sense, journalism training in schools is a type of learned incapacity.[28] By way of summing up, journalism education has historically emphasized the applied skills that are necessary for good storytelling. At the same time, journalists have historically been poorly trained to cover scientific matters. These facts limit journalists' ability to critically analyze and evaluate scientific literature, particularly in instances where world events lead scientific research to constantly shift and evolve in its understanding of scientific phenomenon.[29]

News Media Framing

Generally speaking, a frame is "a central organizing idea for making sense of relevant events and suggesting what is at issue."[30] Frames have been demonstrated to make some facts more salient to an audience than others, and act to define problems, diagnose causes, and suggest remedies; they also influence moral/ethical evaluations.[31] Of note, they "are located in the communicator, the text, the receiver, and the culture at large. Frames are central organizing ideas within a narrative account of an issue or event; they provide the interpretive cues for otherwise neutral facts."[32] Importantly, they also provide consistent meanings through time, since once established they help to guide the interpretive process. As a process, framing occurs through "the presence or absence of certain keywords, stock phrases, stereotyped images, sources of information, and sentences that provide thematically reinforcing clusters of fact or judgments."[33] To this list we can also add metaphors, concepts, images, labels, and symbols. All these and more act to highlight some features of reality over others. In the case of the MSM, journalists cannot help but frame issues and events in their news stories through both the conscious and unconscious language choices they make. "For instance," asks Jim A. Kuypers, "how often are words such as 'budget cuts' versus 'controlling costs' used across time by journalists when describing Republican efforts to construct a balanced budget? Or using 'undocumented migrant' or 'undocumented citizen' instead of 'illegal alien' or 'illegal immigrant'? Or writing 'anti-abortion' instead of 'pro-life'? Or writing 'single payer healthcare' instead of 'tax-payer funded healthcare'?"[34] Importantly, frames work to highlight some features of reality over others. This works since frames give facts their meaning; they offer a particular understanding, with some facts made more salient than others once an issue has been framed. We see this process of framing operating in the news media discussion of hydroxychloroquine.

HYDROXYCHLOROQUINE AND A RETRACTION

For our case study we examine the May 21, 2020, release of a major study published in the *Lancet* medical journal through to its June 4, 2020, retraction. We examine the following MSM publications as examples of mainstream news sources purporting to provide unbiased, fact-based, neutral reporting: NBC News, ABC News, CBS News, the *New York Times*, *Washington Post*, the *Wall Street Journal,* CNN, Fox News, and MSNBC. We then look at one left-leaning publication, the *Huffington Post*, and one right-leaning publication, Breitbart News, during the same time frame. The idea is to compare the reporting and frames of the self-described left and right publications with the self-described neutral MSM publications. We took for our sample all online published articles that contained the words "hydroxychloroquine" and "Lancet" during the date window above which resulted in 77 articles.

Once articles were collected, in order to determine both what was framed and how, we looked for themes in the news stories. As David Levin articulated, "The reason themes [are] taken as a measure of the presence of frames [is] the difficulty of finding a completely developed frame in a single press release. [Frames] are built across a series of news media articles, and not all elements are present in any single article."[35] We next looked to see how the dominant themes were framed in the news stories and across time, and then compared each publication with the other. Keep in mind that "a theme is the subject of discussion, or that which is the subject of the thought expressed. The frame . . . is suggesting a particular interpretation of the theme."[36] We used no pre-established themes or frames; instead, we engaged in a close-textual reading to determine what the news reports *offered* as themes and frames, thereby making this an inductive style-framing analysis.[37]

We view news stories here collectively as a composite framing event.[38] Looking for points of overlap among single news articles on the announcement of the *Lancet* study, we can detect the major themes and collective framing of those themes as they exist across MSM coverage of the issue. In the case of our *Lancet* study, although individually stories could present independent themes, looked at aggregately, we found that there were two main themes expressed through the flow of coverage: the effects of hydroxychloroquine on COVID-19 sufferers, and results of the study vis-à-vis President Trump.

The Study's Conclusions on the Effects of Hydroxychloroquine

The *Lancet* is a premier and popular medical journal. The study published was focused on the administration of hydroxychloroquine to *hospitalized* COVID-19 patients, with no mention of zinc, a major consideration in studies showing the effectiveness of hydroxychloroquine. The original study was quite clear in not overstating its results:

> We were unable to confirm a benefit of hydroxychloroquine or chloroquine, when used alone or with a macrolide, on in-hospital outcomes for COVID-19. Each of these drug regimens was associated with decreased in-hospital survival and an increased frequency of ventricular arrhythmias when used for treatment of COVID-19.[39]

Variations away from this statement are interpretations from the press, and we found that the results of the study were used to frame hydroxychloroquine as a dangerous drug that was harmful if used by those who have COVID. The results stressing higher rates of death and harmful effects were pushed in almost all articles examined. What was not stressed is that the study was focused on *hospitalized patients*, who are therefore *severely ill,* thus making it seem as if *all* with COVID were at the same risk. This ran across all the news sources examined:

- *CBS* provides a common example of this type of framing: "Malaria drugs pushed by President Donald Trump as treatments for the coronavirus did not help and were tied to a greater risk of death and heart rhythm problems in a new study."[40]
- *NBC* led with this: "hydroxychloroquine does not help COVID-19 patients, and indeed may increase deaths, according to a large, international study published Friday in The Lancet."[41]
- *Breitbart* news, although offering more precise reporting, offered: "Chloroquine and hydroxychloroquine offer no clinical benefit for people with COVID-19 and might cause serious heart-related side effects, according to a study published Friday in The Lancet. People with severe illness caused by the new coronavirus, SARS-CoV-2, treated with either drug—either alone or with an antiviral medication—were up to twice as likely to die than those in the control group."[42]

- *The Wall Street Journal* wrote, "Antimalaria drugs didn't help patients fight Covid-19, while raising the risk for heart problems and death."[43]

Although generally in keeping with the results of the published study, through reportorial interpretation and the picking of sources, the framing of this information was made most dire:

- "this drug combination, whichever way you slice it or dice it, does not show any evidence of benefit and in fact, is immutably showing a signal of grave harm."[44]
- "It's one thing not to have benefit, but this shows distinct harm. . . . If there was ever hope for this drug, this is the death of it."[45]
- The drug "is harmful, and . . . no one should be taking it outside of a clinical trial."[46]
- "another nail in the coffin for hydroxychloroquine."[47]
- "there's no evidence whatsoever in this study . . . of any benefit from hydroxychloroquine and there are really substantial risks."[48]
- "the first principle of medicine is to do no harm, and when you see evidence of a clear signal of harm, one has to take a step back and correct a wrong we may have done."[49]
- "there is no benefit, but . . . a very consistent signal of harm."[50]

Additionally, an important qualifier for the study was that it looked at "hospitalized" patients, thus those who by implication were already seriously ill whether from the disease or pre-existing conditions. This important qualifier was omitted or mentioned only *after* the first five or more paragraphs by approximately 58 percent of the articles examined.

A TRUMP "SANDWICH"

In its coverage of the *Lancet* study, we found that the news media emphasized both numbers of deaths associated with hydroxychloroquine and President Trump as a proponent; moreover, it did not contextualize the study (i.e. hospitalized patients), but rather used a technique called sandwiching to pillory Trump over advocacy of the drug. Sandwiching is a term used to describe a means whereby bias, often political, is introduced into news stories. It is a reportorial framing practice that mimics a sandwich in that it involves the placement of something in between two other items of a different nature. As explained by Jim A. Kuypers, the technique involves one element of a story "sandwiched" in between two other elements. [T]here is a "fairness and balance" bias inherent within the American press, so the press often thinks it is being "fair" by presenting "both sides" of an issue. However, even though the "other side" is often presented in a story, the way that a reporter places the sides can change their meaning or interpretation. Often this takes the form of journalists placing explanation or support for whatever "side" of the issue they disagree with in between complimentary points of view, and these views tend to agree with the position espoused by the journalists. So, whatever positions journalists dislike are made to seem weaker than those they support. This is often accomplished by journalists writing a summation of the story (with or without quotes) that supports a point of view (side 1) and then presentation of the other point of view (side 2), and then quotes supporting the journalists' point of view (side 1). Although on its face balanced (since "both" sides are presented), in practice the story is biased toward one side.[51]

We see this practice throughout the reporting of the *Lancet* study with President Trump the inner portion of the press "sandwich." Generally speaking, examples of this technique can range from pithy[52] to lengthy, as were those in our case study here. They took a form that conveyed an attempt to confront and damage President Trump, making the press into adversaries, not objective reporters—thus, presentation of facts, but in such a way as to take sides. For instance, CBS provided three paragraphs stressing the high risk of using hydroxychloroquine to treat COVID-19 [side 1], ending with the paragraph,

> Side 1: "'It really does give us some degree of confidence that we are unlikely to see major benefits from these drugs in the treatment of COVID-19 and possibly harm.'"

Then the Trump paragraph:

> Side 2: "President Trump has repeatedly pushed the malarial drugs, and has said he is taking hydroxychloroquine to try to prevent infection or minimize symptoms from the coronavirus."

After which the story has two paragraphs again stressing the high risk and dangers:

> Side 1: "no large rigorous tests have found them safe or effective for preventing or treating COVID-19. These drugs also have potentially serious side effects."[53]

The *New York Times* provides an example of this as well:

Side 1: "The drugs did not help coronavirus patients, and should not be used outside clinical trials, researchers said. The malaria drugs hydroxychloroquine and chloroquine did not help coronavirus patients and may have done harm, according to a new study based on the records of nearly 15,000 patients who received the drugs and 81,000 who did not."

Side 2: "hydroxychloroquine is the drug that President Trump has advocated, and that he said he has been taking in hopes of preventing coronavirus infection."

Side 1: "People who received the drugs were more likely to have abnormal heart rhythms. . . . They were also more likely to die."[54]

CNN represents a particularly aggressive use of the technique, beginning its article with a clearly mocking montage video of President Trump saying, dozens of times, the word "hydroxychloroquine" and placing this immediately following its headline—for viewing prior to reading the story. With this in mind, we find the following sandwiching sequence:

Side 1: Headline: "Drug touted by Trump as Covid-19 treatment linked to a greater risk of death, study finds."

Side 1: Mocking video montage

Side 1: "Seriously ill Covid-19 patients who were treated with hydroxychloroquine or chloroquine were more likely to die or develop dangerous irregular heart rhythms. . . .

Side 2: "President Donald Trump has been a frequent cheerleader for a combination of the antimalarial hydroxychloroquine and the antibiotic azithromycin as a Covid-19 treatment. He promoted the drugs nearly 50 times, despite pleas from scientists to let studies decide if the treatment worked or not."

Side 1: The lead author of the study, "told CNN that he would recommend hospitals stop using these drugs to treat Covid-19. 'Our data has very convincingly shown that across the world in a real-world population that this drug combination . . . does not show any evidence of benefit, and in fact, is immutably showing a signal of grave harm.'"[55]

The framing of this theme was made to mock the President, and turned the reporting of the study into a blow against the President, thus politicizing what should have been a scientific presentation of the merits and demerits of the study. Instead, with President Trump used as a foil, the study's findings were artificially enhanced to such a degree, and the press frame so strengthened, that stray contrary facts, such as other studies showing the effectiveness of hydroxychloroquine, were omitted. The aggregate strength of this frame was so strong that 50 percent of the articles examined place "Trump" in the title of the article, as in this example from *The New York Times*: "Malaria Drug Taken by Trump Is Tied to Increased Risk of Heart Problems and Death in New Study."[56]

ALTERNATE FRAMING

Any given theme may be framed in different ways, and the stories on the *Lancet* study could have offered alternate frames, especially given the various news sources. Yet such was not the case. Only four outlets of the 11 included any information touching upon alternate explanations for the initial *Lancet* study: *CBS, NBC, ABC,* and *Breitbart News. CBS*, at the very end of one of its articles quoted White House Corona Virus Response Coordinator Deborah Birx who stressed that "many of the patients in the study had other underlying health conditions."[57] And also touched upon shortcomings of observational studies of this type. *ABC* also quoted Birx, thus putting attention on the idea of "comorbidities."[58] *NBC* included comments from a pulmonologist not part of the study who stated, "'If we gave the hydroxychloroquine to less sick patients, maybe we'd see a benefit.'"[59] *Breitbart News* also mentioned that the authors cautioned that "it is not possible to exclude the possibility that other, unmeasured factors were responsible for the apparent link between treatment with these drugs and the decrease in patient survival," and importantly, that "randomized clinical trials are needed before any conclusion can be reached regarding benefit or harm of these agents in COVID-19 patients."[60] Of course, none of these instances rise to the level of a frame, only hint at the possibility, and collectively offer no counter balance to the overall trajectory of the MSM frames; their salience was minimized by the power of the overall frame.

Dominant frames are also supported by omitted information.[61] Frames both increase and decrease the saliency of certain information, "but they also make it easier for those writing stories to leave out contradictory information that does not 'fit' in the frame the journalist is constructing."[62] This "reinforcement of existing attitudes through omission is far from the trivial effect that many scholars imply. Holding support under adverse new conditions is a crucial goal in politics, not just winning over new supporters. So one way the media wield influence is by omitting or de-emphasizing information, by excluding data about an altered reality that might otherwise disrupt existing support."[63]

Looking at the reporting about the *Lancet* study we find that the media tend to simplify the research around hydroxychloroquine that was going on at the time. For example, there were a number of more tightly controlled field trials testing the drug that could yield more definitive results than the observational data in the *Lancet* study. In addition, all media accounted for here failed to mention ongoing research about zinc's important role in recovery and effectiveness, and none mentioned that it was already known that hydroxychloroquine results have been best with mild to moderate cases that include zinc treatment as well. Essentially all positive or ongoing work with hydroxychloroquine was omitted from reporting of the study. *Breitbart News*, for example, went so far as to write: "Their praise [President Trump, Elon Musk, others] has come despite a lack of scientific evidence."[64] Yet this completely ignores the successes of physicians such as Didier Raoult, whose work with hydroxychloroquine and zinc against COVID shows enormous promise. In a sense, it would have been easy for the reporters to mention that advocates of hydroxychloroquine treatment for COVID have never suggested that hospitalized COVID patients were good candidates for treatment. Instead, they have primarily advocated a regimen of hydroxychloroquine with zinc for treatment in the initial onset and early stage of COVID symptoms. The reason for this is that hydroxychloroquine enables easier absorption of zinc into the cells where the viral replication is then disrupted by the zinc. In short, the *Lancet* study reporting simply told what was already known by those against hydroxychloroquine's use and ignored how it was being successfully administered. Such admissions are unconscionable.[65] Of note is that although in general *Fox News* and *Breitbart News* often offer alternate frames to political topics, there was only limited evidence of that with scientific reporting.[66]

THE OFFICIAL RETRACTION

On June 4, 2020, the authors of the *Lancet* study voluntarily retracted it due to issues with the validity of the database used, in particular because they did not feel that they could verify the data which was provided by a third party and because it received significant criticisms from the scientific community. Ten of the eleven news outlets offered stories specifically on the retraction. This lead paragraph by *ABC News* (which was also quoted by *Brietbart News*)[67] sums well the frame used by the press with the retraction: "Several authors of a large study that raised safety concerns about malaria drugs for coronavirus patients have retracted the report, saying independent reviewers were not able to verify information that's been widely questioned by other scientists."[68] *NBC News* explained it this way: "A first-year statistics major could tell you about major flaws in the design of the analysis," one expert said. "Thursday's retraction doesn't mean that the drug is helpful—or harmful—with respect to the coronavirus. Rather, the study authors were unable to confirm that the data set was accurate."[69] In short, media reports suggested that nothing they said before changes, just that this study was removed from the discussion. We note here, though, that the study was clearly used to push the alleged dangers of the drug; importantly, the framing of the retraction was for that study, but the original tone and anti-hydroxychloroquine reporting of the previous articles mentioning the study were allowed to stand.

The New York Times, Brietbart News, and *Fox News* were the only news organizations that offered more than a simple retraction, yet still maintained the overall press framing of hydroxychloroquine. *Fox News*, for example, offered that "Controversial research into the effectiveness of COVID-19 drug hydroxychloroquine is coming under scrutiny as experts raise serious scientific questions"[70] about the data used, thus continuing the frame and the overall uncertainty about its effectiveness, even as it failed to denote well the difference between hospitalized and initial COVID infection uses for the drug.

The New York Times offered that

> The retractions may breathe new life into the antimalarial drugs hydroxychloroquine and chloroquine, relentlessly promoted by Mr. Trump as a remedy for Covid-19 despite a lack of evidence. But the retractions also raise troubling questions about the state of scientific research as the pandemic spreads. Thousands of papers are being rushed to online sites and journals with little or no peer review, and critics fear long-held standards of even the most discerning journals are eroding as they face pressure to rapidly vet and disseminate new scientific reports.[71]

Important questions, but note that the *New York Times* still refuses to acknowledge studies showing the effectiveness when combined with zinc in early stages of the disease. The *Washington Post*, too, mentioned that the controversy with hydroxychloroquine would continue, as well that there are questions from "the medical and scientific community that researchers and prestigious medical journals are lowering their standards in a rush to publish during the pandemic."[72]

FRAMING, POLITICS, SCIENTIFIC KNOWLEDGE, AND REPORTORIAL PRACTICES

In this section, we look at where journalists failed in their reporting of the *Lancet* study. We highlight several fundamental deficiencies in the reporting that could have been avoided had journalists been better equipped and willing to analyze the science behind the study, and had they engaged in more critical reflection of their own biases. Perhaps most troubling is the observation that the *Lancet* study reporting had significant consequences on both future research and public opinion that was founded upon flawed scientific data. For example, Reuters reported that after coverage of the study, patients in field trials with hydroxychloroquine began to fear the effects of the drug and withdrew their participation; even the World Health Organization stopped all studies.[73] Perhaps most concerning is the fact the other researchers who were unaware of the retraction continued to reference the findings in the *Lancet* study as stated fact, thus furthering the spread of misinformation and public confusion.[74] Adding to the confusion was the fact that of the initial May 22 and 23 stories focusing on the release of the *Lancet* study, only three, CBS, *The New York Times*, and the *Washington Post* mentioned the subsequent June retraction of the study as a note in their original stories. None of the stories that mention the study that fell between the initial report and the stories of the retraction were subsequently modified to include the retraction, meaning that, except for the three mentions above of the retraction, all stories up to the stories on the retraction advanced the original illegitimate *Lancet* study results as if they were not retracted. In short, news sources, although offering a retraction article, allowed the original reported results and framing to stand. Certainly journalists must make every effort to ensure accuracy in their reporting, even at times when the facts themselves can change.

A FAILURE TO CONTEXTUALIZE SCIENTIFIC RESEARCH

The events that unfolded around the *Lancet* study suggest there are a number of actions that journalists could take to avoid such catastrophes in reporting in the future. First, there is a tendency in journalism to report on each new ground-breaking discovery as if it were conclusive, but scientists themselves recognize that it often takes numerous studies and years, even decades, of research to reach any formal conclusion about a matter. Given this reality, journalists would do well to contextualize studies within the body of literature surrounding any given finding. In other words, any area of scientific research has background contexts that are often discussed in the study itself. This background and context are often essential to understanding the degree to which a set of findings could be generalized to a given population. When journalists fail to explain how a given study is situated within this context, they also fail at their mission of informing the public. Whereas scientists see research as a conversation with results that are often flawed and nuanced, journalists often try to simplify these findings, and such reports often only lead to an increase in misinformation and a more confused public.

A FAILURE TO UNDERSTAND GOOD SCIENTIFIC PRACTICES

Journalists covering scientific research often fail to take into consideration the research methodologies of any given study and how these methodologies present certain limitations to any given finding; they should know the basic differences between surveys, observations, and experiments, and how each approach used by a researcher places certain limits on a finding. For example, researchers have often known that experimental studies, particularly in medical research, are critical for testing the effects of any drug because these methodologies make use of randomized sampling techniques and controlled laboratory conditions that allow researchers to rule out other influences also known as confounds. The *Lancet* study in contrast relied on observational data, a considerably more imperfect approach to medical research, and although a few outlets mentioned this, fewer still adequately explained its full meaning.

There are other methodological issues, such as the quality of the sample in a study, that place limits on the validity of any piece of research. In the *Lancet* study, researchers garnered a seemingly impressive sample of over 90,000 patients, but the study fell short in that there could be wildly different conditions under which hospitalized patients were administered hydroxychloroquine. Other sampling issues may have been complicated by the hospital conditions and policies that determined uses and doses of hydroxychloroquine. Each of these variations in sampling can introduce error in any research study. Journalists, however, who in the main are ill equipped to analyze research for such problems, far too often report findings with an uncritical eye, as they did here.

In addition, given the scrutiny that science is often under today, scientists are increasingly called upon to be more transparent in their processes. In practice this means documenting their practices through the entire research project. This could include documentation on how the data was analyzed (e.g. statistic formulas and software used) and access to that data for secondary analysis so that future researchers can verify its accuracy. The Open Science Foundation, an advocate for transparency in research, notes a number of standards for good transparency practice. These could include preserving versions and revisions of a research document, listing outside sources of funding and conflicts of interest, and providing consumers with direct access to review key research claims.[75] Yet the *Lancet* study failed to use such standards in their report. In fact, the organization that housed the data refused to provide both their analysis and the raw data that was used so that it could be checked for accuracy. Although it is true that a journalist covering a new study may not be able to do all of the heavy analysis needed to verify claims in a given study, with proper training and a little effort they are more than capable of verifying that the information is available to experts should the need arise. Yet in none of our news stories do we see journalists exacting this level of scrutiny on the *Lancet* study. Further, in none of their news reports do we see journalists caution publics about the lack of transparency that was provided.

Patterson has provided a way for journalists to investigate questions around transparency by suggesting that journalists can move beyond basic reports about science and serve as "knowledge brokers" who help publics in understanding scientific processes. Referring to Patterson's ideas, Nisbet argues that "journalists [should] play an essential role as 'knowledge brokers,' unpacking the process of expert knowledge production for their readers, examining how and why scientific research was done, sometimes positing alternative interpretations or drawing connections to ongoing debates about a complex problem. Through this perspective, readers learn not only about the basic facts of science, but also how scientific research is conducted, interpreted, communicated, and contested."[76]

A Failure to Do Basic Good Journalism

A week after the *Lancet* study was published over 100 scientists signed their name to an open letter which heavily criticized the study for a number of problematic issues, some of which have already been noted above.[77] The scientists observed that the hydroxychloroquine study failed on a number of *basic* levels, noting, for example, that the study had some elementary math issues. Among those issues were common concerns about statistics used in the study, and in one instance some of the COVID cases reported by hospitals in the countries under study exceeded the numbers of cases reported by governments in those countries at the time. Failure to check such basic facts is perhaps among the more glaring examples of how journalists could have been more critical of the study. This is not a failure to understand science, but a failure to engage in due diligence by fact-checking claims. The Society of Professional Journalists clearly states this expectation to verify when it notes that journalists must "take responsibility for the accuracy of their work [and] verify information before releasing."[78] So embedded in professional expectations are these simple steps that Bill Kovach and Tom Rosenstiel, in the *Elements of Journalism*, dedicate an entire chapter to the verification of facts, and note that "in the end, the discipline of verification is what separates journalism from entertainment, propaganda, fiction or art."[79] Yet in the coverage of the *Lancet* study, journalists seem to lose these critical abilities.

In addition to this failure to check basic facts, in the *Lancet* study we see journalists deviate from other ethical concerns. Beyond the Society of

Professional Journalists Code of Ethics, the Radio Television Digital News Association (RTDNA) suggest that journalists are obligated to reflect on their failures of coverage and vigorously correct them:

> Effectively explaining editorial decisions and processes does not mean making excuses. Transparency requires reflection, reconsideration and honest openness to the possibility that an action, however well intended, was wrong. Ethical journalism requires owning errors, correcting them promptly and giving corrections as much prominence as the error itself had.[80]

In the coverage of the *Lancet* study, we clearly do not see journalism engage in any significant reflection of how it got things so wrong, nor do we see equal prominence given to the retraction. For example, in the previously mentioned retraction from *The New York Times*, we see not only a failure to reflect on how they could do better and where they got it wrong, but also a diverting of the blame to other concerns in scientific research:

> The retractions also raise troubling questions about the state of scientific research as the pandemic spreads. Thousands of papers are being rushed to online sites and journals with little or no peer review, and critics fear long-held standards of even the most discerning journals are eroding as they face pressure to rapidly vet and disseminate new scientific reports.[81]

Although this observation may be true, it is a self-serving, overly broad indictment of scientific research. The *Lancet* medical journal, for example, has a fairly rigorous set of standards and ranks among the highest cited medical journals in the world. And although cases like this provide examples of times when even some of the best journals fail to get it right, for journalists of *The New York Times* to provide this argument as a rationale for their basic failure to do good journalism evades the more critical question of why they did not engage in more scrutiny of themselves.

A Failure to Report Retractions in an Ethical Manner

We see other good journalistic practices break down concerning the *Lancet* study, especially when we turn our attention to ethical issues in journalism. In many instances, news organizations left original reports of the *Lancet* study up on their websites without providing addendums that indicated that the study had been retracted, and when journalists did cover retractions they dedicated much less coverage to the topic. Moreover, those stories referencing the *Lancet* study that were published between the original story on the study through to the stories on the retraction did not contain a retraction. Thus, numerous stories cited the original *Lancet* study as true, even after it was retracted. This is a basic breakdown in transparency practices advocated by most professional journalism organizations that mistakes be corrected "prominently" and explained "clearly."[82] The RTDNA code of ethics is even more clear about such practices and states that "ethical journalism requires owning errors, correcting them promptly and giving corrections as much prominence as the error itself had."[83] Yet in the coverage of the *Lancet* study and its retraction we see journalists fail their basic obligation to correct and document misinformation promoted by their organization.

HOW THE PANDEMIC IMPACTED OR WILL IMPACT THE TEACHING OF JOURNALISM AND MASS COMMUNICATION

Since the 1930s, science coverage has been typically treated as just one of the types of stories journalists covered in any given day. In other words, journalists have rarely seen themselves as wholly dedicated to the coverage of science and have largely treated its coverage like other types of news.[84] Sharon Dunwoody notes that coverage of science has largely followed journalistic norms rather than scientific ones. For example, stories on science rarely explore methods or processes that have led to scientific discoveries. Instead they focus on other journalistic norms that typically dictate coverage such as whether a scientific discovery is timely, unusual, novel, or dramatic.[85] Science, however, is often the opposite, with slow progress toward definitive results. It is sometimes mundane, yet important. Scientific discoveries are often quite complex to interpret, and quite often limited in scope. Today these truths are often glossed over by reportorial standards in the interest of constructing a simple narrative that could be packaged for television or a quick scan on the web. The problem with such coverage, of course, is that when journalists get the coverage wrong they contribute to the streams of misinformation and confusion that often plague news reports today. Many aspects of life have changed as a result of the global pandemic brought about by COVID-19, and to that end we suggest that journalism education itself reflect on the ways that it could improve reporting norms and practices in the future. As a result, we offer the following suggestions.

First, journalism curriculums must do better at helping journalists deal with scientific coverage. A curriculum must emphasize the importance of covering science according to standards set by science and not by journalism. As we have noted, scientists cover each new scientific discovery with a certain degree of skepticism. They acknowledge the limits of a scientific finding and they contextualize each scientific discovery in the historical contexts in which that study had taken place. These are just a few of the standing practices that should be emphasized in science reporting.

Second, journalism education should develop a special set of ethics and practices for retractions when science reporting fails. These might include requiring students to examine case studies on "science reporting failures" and considerations of how students might avoid such pitfalls in the future. In addition, students should be encouraged to develop standards for retractions in terms of how these are publicized and corrected on the mediums in which they were created. For websites, this might mean giving more prominent coverage to retractions. At the very least, it should include the removal of false reports or footnotes indicating the errors in coverage.

Third, journalism education must acknowledge that biases, including the political, exist in news reporting, and adopt standards of education that address these biases[86] in such a manner that students have realistic expectations of the challenges they will soon face. For instance, in this chapter we have seen how journalists reported on the *Lancet* study without properly considering studies that fell outside of the MSM accepted narrative about hydroxychloroquine, and by omitting those studies, diminished a fuller understanding of the *Lancet* study in the overall discussion. Journalists' antipathy toward President Trump also contributed to a sense of "gotcha!" in the reporting, thus contributing to contextualizing the study in a political as opposed to scientific manner. Unconscious biases are a well-known and accepted norm in psychology,[87] yet far too many journalists refuse to acknowledge their own unconscious biases for or against certain policies and politicians. Identification of such biases and how to act to mitigate them should be part of basic journalistic education.

FUTURE SUGGESTIONS FOR RESEARCH IN JOURNALISM AND MASS COMMUNICATION

Obviously one case study such as the *Lancet*'s retraction of hydroxychloroquine research is not definitive proof that science journalism is always poorly done and our analysis here is limited to some of the more popular mainstream news sites that are read by mass audiences and liberal and conservative groups. Other research might cast a wider net and consider how some of the more niche publications that are dedicated to science might cover complicated scientific matters. There are also a number of studies both empirical and humanistic that academic researchers might conduct to explore the concerns we have raised further. For example, Anders Hansen has suggested that it is time for journalism studies to specifically look again at questions of accuracy around scientific reporting.[88] Studies in this area were popular in the 70s and 80s but have since become less of a focus despite the proliferation of misinformation widely available on the internet and that is easier to generate with modern digital publishing platforms. Content analytic approaches that explore track records of accuracy in scientific matters across newsrooms might be one way to explore this topic. Another approach might consider the degree to which newsrooms make publics aware of scientific retractions and corrections. Research might ask if corrections are given the same prominence and linked to original stories or whether they are instead relegated to the "back page" section of the internet where they are less visible to the public.

In other areas, an excellent case study that might explore differences in reporting coverage, including reporting on scientific nuances, would be the comparison of the lockdown protests in late spring and the summer of 2020 with the Black Lives Matter protests occurring at roughly the same time. Researchers might consider how media framed the wearing of masks and the degree of risks that were involved with public gatherings in public spaces at a time when COVID-19 cases were on the rise in the United States. Other case studies might also take a comparative approach and look at coverage of controversial and noncontroversial science topics. For example, researchers might consider how journalists cover a heavily politicized topic such as climate change versus nonpolitical topics such as a study on how to fend off black widow spiders.[89] When so doing, they could examine how such studies were framed and ask how any retractions were handled. By comparing political topics to nonpolitical topics, one could detect the injection of bias into reportorial practices.

Researchers could also consider examining how journalists use social media to report on science, and how those platforms enhance or diminish thoughtful and informed reporting. For instance, NBC correspondent Ken Dilanian, who covers national security and intelligence issues tweeted this out with no context or explanation: "New data suggests that fully vaccinated individuals are not just contracting COVID, but could be carrying higher levels of virus than previously understood, facilitating spread, my *NBC News* colleagues are reporting. New indoor masking guidance expected today."[90] No further explanation, no link to the sources or to the "new data" mentioned. No explanation why a national security reporter was conveying medical/scientific content. No mention of differences among variants of COVID, or that the different variants have different viral loads (for instance, the Delta variant, which as of this writing is driving the increase in both general infections and cases of those vaccinated, has around 1000 times more of a load than the original viral strain, yet considerably less chance of death). How do such reckless social media posts contribute to the public's misinformation and confusion about science issues?

Finally, studies might turn their focus to journalism education itself and consider how journalists today are prepared for scientific coverage. An analysis of the accredited journalism programs in the country that examine the degree to which students are immersed in science culture and practices could yield useful insights into how well journalism education is preparing students for coverage of these complex topics.

FINAL THOUGHTS

It has often been said that journalists write the first draft of history. It no doubt remains to be seen how history will describe the Global Pandemic of 2020–2022, but it is almost certain that historians of the future will see that journalists made their fair share of mistakes. The question that we raise in this chapter is not what to do when journalists get things wrong, but how do we help them do better at getting things right? To this end we have offered a few suggestions for journalism. Specifically, we observe that journalists were perhaps too eager to publish scientific findings that aligned with their own assumptions. In this instance, Trump, who has had a history of being combative with the media, became too much the focus in the coverage of a study because he supported research contrary to the findings. It seemed as if proving Trump wrong became of greater interest in the reports than scrutinizing the study itself.

In light of this, we suggest that both working journalists and journalism students seek ways to combat their own biases in their reporting by surrounding themselves with more ideologically diverse voices. In the classroom, this may happen through dialogue about the assumptions implied in the frames chosen for a story; in the newsroom it may look more like editorial oversight or observations from ombudsmen who are tasked with the job of thinking about such things. Sadly, it appears that newsrooms are doing the exact opposite in recent years. In 2017, *The New York Times* fired Liz Spayd and eliminated her position as public editor for simply challenging some of what she saw as left-leaning biases in reporting. Spayd once wrote about the liberal bias of *The New York Times* in a column and said, "A paper whose journalism appeals to only half the country has a dangerously severed public mission."[91] In another instance, Glen Greenwald, the Pulitzer Prize winning journalist and founder of the *Intercept*, resigned from that company, claiming, in part, that the media company censored a report that was critical of Joe Biden and his son Hunter. Lara Logan, a former correspondent for *60 Minutes* also recently suggested that mainstream media is increasingly ideological. In an interview reported by *RealClearPolitics*, she said, "We've become political activists in a sense. And some could argue, propagandists, right? . . . The media everywhere is mostly liberal. Not just in the U.S. But in this country,

85 percent of journalists are registered Democrats. So that's just a fact, right? . . . Most journalists are left or liberal or Democrat or whatever word you want to give it."[92]

Although these are just anecdotal examples, prior research has suggested that journalists as a group are overwhelmingly liberal or progressive. This is a longstanding situation, one beginning with a shift from more balanced newsrooms to the left in the late 1950s.[93] Studies show that the percentage of journalists voting for the Democrat candidate for president consistently hovers between 75 and 80% since the 1960s, and other studies have found that when journalists donate to a political campaign, support almost always goes to Democrats.[94]

This type of party and ideological identification is also present among journalism educators. As reported in one study: "One recent study of college professors found that in the communication majors, which tends to be where journalists earn their degrees, the number of Republicans on average approaches zero. Keep in mind that the number of Americans who lean toward or identify as Republican is around 40%, plus or minus a few percentage points."[95] This plays out in the classroom as well, with conservative students feeling pressure to conform with the political views of liberal-minded faculty.[96] All of this, of course, leads to a disconnect between journalists and the public they are to serve, with the lack of viewpoint diversity among journalists contributing to a narrow band of correct reporting, lacking the rich diversity of thought held by the general American public.[97]

Our criticism of the current political and ideological leanings in journalism is not intended to suggest that it is problematic for journalists to have a point of view, but rather to suggest that it is problematic for them to work in silos. Moreover, we point out that the homophilous nature of the current state of news is grossly out of sync with the political and ideological composition of the country. Such practices limit journalists' credibility among over half the public and reduce their trustworthiness when they are called upon to report on matters of scientific importance.

In their recent essay Jose Duarte and his colleagues discuss the inherent problems of this type of groupthink.[98] First, they observe that organizations that lack diversity in thought run the risk of engaging in in-group/out-group behaviors that do not fairly represent the views of individuals who are perceived to be outside of their chosen group affiliation. Given their limited ability to understand the thinking of those groups and their limited interactions with them, any representation of those views will likely be shallow in depth, sophistication, and nuance.

Scholarship has also pointed out that groups that have limited viewpoint diversity often fail to ask the right questions or the most critical questions about the nature of a scientific findings. Our world views shape the ideas that we see as important, and also can serve as blinders to asking questions not deemed as relevant.[99] The *Lancet* study serves as one example of how journalists may be susceptible to *not* asking critical questions about science when the findings align with pre-existing beliefs. Related to this is the problem of confirmation bias. Newsrooms that lack ideological diversity run the risk of accepting certain findings without question. As a case in point, in 2018 The Oxford Internet Institute released a press release that noted that the majority of misinformation shared on social media came from Trump supporters.[100] Many mainstream news outlets, including the *Guardian* and the *Washington Post* shared the story. Several days later, the *Washington Free Beacon*, a conservative-leaning news outlet, noted certain concerns with the data analysis mentioned in the study.[101] Among them included the observation that the majority of the news shared in the study was of a pro-Trump orientation reducing the likelihood that it would be shared by non-Trump supporters. Such observations severely limit the generalization of these findings and represent the types of critical questions that can be asked when newsrooms seek ways to combat their own biases.

It is difficult to tell what motivated the mainstream media to become so blindly uncritical of the *Lancet* report. Perhaps it was motivated by their political orientation, perhaps it was a reaction to a presidential administration that had often singled them out as an "enemy of the people."[102] In either case, it seems clear that the MSM injected its values and own biases into its crisis reporting, and our informal observations lead us to believe it was injected beyond that single study into the general pandemic reporting. As such, we agree with Joe Allsop that in "the absence of hard facts, many journalists, especially on TV, elide doubts, or filter the story of the pandemic through the familiar certitudes of partisan politics—casting scientific debates as partisan fights, and lavishing outsized attention on the risky behavior of Trump and some of his supporters."[103] In the *Lancet* study this became obvious where a press system seemed more intent on proving a president wrong than examining the science behind the study. Such practices fail miserably at helping citizens separate scientific fact from fiction, yet they go far in exacerbating political divides.

Thomas Patterson, echoing Walter Lippmann's admonition, succinctly makes the case that the news media

> cannot provide the guidance that citizens need. The function of news . . . is to signalize events. In carrying out this function properly, the press contributes to informed public opinion. However, politics is more a question of values than of information. To act on their interests, citizens must arrive at an understanding of the relationship of their values and those at stake in public policy. Political institutions are designed to help citizens make this connection. The press is not.[104]

We agree with Patterson. Only by culling out political and other biases, and dedicating the industry to knowledge-based reporting stressing sound *scientific standards* instead of *journalistic standards* when reporting science can the industry rise itself out of its last place credibility finish.

NOTES

1. Sharon Dunwoody, "Science Journalism: Prospects in the Digital Age." In *Routledge Handbook of Public Communication of Science and Technology* (Routledge, 2021), 14–32.

2. For a late December, 2020 snapshot see this Franklin Templeton-Gallup survey: Jonathan Rothwell and Sonal, "How Misinformation is Distorting COVID Policies and Behaviors," *Brookings*, December 22, 2020, https://www.brookings.edu/research/how-misinformation-is-distorting-covid-policies-and-behaviors/

3. See as examples: Meghan Roos, "COVID-19 Vaccine Maps Reveal Political Divide, Public Health Service Disparities," *Newsweek*, June 2, 2021, https://www.msn.com/en-us/news/us/covid-19-vaccine-maps-reveal-political-divide-public-health-service-disparities/ar-AAKE1Zh. In October 2020 *Scientific America* firmly stated that it was an "insidious" "myth" that the virus was created in a Wuhan lab (Tanya Lewis, "Eight Persistent COVID-19 Myths and Why People Believe Them," *Scientific America*, October 12, 2020, https://www.scientificamerican.com/article/eight-persistent-covid-19-myths-and-why-people-believe-them/) yet as more news leaks out, increasing numbers of Americans believe that it did: Alice Miranda Ollstein, "POLITICO-Harvard poll: Most Americans believe Covid leaked from lab," *Politico*, July 9, 2021, https://www.politico.com/news/2021/07/09/poll-covid-wuhan-lab-leak-498847

4. Dunwoody, "Science Journalism."

5. Robert W. McChesney and John Nichols. *The Death and Life of American Journalism: The Media Revolution That Will Begin the World Again* (Bold Type Books, 2011).

6. Michael Schudson, *Discovering the News: A Social History of American Newspapers* (Basic Books, 1978).

7. Everett Rogers, *A History of Communication Study: A Biographical Approach* (New York: The Free Press, 1994).

8. "Nine Accrediting Standards," Accrediting Council on Education in Journalism and Mass Communications, https://www.acejmc.org/policies-process/nine-standards/

9. Schudson, *Discovering the News.*

10. David Dunlap, "1896: Without Fear of Favor," *The New York Times*, August 14, 2015, https://www.nytimes.com/2015/09/12/insider/1896-without-fear-or-favor.html

11. Code of Ethics, Society for Professional Journalists http://spj.org/ethics/code.htm

12. Numbering is ours. For the complete listing of the Associated Press's code of ethics, see http://www.asne.org/ideas/codes/apme.htm.

13. American Society of Newspaper Editors Statement of Principles. "ASNE's Statement of Principles was originally adopted in 1922 as the 'Canons of Journalism.' The document was revised and renamed 'Statement of Principles' in 1975." The full document can be obtained at https://members.newsleaders.org/asne-principles

14. Jim A. Kuypers, *President Trump and the News Media: Moral Foundations, Framing, and the Nature of Press Bias in America* (Lanham, MD: Lexington Books, 2020), 179. Italics removed.

15. Thomas E. Patterson, *Informing the News: The Need for Knowledge-Based Journalism* (Vintage, 2013), 61.

16. James Curran, *Media and Democracy* (New York City, New York: Routledge, 2011), 3.

17. David Broder, *Beyond the Front Page: A Candid Look at How the News Is Made* (New York City, New York: Simon & Schuster, 1987), 19.

18. See, for instance, Jill Filipovic, "Thank God for Andrew Cuomo," *CNN*, March 25, 2020, https://www.cnn.com/2020/03/24/opinions/thank-god-for-andrew-cuomo-filipovic/index.html

19. Jackie Salo, "New Studies Claim COVID-19 Immunity May Last Years," *New York Post*, May 27, 2021, https://nypost.com/2021/05/27/new-studies-claim-covid-19-immunity-may-last-years/. Italics ours.

20. Although slanted to impugn non-left points of view, we see this press behavior reported here: https://www.cjr.org/the_media_today/herd_immunity_vaccines_coronavirus.php

21. Jim A. Kuypers, *Partisan Journalism: A History of Media Bias in the United States.* (Lanham, MD: Rowman & Littlefield, 2014). See also Dunwoody, Sharon. "Science Journalism: Prospects in the Digital Age." In *Routledge Handbook of Public Communication of Science and Technology*, pp. 14–32. Routledge, 2021, for a discussion on the degrees to which journalism has debated a need for more science education in the curriculum to promote better scientific understanding.

22. Walter Lippmann, *Liberty and the News* (Forgotten Books, 2020) 41–42. Reprint of New York City, New York; Harcourt, Brace and Howe, 1920.

23. Patterson, 65–66.

24. C.W. Anderson, Emily Bell, and Clay Shirky, "Post-Industrial Journalism: Adapting to the Present," Tow Center for Digital Journalism, (2014): 23. https://academiccommons.columbia.edu/doi/10.7916/D8N01JS7

25. Patterson, *Informing the News*, 72.

26. Cristine Russell, "Covering Controversial Science: Improving Reporting on Science and Public Policy," quoted in Patterson, *Informing the News*, 86.

27. Patterson, *Informing the News*, 79.

28. See, for instance, the Investigative Reporters and Editors who founded the National Institute for Computer-Assisted Reporting in 1989. https://www.ire.org/

29. Matthew Nisbet, "Models of Knowledge-Based Journalism: Brokering Knowledge, Dialogue, and Policy Ideas," Personal Web page, April 1, 2017, https://web.northeastern.edu/matthewnisbet/2017/04/01/models-of-knowledge-based-journalism/

30. William A. Gamson, "News as Framing: Comments on Graber," *American Behavioral Scientist* 33 (1989): 157.

31. For an overview of the moral components of news frames that challenges accepted notions of their presence, see: Kuypers, *President Trump and the News Media*.

32. Jim A. Kuypers, "Framing Analysis," *Rhetorical Criticism: Perspectives in Action*. Jim A. Kuypers, ed. (Lanham, MD: Lexington Books, 2009), 182.

33. Peter A. Kerr and Patricia May, "Newspaper Coverage of Fundamentalist Christians, 1980–2000," *Journalism and Mass Communications Quarterly* 79, (2002), 54–72.

34. Kuypers, *Partisan Journalism*, 101. Some of these liberal privileging of usages are institutionalized in the Associated Press Stylebook. See, Ryan Saavedra, "Associated Press Now Refers To Illegal Aliens As 'Undocumented Citizens,'" *The Dailywire*, September 7, 2017, https://www.dailywire.com/news/associated-press-now-refers-illegal-aliens-ryan-saavedra

35. David Levin, "Framing Peace Policies: The Competition for Resonate Themes," *Political Communication* 22 (2005): 89. This argument is also made by Kuypers in *Bush's War* and Jim A. Kuypers and Stephen Cooper, "A Comparative Framing Analysis of Embedded and Behind-the-Lines Reporting on the 2003 Iraq War," *Qualitative Research Reports in Communication* 6., no. 1 (2005), 1–10.

36. Jim A. Kuypers, "Framing Analysis," *Rhetorical Criticism: Perspectives in Action*. Jim A. Kuypers, ed. (Lanham, MD: Lexington Books, 2009), 182.

37. More details on using themes in framing analyses is found in Jim A. Kuypers, *Bush's War: Media Bias and Justifications for War in a Terrorist Age* (Lanham, MD: Rowman and Littlefield, 2006).

38. This is not dissimilar to the idea of a composite narrative. See, Jim A. Kuypers, Marilyn J. Young, and Michael K. Launer, "Composite Narrative, Authoritarian Discourse, and the Soviet Response to the Destruction of Iran Air Flight 655," *Quarterly Journal of Speech* 87, no. 3, (2001), 307; Marilyn J. Young and Michael K. Launer, *Flights of Fancy, Flight of Doom: KAL 007 and Soviet-American Rhetoric* (Lanham, MD: University Press of America, 1988): 19–22.

39. Mandeep R. Mehra, Sapan S. Desai, Frank Ruschitzka, and Amit N. Patel, "Hydroxychloroquine or Chloroquine With or Without a Macrolide for Treatment of COVID-19: A Multinational Registry Analysis," *The Lancet*, May 22, 2020, https://www.thelancet.com/journals/lancet/article/PIIS0140-6736(20)31180-6/fulltext

40. CBS, "Large study finds drug touted by Trump is 'not useful and may be harmful' for COVID-19 patients," *CBS News*, May 22, 2020, https://www.cbsnews.com/news/hydroxychloroquine-coronavirus-drug-study-not-helpful-harmful-heart-risks-trump/

41. Erica Edwards, "Another large study finds no benefit to hydroxychloroquine for COVID-19: The medication may, in fact, lead to an increased risk of death," *NBC News*, May 22, 2020, https://www.nbcnews.com/health/health-news/another-large-study-finds-no-benefit-hydroxychloroquine-covid-19-n1212886

42. UPI, "Chloroquine, hydroxychloroquine linked to higher death risk in COVID-19," *Breitbart News*, May 22, 2020, https://www.breitbart.com/news/chloroquine-hydroxychloroquine-linked-to-higher-death-risk-in-covid-19/

43. Jared Hopkins, "hydroxychloroquine Provides No Covid-19 Help, Increases Risk, Study Finds; The study found drug and similar malarial treatment in 15,000 patients raised the risk of heart problems," *Wall Street Journal*, May 22, 2020, https://www.proquest.com/newspapers/hydroxychloroquine-provides-no-covid-19-help/docview/2405705460/se-2?accountid=14826

44. Jamie Gumbrecht and Elizabeth Cohen, "Large study finds drug Trump touted for Covid-19 is linked to greater risk of death and heart arrhythmia," *CNN*, May 22, 2020, https://www.cnn.com/2020/05/22/health/hydroxychloroquine-coronavirus-lancet-study/index.html

45. Ariana Eunjung Cha and Laurie McGinley, "Antimalarial drug touted by Trump linked to increased risk of death in coronavirus patients, study says," *The Washington Post*, May 22, 2020, Gale In Context: Biography, link.gale.com/apps/doc/A624637777/BIC?u=viva_vpi&sid=BIC&xid=9002526e.

46. Ariana Eunjung Cha and Laurie McGinley, "Antimalarial drug touted by Trump linked to increased risk of death in coronavirus patients, study says," *The Washington Post*, May 22, 2020, Gale In Context: Biography, link.gale.com/apps/doc/A624637777/BIC?u=viva_vpi&sid=BIC&xid=9002526e.

47. Ariana Eunjung Cha and Laurie McGinley, "Antimalarial drug touted by Trump linked to increased risk of death in coronavirus patients, study says," *The Washington Post*, May 22, 2020, Gale In Context: Biography, link.gale.com/apps/doc/A624637777/BIC?u=viva_vpi&sid=BIC&xid=9002526e.

48. Jared Hopkins, "hydroxychloroquine Provides No Covid-19 Help, Increases Risk, Study Finds; The study found drug and similar malarial treatment in 15,000 patients raised the risk of heart problems," *Wall Street Journal*, May 22, 2020, https://www.proquest.com/newspapers/hydroxychloroquine-provides-no-covid-19-help/docview/2405705460/se-2?accountid=14826

49. Jared Hopkins, "hydroxychloroquine Provides No Covid-19 Help, Increases Risk, Study Finds; The study found drug and similar malarial treatment in 15,000 patients raised the risk of heart problems," *Wall Street Journal*, May 22, 2020, https://www.proquest.com/newspapers/hydroxychloroquine-provides-no-covid-19-help/docview/2405705460/se-2?accountid=14826

50. CBS, "Large study finds drug touted by Trump is 'not useful and may be harmful' for COVID-19 patients," *CBS News*, May 22, 2020, https://www.cbsnews.com/news/hydroxychloroquine-coronavirus-drug-study-not-helpful-harmful-heart-risks-trump/

51. Jim A. Kuypers, *President Trump and the News Media: Moral Foundations, Framing, and the Nature of Press Bias in America* (Lanham, MD: Lexington Books, 2020), 171.

52. For examples see; ABC News, "Coronavirus government response updates: Trump declares houses of worship 'essential,' threatens to override governors," May 22, 2020, https://abcnews.go.com/Politics/coronavirus-government-response-updates-trump-declares-churches-provide/story?id=70832416; Ariana Eunjung Cha

and Laurie McGinley, "Antimalarial drug touted by Trump linked to increased risk of death in coronavirus patients, study says," *The Washington Post*, May 22, 2020, Gale In Context: Biography, link.gale.com/apps/doc/A624637777/BIC?u=viva_vpi&sid=BIC&xid=9002526e; Alexandria Hein, "hydroxychloroquine, Chloroquine Linked to Increased Risk Of Death in Hospitalized Coronavirus Patients, Study Finds," *Fox News*, 22 May 2020, https://www.foxnews.com/health/hydroxychloroquine-chloroquine-linked-to-increased-risk-of-death-in-hospitalized-coronavirus-patients-study-finds

53. CBS, "Large study finds drug touted by Trump is 'not useful and may be harmful' for COVID-19 patients," CBS News, May 22, 2020, https://www.cbsnews.com/news/hydroxychloroquine-coronavirus-drug-study-not-helpful-harmful-heart-risks-trump/

54. Denise Grady, "Malaria Drugs Raised Risks Of Heart Issues In New Study," *The New York Times*, May 23, 2020, link.gale.com/apps/doc/A624671063/BIC?u=viva_vpi&sid=BIC&xid=946211c5.

55. Jamie Gumbrecht and Elizabeth Cohen, "Large study finds drug Trump touted for Covid-19 is linked to greater risk of death and heart arrhythmia," *CNN*, May 22, 2020, https://www.cnn.com/2020/05/22/health/hydroxychloroquine-coronavirus-lancet-study/index.html

56. Denise Grady, "Malaria Drug Taken by Trump Is Tied to Increased Risk of Heart Problems and Death in New Study," *The New York Times*, May 22, 2020, https://www.nytimes.com/2020/05/22/health/malaria-drug-trump-coronavirus.html

57. CBS, "Large study finds drug touted by Trump is 'not useful and may be harmful' for COVID-19 patients," CBS News, May 22, 2020, https://www.cbsnews.com/news/hydroxychloroquine-coronavirus-drug-study-not-helpful-harmful-heart-risks-trump/. Note that while the *Lancet* study did in fact account for comorbidities and found that this was not a significant contributing factor, other research published at the time was finding comorbidities to be associated with a greater likelihood of death. See CDC guidelines for more information at https://www.cdc.gov/coronavirus/2019-ncov/need-extra-precautions/people-with-medical-conditions.html.

58. ABC News, "Coronavirus government response updates: Trump declares houses of worship 'essential,' threatens to override governors," May 22, 2020, https://abcnews.go.com/Politics/coronavirus-government-response-updates-trump-declares-churches-provide/story?id=70832416

59. Erica Edwards, "Another large study finds no benefit to hydroxychloroquine for COVID-19: The medication may, in fact, lead to an increased risk of death," *NBC News*, May 22, 2020, https://www.nbcnews.com/health/health-news/another-large-study-finds-no-benefit-hydroxychloroquine-covid-19-n1212886

60. UPI, "Chloroquine, hydroxychloroquine linked to higher death risk in COVID-19," *Breitbart News*, May 22, 2020, https://www.breitbart.com/news/chloroquine-hydroxychloroquine-linked-to-higher-death-risk-in-covid-19/

61. Bias by omission is a well-known press characteristic. See the concluding chapter of Kuypers, *Press Bias and Politics*; Abe Aamidor, Jim A. Kuypers, and Susan Wiesinger, *Media Smackdown: Deconstructing the News and the Future of*

Journalism (New York, Peter Lang Publishing, 2013); and the Media Research Center (mrc.org) routinely publishes examples of MSM omissions.

62. Jim A. Kuypers, *President Trump and the News Media: Moral Foundations, Framing, and the Nature of Press Bias in America* (Lanham, MD: Lexington Books, 2020), 173.

63. Robert M. Entman, "How the Media Affect What People Think: An Information Processing Approach," *The Journal of Politics* 51, no. 2 (1989): 367.

64. UPI, "Chloroquine, hydroxychloroquine linked to higher death risk in COVID-19," *Breitbart News*, May 22, 2020, https://www.breitbart.com/news/chloroquine-hydroxychloroquine-linked-to-higher-death-risk-in-covid-19/

65. Only *The Washington Post* mentioned zinc's link with hydroxychloroquine and it was done to belittle the connection, ignoring all evidence to the contrary: Ariana Eunjung Cha and Laurie McGinley, "Antimalarial drug touted by Trump linked to increased risk of death in coronavirus patients, study says," *The Washington Post*, May 22, 2020, Gale In Context: Biography, link.gale.com/apps/doc/A624637777/BIC?u=viva_vpi&sid=BIC&xid=9002526e.

66. For example, see Adria Y. Goldman, and Jim A. Kuypers, "Contrasts in News Coverage: A Qualitative Framing Analysis of 'A' List Bloggers and Newspaper Articles Reporting on the Jena 6," *Relevant Rhetoric* 1.1 (2010). http://relevantrhetoric.com/Contrasts%20in%20News%20Coverage.pdf. Goldman and Kuypers find that self-describe right-leaning outlets offer additional information and suggestions for frames that self-described left-leaning outlets and the MSM do not.

67. AP, "Study on safety of malaria drugs for coronavirus retracted," *Breitbart News*, June 4, 2020, https://www.breitbart.com/news/study-on-safety-of-malaria-drugs-for-coronavirus-retracted/

68. Marilynn Marchione, "Study on safety of malaria drugs for coronavirus retracted," *ABC News*, June 4, 2020, https://abcnews.go.com/Health/wireStory/study-safety-malaria-drugs-coronavirus-retracted-71075176

69. Erica Edwards, "The Lancet retracts large study on hydroxychloroquine," *NBC News*, June 4, 2020, https://www.nbcnews.com/health/health-news/lancet-retracts-large-study-hydroxychloroquine-n1225091

70. James Rogers, "Controversial COVID-19 papers retracted from the Lancet, New England Medical Journal amid backlash," *Fox News*, June 4, 2020, https://www.foxnews.com/science/covid-19-papers-retracted-lancet-new-england-medical-journal

71. Roni Caryn Rabin and Ellen Gabler, "Two Huge Covid-19 Studies Are Retracted After Scientists Sound Alarms," T*he New York Times*, June 4, 2020, https://www.nytimes.com/2020/06/04/health/coronavirus-hydroxychloroquine.html

72. Laurie McGinley, "Researchers retract study that found big risks in using hydroxychloroquine to treat covid-19," *The Washington Post*, June 4, 2020, link.gale.com/apps/doc/A625748380/BIC?u=viva_vpi&sid=BIC&xid=79ee2406. Accessed 21 May 2021.

73. Michael Erman and Kate Kelland, "'Truly sorry': Scientists pull panned Lancet study of Trump-touted drug," *Reuters*, June 4, 2020, https://www.reuters.com/article

/us-health-coronavirus-hydroxychloroquine/truly-sorry-scientists-pull-panned-lancet-study-of-trump-touted-drug-idUSKBN23B31W

74. Charles Piller, "Many scientists citing two scandalous COVID-19 papers ignore their retractions," *Science,* January 15, 2021, https://www.sciencemag.org/news/2021/01/many-scientists-citing-two-scandalous-covid-19-papers-ignore-their-retractions

75. https://www.cos.io/about/mission

76. Matthew Nisbet, "Models of knowledge-based journalism: Brokering knowledge, dialogue, and policy ideas," Personal Web page, April 1, 2017, https://web.northeastern.edu/matthewnisbet/2017/04/01/models-of-knowledge-based-journalism/

77. Chris Dall, "Controversy over data in hydroxychloroquine COVID-19 study grows," *CIDRAP*, June 3, 2020, https://www.cidrap.umn.edu/news-perspective/2020/06/controversy-over-data-hydroxychloroquine-covid-19-study-grows

78. "SPJ Code of Ethics," https://www.spj.org/ethicscode.asp

79. Bill Kovach and Tom Rosenstiel, *The Elements of Journalism, Revised and Updated 4th Edition: What Newspeople Should Know and the Public Should Expect* (New York: Crown Publishing Group, 2021).

80. "Code of Ethics," RTDNA, https://www.rtdna.org/content/rtdna_code_of_ethics

81. Roni Caryn Rabin and Ellen Gabler, "Two Huge Covid-19 Studies Are Retracted After Scientists Sound Alarms," *The New York Times*, June 4, 2020, https://www.nytimes.com/2020/06/04/health/coronavirus-hydroxychloroquine.html

82. "SPJ Code of Ethics," https://www.spj.org/ethicscode.asp

83. "Code of Ethics," RTDNA, https://www.rtdna.org/content/rtdna_code_of_ethics

84. Sharon Dunwoody, "Science journalism: Prospects in the digital age," *Routledge handbook of public communication of science and technology* (Routledge, 2021),14–32.

85. See Dunwoody.

86. For a listing and discussion of a range of biases see: Abe Aamidor, Jim A. Kuypers, and Susan Wiesinger, *Media Smackdown: Deconstructing the News and the Future of Journalism* (New York, Peter Lang Publishing, 2013), 127–154.

87. For example, see Elizabeth R. Thornton, "You Can't Be Mad At Your Mind for Having Unconscious Biases," *Psychology Today*, November 15, 2017, https://www.psychologytoday.com/us/blog/the-objective-leader/201711/you-cant-be-mad-your-mind-having-unconscious-biases

88. Anders Hansen, "The changing uses of accuracy in science communication." *Public Understanding of Science* 25, no. 7 (2016): 760–774.

89. Andreas Fischer, Yerin Lee, T'ea Dong, and Gerhard Gries, "Know your foe: synanthropic spiders are deterred by semiochemicals of European fire ants," *Royal Society Open Science*, 8: 210279 (May 19, 2021). https://doi.org/10.1098/rsos.210279

90. Ken Dalanian, Twitter Post, July 27, 2021, 10:12a.m., https://twitter.com/KenDilanianNBC/status/1420024393263206407

91. Kyle Smith, "At the *New York Times*, a Public Execution," *The National Review*, June 1, 2017, https://www.nationalreview.com/2017/06/new-york-times-public-editor-liz-spayd-fired-media-bias/

92. Tim Harris, "Lara Logan Slams Media For Becoming Left-Wing 'Propagandists' With 'Horseshit' Low Standards," *RealClear Politics*, February 19, 2019, https://www.realclearpolitics.com/video/2019/02/19/lara_logan_hits_media_for_becoming_left-wing_propagandists_horseshit_low_standards.html

93. Kuypers, *Partisan Journalism*.

94. Dave Levinthal and Michael Beckel, "Journalists Shower Hillary Clinton With Campaign Cash," *The Center for Public Integrity*, October 17, 2016, https://publicintegrity.org/politics/journalists-shower-hillary-clinton-with-campaign-cash/

95. Michael Horning and Jim A. Kuypers, "Media Bias and Talking of War," *Vietnam: Veterans for Factual History* (Spring, 2019).

96. Colleen Flaherty, "Students, Professors and Politics," *Inside Higher Education*, March 3, 2020, https://www.insidehighered.com/news/2020/03/03/some-students-do-feel-political-pressure-their-professors-few-change-their-views

97. Jim A. Kuypers, *Press Bias and Politics: How the Media Frame Controversial Issues* (Westport, CT: Praeger, 2002).

98. Duarte, José L., Jarret T. Crawford, Charlotta Stern, Jonathan Haidt, Lee Jussim, and Philip E. Tetlock. "Political diversity will improve social psychological science 1." *Behavioral and brain sciences* 38 (2015).

99. These findings are also echoed in Kuypers, *President Trump and the News Media*.

100. "Trump Supporters and extreme right 'share widest range of junk news,'" Oxford University, accessed September 8, 2021 https://www.ox.ac.uk/news/2018-02-06-trump-supporters-and-extreme-right-share-widest-range-junk-news

101. Eliabeth Harrington, "*The Oxford Study Saying Trump Supporters Share More Fake News Is Fake News,*" *The Washington Free Beacon*, September 8, 2021 https://freebeacon.com/issues/the-oxford-study-saying-trump-supporters-share-more-fake-news-is-fake-news/

102. Samuels, Brett. "Trump Ramps up Rhetoric on Media, Calls Press 'the enemy of the people." *The Hill,* April 5, 2019, https://thehill.com/homenews/administration/437610-trump-calls-press-the-enemy-of-the-people

103. Joe Allsop, "On 'herd immunity,' Vaccines, and Pandemic Whiplash," *Columbia Journalism Review*, October 21, 2020, https://www.cjr.org/the_media_today/herd_immunity_vaccines_coronavirus.php

104. Thomas Patterson, "The News Media: An Effective Political Actor?" *Political Communication* 14 (1997): 445.

Chapter 3

The Politicization of Protests and Protection

The Major Free Speech Issues during COVID-19 Pandemic

Benjamin Medeiros, Ann E. Burnette,
Rebekah L. Fox, and David R. Dewberry

In this chapter we examine the major conflicts around freedom of expression that have emerged during the COVID-19 pandemic. These conflicts have primarily concerned the application of gathering restrictions to different kinds of expressive activity, and thus the chapter covers three important and interanimated considerations: the appropriate standard of constitutional review generally, the impact of gathering restrictions on religious expression, and perceptions of selective enforcement regarding physical protest. A secondary but still important area of debate concerned the free speech implications of mask mandates, which we also cover below.

Restrictions on physical gathering have been among the central tools in the fight against the coronavirus pandemic, but they have also generated immense backlash. Concerns about the psychological and practical impact of curtailing in-person school, work, and socializing have understandably garnered the majority of the attention in the press. Yet the restrictions have also prompted questions about where the government's ability to restrict activity in the name of public health ends and the First Amendment guarantees of freedom of speech, religion, and assembly begin. This backlash has forced courts to consider a fundamental threshold question: what legal standard should be used in the evaluation of the effects of the pandemic restrictions on civil liberties? Specifically, in numerous lawsuits that began almost immediately in response to the state-issued stay-at-home orders, the courts have grappled with the applicability of the test outlined more than 100 years ago in *Jacobson v. Massachusetts* (1905) and its relationship to more modern First Amendment standards of review. Courts have approached this question with some variation, and this therefore highlights one way in which novel, even cataclysmic events such as the pandemic provide an opportunity to confront some previously latent legal questions.

A second key area of consideration is that the gathering restrictions have had an acute impact—and to some, a disproportionate one—on religious institutions. Although the religion cases represent a subset of the challenges to gathering restrictions, their subject matter has prompted distinct debates. First, they have forced courts to consider whether the exceptions made for "essential" businesses in the various gathering restrictions make insufficient accommodation for religious expression given its explicit protection in the First Amendment. The impact on religious institutions has also brought into sharper relief the perceived importance of physical interaction in the exercise of expressive rights.

The third area of consideration involves the eruption of the protests in response to the murder of George Floyd in May 2020 further complicated the application of First Amendment law in the pandemic. Specifically, it prompted interesting questions about how the meaning (and, ultimately, the constitutionality) of a law is affected by the behavior and rhetoric of those responsible for crafting and executing it. News commentary offering a conservative point of view during the summer of 2020 commonly alleged that the gathering restrictions were being selectively enforced, and this argument was advanced in several lawsuits that met with mixed success. Even though the results resist clear-cut conclusions about political bias, they illustrate the general difficulty of disentangling abstract First Amendment principles from the particular political context in which they are applied.

Finally, the fourth area of consideration involves the First Amendment issues implicated by the ubiquitous mask mandates that have become another staple of life during the coronavirus pandemic. Traditionally, masks have become a First Amendment issue in situations where the wearer *wants* to be wearing a mask in pursuance of some expressive goal, but has been prevented from or punished for doing so. The pandemic thus reverses this scenario, with the *mandate* to wear a mask providing an opportunity to explore new dimensions of the ways in which masks can function as "symbolic speech." In order to effectively cover each of these concerns we cover the following areas in the pages that follow: Gathering Restrictions and the Speech and Assembly Clauses: General Challenges; Gathering Restrictions and Freedom of Religion; Gathering Restrictions and the Politics of Protest; Masks and the Freedom of Speech; The Courts on Masks as a Free Speech Issue; Case

Law Applied to COVID Masks; Implications for Teaching and Research; Conclusion.

GATHERING RESTRICTIONS AND THE SPEECH AND ASSEMBLY CLAUSES: GENERAL CHALLENGES

Many courts and legal commentators have looked instinctively to *Jacobson v. Massachusetts* for guidance. *Jacobson* concerned the constitutionality of a Massachusetts law that compelled smallpox vaccination with some exceptions for health risks. Justice Harlan's majority opinion hinged on the scope of the "police power," or a state's responsibility to pass laws to safeguard the health and welfare of its population. The majority ruled in favor of Massachusetts, and *Jacobson* thus represents the general idea that "democratically elected officials [are granted] discretion to pursue innovative solutions to hard social problems."[1]

Yet the deference that the *Jacobson* Court granted to elected officials was not absolute. In the style of the balancing tests that the Court would come to adopt in later cases, the Jacobson majority articulated a four-part test for determining the constitutionality of restrictions in the name of public health. For a regulation to be valid, lawmakers must first demonstrate that there is a significant health threat which demands action; that the action taken is a "reasonable means" of actually accomplishing the health objective; that it is proportional, meaning that it strikes a "reasonable balance between the public good to be achieved and the degree of personal invasion," and finally, that exemptions are made in cases where the regulation might actually do harm (e.g. vaccinations for those at risk of serious health complications).[2] Overall, the Court thus established a standard that was "permissive of public health intervention" while it "nevertheless required a deliberative governmental process to safeguard liberty."[3]

The *Jacobson* case has been cited in at least 77 subsequent Supreme Court decisions. It has been most commonly cited (in 60 of those cases) in support of what legal scholar Lawrence Gostin calls its "social compact theory" of deference to public health imperatives: the notions that the "state can regulate individuals and businesses to protect public health and safety," and that "questions of policy and science are for the legislature, not the courts."[4] Given this legacy, it is understandable that the case would be invoked in the present to evaluate state restrictions on individual liberty in the name of protecting public health in a pandemic.

In the initial months of the pandemic, challenges to the gathering restrictions were predominantly brought by religious institutions (covered in a subsequent section of this chapter), with only a handful of lawsuits brought on speech and assembly clause grounds. As one review of the extant cases conducted by the ACLU noted, as of May 27th, 2020, only six such cases had been filed, and none had succeeded.[5] Importantly, Jacobson's "deferential standard" for public health restrictions was cited in each instance as guiding precedent to frame the overall balancing analysis.[6]

In an early decision regarding a challenge to California's restrictions as they applied to religious gatherings, *South Bay Pentecostal Church v. Newsom* (I), Chief Justice Roberts framed *Jacobson*'s relevance specifically in terms of its pronouncement on judicial restraint. Given the fact-intensive, fluid nature of decisions regarding the protection of public health in a pandemic, Roberts reasoned, it was especially important to grant the legislature broad latitude to determine the best course of action. The Supreme Court's seminal decision on the constitutionality of the gathering restrictions therefore did not even reach the stage of analysis in which it would have applied the *Jacobson* four-factor test. Because the legislature should be given "especially broad latitude" when it "act[s] in areas fraught with medical and scientific uncertainties," Roberts reasoned that it was unlikely that the petitioners could make the requisite demonstration that it was "indisputably clear" that their rights were being violated in order to satisfy the requirement for the injunctive relief they sought.[7]

Following this approach in the *South Bay* case, courts supplemented a foundational grounding in *Jacobson* by also applying the more modern standards of First Amendment analysis that revolve around the question of "content neutrality" in evaluating the merits of the challenges to gathering restrictions. Generally, in assessing the threshold question of "content neutrality" in this First Amendment framework, courts typically evaluate whether the restrictions were crafted to apply to particular categories of speech or to discriminate against particular speakers. If the answer is yes, then the restriction in question receives "strict scrutiny," meaning that the government in defense must demonstrate that the restriction serves a "compelling state interest" and that it is "narrowly tailored" to achieve that interest by representing the least-restrictive means of doing so. If the regulation is deemed content-neutral, then it is assessed using the "intermediate scrutiny" standard for "time, place, and manner" restrictions, which only requires that the law serve a significant state purpose, be tailored to achieving this purpose (even if not the least-restrictive alternative), and leaves open sufficient alternative channels of communication for speakers.

The early gathering restrictions were typically found to be content-neutral for the purposes of the speech and assembly clause analysis. In one case involving an application to protest at the California state capitol, for instance, the District Court concluded that "the State's order, and the resulting moratorium on permits, are, beyond question, content-neutral," as "the CHP is temporarily denying all permits for any in-person gatherings at the State

Capitol."[8] While the narrow-tailoring prong of the intermediate scrutiny test might seem challenging in situations where the state has banned *all* gatherings (or even all gatherings above a certain size), the Court in *Givens* reasoned that a ban on all gatherings was nonetheless appropriate to the situation because it was necessary to accomplish the state's very weighty interest in preventing the rapid transmission of coronavirus: it "advances the only fool-proof way to prevent the virus from spreading at in-person gatherings: prohibiting in-person gatherings."[9] Further, ample alternative channels existed through which the plaintiffs may safely broadcast their message—namely social media and other virtual platforms, as well as novel adaptations such as in-car protests.[10] Finally, even as it engaged in the intermediate scrutiny analysis, the Court also grounded its general approach in *Jacobson*—specifically the idea that "in the context of this public health crisis, the judiciary must afford more deference to officials' informed efforts to protect all their citizens."[11]

Even following the decision in *South Bay*, however, some courts adopted an approach not grounded in *Jacobson*. In late May of 2020, for instance, the District Court of Maine bemoaned how the *Jacobson* framework "floats about in the air as a rubber stamp for all but the most absurd and egregious restrictions on constitutional liberties."[12] In this view, the establishment of the tiers of scrutiny rendered *Jacobson* entirely obsolete. Adopting this approach in a subsequent case, the District Court of the Western District of Pennsylvania determined in September 2020 that Pennsylvania's gathering restrictions even failed intermediate scrutiny. Specifically, the court argued that the order was not narrowly tailored because it featured both a strict numerical cap on congregate gatherings as well as a proportional cap based on maximum facility occupancy for commercial gathering that were both designed to achieve the same government interest (controlling the transmission of the coronavirus). The latter rule, the court argued, applies "in a manner that is far less restrictive of the First Amendment right of assembly than the orders permit for activities that are more traditionally covered within the ambit of the Amendment—political social, cultural, educational, and other expressive gatherings [i.e. the latter restriction on congregate gatherings]."[13]

The Supreme Court issued another ruling on gathering restrictions in November 2020 that addressed the relationship between the *Jacobson* framework and the modern constitutional tiers of scrutiny. The case before the Court again involved a religious institution challenging the neutrality of a gathering restriction, not a speech clause challenge per se, and the Court's per curiam opinion concerned only whether enforcement of the law should be enjoined while the case was decided on the merits in the 2nd Circuit Court of Appeals. At the heart of the dispute was the way in which New York's revised gathering restrictions expressly singled out houses of worship for more stringent restrictions than different kinds of essential (and in some places even nonessential) commercial businesses. The Court granted the injunction because the law was not neutral with respect to religion and not likely to pass strict scrutiny because of its lack of narrow tailoring. (The Court's reasoning regarding the religious freedom element of the case will be discussed in detail in the later section on freedom of religion issues during the pandemic.)

A concurring opinion by Justice Gorsuch, however, also squarely addressed the role of the *Jacobson* framework in the analysis of pandemic restrictions. Gorsuch vehemently challenged what he saw as the misapplication of *Jacobson* by lower courts in light of the Supreme Court's earlier decision in *South Bay*. Noting that while *South Bay* did not explicitly preclude the application of the modern tiers of scrutiny, Jacobson "was the first case it cited," and "the only one involving a pandemic." As a result, he argued, "many lower courts quite understandably read its invocation as inviting them to slacken their enforcement of constitutional liberties while COVID lingers."[14]

But Gorsuch contended that read properly, *Jacobson* does not actually represent an "invitation to slacken enforcement of constitutional liberties" for the sake of public health regulation. To Gorsuch, the *Jacobson* case essentially applied a form of protorational basis review, meaning that it merely "applied what would become the traditional legal test associated with the right at issue" (since the vaccination law at issue offered opt-out provisions and did not involve different treatment based on suspect classifications). From this perspective, the approach in *Jacobson* therefore stands for *not* "depart[ing] from the normal legal rules during a pandemic."[15] In the case of adjudicating the New York gathering restrictions, then, this would mean applying strict scrutiny given the disparate treatment of religious institutions.

The *Roman Catholic Diocese of Brooklyn* decision did not necessarily clarify the matter for lower courts, however, because it did not explicitly overturn *Jacobson*. Disagreement about how the case should apply in different circumstances has thus persisted. In December of 2020, for instance, in *Let Them Play v. Walz*, the Minnesota District Court decided a case involving much the same issues. Yet because the 8th Circuit (which covers Minnesota) had not formally decided a case using the updated framework outlined in *Brooklyn Diocese*, the court thus analyzed the challenge to Minnesota's restrictions under both the *Jacobson* test and the intermediate scrutiny test for content-neutral regulations.[16] When the 8th Circuit affirmed the denial of Let Them Play's request for an injunction soon after, however, it did not address the underlying question of which standard of review to apply. In a subsequent case, the District Court was therefore left once again to determine how to review the claims in light of *Brooklyn Diocese*. Because the claims before it were unlikely to survive even the rational basis-esque review of the *Jacobson* framework, however, the court was able to dodge a definitive statement on which standard to apply.

Other trial courts have chosen to continue applying *Jacobson* on the notion that *Diocese* specifically addressed free exercise claims. In *Forbes v. County of San Diego*, the court reasoned that because "*Jacobson* remains good law" and "[the case before them] does not involve the Free Exercise Clause," it would apply Jacobson's "deferential standard of review" to the plaintiff's challenge.[17] Again, however, the court found that the challenge would not succeed under rational basis review in the event that the tiers of scrutiny-approach were applied, and thus the result would have been the same regardless.

The overall arc in the adjudication of challenges to the gathering restrictions thus illuminates how novel contexts provide an opportunity to address latent doctrinal questions in law. Specifically, the conflicts arising from the exercise of state power to combat the pandemic provided an occasion for courts to consider how exactly to reconcile an old but influential case like *Jacobson* with the more modern tiers of scrutiny analysis. The continuing variability in the ways in which lower courts have interpreted the Supreme Court's guidance in *Brooklyn Diocese* provide a useful window on the iterative, discursive nature of this process. At the same time, the degree to which those challenging the gathering restrictions have been largely unsuccessful perhaps also indicates that even though the analytical framework for evaluating such restrictions has evolved, the latitude that they provide for governments to restrict liberties in a content-neutral manner for the sake of public health has not radically changed.

GATHERING RESTRICTIONS AND FREEDOM OF RELIGION

> But when you pray, go into your room, close the door and pray to your Father, who is unseen. Then your Father, who sees what is done in secret, will reward you.—Matthew 6:6

> "It's not right," Trump said. "I'm calling houses of worship essential. If there's any question, they're going to have to call me, but they're not going to be successful in that call. The governors need to do the right thing and allow these very important essential places of faith to open right now, for this weekend. If they don't do it, I will override the governors."[18]

The gathering restrictions at the heart of the public health response to COVID-19 have also prompted questions about how their impact on religious institutions might conflict with the First Amendment's religion clauses.

The impact of these restrictions on houses of worship has been perceived as particularly onerous by some, with various commentators (both religious and secular) arguing for exemptions for religious gatherings. For example, on June 26, 2020, outside of the Bethel Church in Chehalis, Washington, Sheriff Rob Snaza mocked the state's governor and the mask mandate, imploring his congregation to "[not] be sheep" in acceding to the restrictions.[19] Eric Anderson, pastor of Life Spring Church in Crosby, Minnesota, argued more specifically that masks undermined religious ceremonies in ways that they might not in other circumstances: "Our people are commanded to meet together in fellowship," he stated, but they "can't [engage in] fellowship with masks on their faces."[20] John Whitehead of The Rutherford Institute argued that the restrictions necessitated "the choice between following the law and following one's religious beliefs,' because 'the government (federal or state) has [n]ever attempted to impose such onerous restrictions on the rights of religious individuals as we are seeing play out in response to the COVID-19 pandemic."[21]

Other religious leaders did not find safety restrictions and worship to be incommensurate. Chris Buice, minister of the Tennessee Valley Unitarian Universalist Church, wrote an opinion piece in the Knox News that argued:

> There is a story in the Bible about how Jesus was tempted by the devil, who took him to the highest point of the temple and urged him to jump and trust angels to protect him. "You shouldn't put your Lord God to the test," replied Jesus. Similarly, I am not inclined to take a leap of faith at odds with the good advice given by the Centers for Disease Control and Prevention, which is asking for our help in its efforts to contain the virus, reduce its spread and end the pandemic.[22]

Pope Francis also suggested that those protesting the impact of Covid restrictions on places of worship were simply invoking their faith for selfish reasons:

> You'll never find such people protesting the death of George Floyd, or joining a demonstration because there are shantytowns where children lack water or education, or because there are whole families who have lost their income. You won't find them protesting that the astonishing amounts spent on the arms trade could be used to feed the whole of the human race and school every child. On such matters they would never protest; they are incapable of moving outside of their own little world of interests.[23]

The powerful emotions that animate this small selection of quotes show how passionately people feel about the topic, but they also reveal the terms of the central debate in the pandemic context: how integral is it to the constitutionally protected "right to assemble" and "free exercise of religion" for religious worship to continue in person, and what (if any) modifications of these practices might be mandated without running afoul of the First Amendment?

The eminent First Amendment scholar Eugene Volokh has framed the protection of "[l]iberty of movement and physical association—coming together for political, religious, social, professional, recreational, or other purposes" as "tremendously important" for fulfilling the purpose of the First Amendment.[24] On the other hand, according to First Amendment scholar John Vile, we must also remember that "in times of genuine public health crises, churches, synagogues, and mosques are no more exempt from neutral and generally applicable laws designed to protect health than are any other institutions."[25] And in the context of the coronavirus pandemic specifically, Volokh points out that physical gathering is a particularly fraught activity: "our assembling is a physical threat . . . regardless of how peaceable our intentions."[26]

In particular, religious gatherings often involve singing, which can disperse respiratory particles more widely throughout a room. One incident from early on in the pandemic demonstrates the potential for religious gatherings involving singing to act as "super-spreader" events. In March 2020, leaders of a church in Mount Vernon, Washington, decided to go ahead with their weekly choir rehearsal. There had not been any reported cases of COVID-19 at that point in their county, and at that time there was no nationwide prohibition of large gatherings. None of the choir members who attended showed any symptoms of COVID; they brought their own sheet music, used hand sanitizer, and tried to maintain physical distance. Three weeks later, 45 participants had fallen ill, three had been hospitalized, and two had died.[27] Because three-quarters of the choir was infected, the practice was a "super-spreading event," according to Jamie Lloyd-Smith, a UCLA infectious disease specialist.[28]

Despite these kinds of tragic outcomes, disputes arose immediately in response to the state restrictions affecting religious gatherings. Many of these disputes hinged on the perception that the restrictions improperly singled out religious gatherings while allowing other types of commercial and generally secular gatherings to occur. Illinois Governor J.B. Pritzker, for instance, issued an order on March 20 closing churches but allowing liquor stores and cannabis dispensaries to stay open.[29] When Chattanooga, Tennessee, Mayor Andy Berke banned drive-in church services, the Metropolitan Tabernacle Church filed a lawsuit claiming that the ban violated their First Amendment rights.[30] One supporter of the lawsuit argued that churches were targeted "despite businesses that are not constitutionally protected being allowed to continue drive-in and drive-thru services or allow more than ten people."[31] And in April, Kentucky Governor Andy Beshear said that law enforcement would note the license plate numbers of people who attended large gatherings, including worshipers who attended Easter services, and that those identified would face mandatory quarantine afterward.[32] U.S. Senator Rand Paul (R-KY) tweeted in response, "Someone needs to take a step back here."[33] While some Kentuckians, including Representative Thomas Massie, decried this attack on religious assembly, others defended Beshear's measure, such as a commenter who observed (in reference to the restrictions on larger gatherings), "[i]f we can social distance at the stores, we can social distance at church."[34]

The Supreme Court would subsequently hand down several rulings that attempted to clarify the proper constitutional boundaries for coronavirus restrictions affecting religious gatherings. On July 24, 2020, the Court ruled 5–4 in *Calvary Chapel Dayton Valley v. Sisolak* that the state of Nevada could restrict gatherings in places of worship to no more than 50 people while allowing businesses including bars, restaurants, casinos, gyms, and water parks to operate at 50% capacity. While the majority did not issue an explanation of their opinion, there were several dissents that stressed the difference between the constitutional status of religious expression and more commercial or recreational activity. Associate Justice Samuel Alito expressed the difference starkly, writing, "The Constitution guarantees the free exercise of religion. It says nothing about the freedom to play craps or blackjack."[35] Associate Justice Neil Gorsuch quipped that "there is no world in which the Constitution permits Nevada to favor Caesar's Palace over Calvary Chapel."[36] Chief Justice John Roberts sided with the majority.

The Court reached a conclusion more in line with the *Calvary Chapel* dissents when it adjudicated the unique restrictions that New York Governor Andrew Cuomo had placed on religious gatherings in the aforementioned *Roman Catholic Diocese of Brooklyn v. Cuomo*. While the restrictions had technically already been removed while the case was being argued, the five-Justice majority felt compelled to rule on the matter as a means of reminding observers that "even in a pandemic, the Constitution cannot be put away and forgotten."[37] As discussed previously, the Court in this case judged the more stringent restrictions on religious gatherings in particular "zones" to violate the "minimum standard of neutrality" and thus trigger strict scrutiny. In addressing the substance of New York's defense of the disparate treatment, the majority held that the restrictions were not narrowly tailored. In fact, they were "far more restrictive than any COVID-related regulations that have previously come before the Court, much tighter than those adopted by many other jurisdictions hard-hit by the pandemic, and far more severe than has been shown to be required to prevent the spread of the virus at the applicants' services."[38] The mere notion that religious gatherings might pose a unique risk of spreading the coronavirus, therefore, was not enough to justify the disparate treatment of religious gatherings.

The Court issued another judgment in which a state gathering restriction was found to infringe on religious freedom on February 5, 2021, in a subsequent lawsuit brought by South Bay Pentecostal Church. In this latest iteration of *South Bay Pentecostal v. Newsom*, Justice Gorsuch (writing in concurrence) rejected California's argument that religious gatherings could be restricted based on the kinds of singular risks related to physical proximity and singing discussed above. The state of California had expressed concern about the number of people who gather for religious observances, the physical closeness of interactions among people in religious gatherings, and the amount of time that worshipers might spend together. In each of these dimensions, Gorsuch argued that "California singles out religion for worse treatment than many secular activities."[39] Furthermore, Gorsuch questioned the ban on singing, asserting that "[e]ven if a full congregation singing hymns is too risky, California does not explain why even a single masked cantor cannot lead worship behind a mask and a plexiglass shield."[40] Noting that there were not similar bans against singing in studios, Gorsuch concluded that "[i]t seems California's powerful entertainment industry has won an exemption."[41]

A little more than two months after the *South Bay Pentecostal v. Newsom* decision, the Supreme Court handed down a ruling in another California case, *Tandon v. Newsom*, on April 9, 2021. In this case, instead of challenging government restrictions of gatherings in churches, the petitioners were fighting state restrictions against religious gatherings inside or outside private homes. The Court asserted that Covid regulations necessitated strict scrutiny to ensure that religious assembly was protected to the same degree that secular activities were protected. The Court noted that California's regulations contained "myriad exceptions and accommodations for comparable activities, thus requiring the application of strict scrutiny."[42] Here the majority found that these restrictions did violate the Free Exercise Clause. This illustrates that applicants on behalf of religion were testing time, place, and manner restrictions in a flurry of unrelated cases and the Court was responding on a case-by-case basis.

The recommended COVID-19 risk mitigations from the Centers for Disease Control evolved during the unfolding of the pandemic as new information about transmission and infection were made available. Similarly, the pragmatic legal questions about time, place, and manner restrictions regarding religious assembly and expression, as well as the Supreme Court rulings responding to these questions, evolved too.

GATHERING RESTRICTIONS AND THE POLITICS OF PROTEST

The protests that erupted following the murder of George Floyd in May 2020 would add an additional variable to the discussion around free speech and the pandemic restrictions: that of whether there was a double standard on display in their on-the-ground enforcement. The perception across much of the media offering a conservative viewpoint was that the protests were being tolerated—even encouraged—by the same public officials who had not only issued the gathering restrictions that were technically still in effect to some degree, but who had sometimes previously chastised those who wished to engage in their own protests on other topics (namely, about the restrictions themselves). The question of whether the authorities had indeed violated the First Amendment by selectively allowing and disallowing protests based on their content was explored in several cases decided since the summer of 2020. Some courts in fact found in favor of the plaintiffs, yet others determined that either the practical concerns of the protest situations demanded restraint in enforcing the restrictions, or that the plaintiffs had demonstrated only hypothetical rather than actual violations of their rights.

The "double-standard" narrative was quickly seized on in right-wing media and promoted by President Trump in the days following Floyd's murder. In a Newsmax interview with former press secretary Sean Spicer on June 2, Trump lamented what he perceived as the hypocrisy of "these protesters . . . the ones that are all claiming social distancing, everything else, it's really interesting. They do that, and then they're jumping on top of each other by the thousands when they're screaming and ranting and raving."[43] Two weeks later, Breitbart criticized New York governor Andrew Cuomo for "warn[ing] New Yorkers against triggering a second wave of the coronavirus, singling out bars and restaurants in Manhattan and the Hamptons as the worst offenders" while extending implicit approval to the Black Trans Lives Matter protest in Brooklyn that day, where "[a]erial views posted on social media show[ed] people packed in like sardines."[44] And Fox News's Tucker Carlson, whose show attracts one of the largest audiences on cable news, argued days later that the "very same officials who threatened us with arrest for going outside urged their own voters to flood the streets" in the preceding weeks, amounting to a "ritual humiliation" because the "flagrant double standard [was] not even hidden, [it was] right in your face."[45]

In turn, several lawsuits tested the degree to which this alleged disparate treatment of different kinds of public activity might amount to a constitutional violation. The outcomes in these cases hinged on how the courts would weigh the statements and actions of public officials regarding the George

Floyd protests in light of the existing gathering restrictions in force. While they thus involve fundamentally similar analytical factors as did the above cases adjudicating the restrictions generally, they also implicate the additional issue of how "neutrality" is determined in the first place.

Conservative activist and blogger Pamela Geller brought several lawsuits against New York City alleging that the blanket and subsequent size-based restrictions on nonessential gatherings restricted her First Amendment right to engage in protest.[46] Her first lawsuit came after she purportedly cancelled a protest (against the restrictions themselves) after mayor Bill de Blasio announced at a press conference in early May that summonses would indeed be issued for "substantial gatherings."[47] The District Court for the Southern District of NY rejected Geller's motion for a temporary restraining order, finding that New York's nonessential gathering restriction survived intermediate scrutiny because "[g]iven the severity of the public health crisis, the City has taken measures that are reasonable and narrowly tailored in temporarily prohibiting public gatherings."[48]

The Floyd protests began just as Geller presented her oral argument before the Second Circuit on appeal. Because she raised new arguments before the Second Circuit in response to the Floyd protests, it gave her a chance to "amen[d] her complaint and/or see[k] appropriate relief in the district court in light of facts and arguments articulated for the first time during oral argument."[49] Geller's amended complaint (what the District Court would refer to as "Geller II") focused squarely on the statements and actions of public officials in response to the Floyd protests. Although the court had determined in Geller I that the gathering restrictions were content-neutral, Geller here argued they should now be subject to strict scrutiny because city and state officials' subsequent actions amounted to "selectively suspending the First Amendment for some protests while 'encouraging' the BLM protests." The amended complaint pointed to a number of statements by Governor Cuomo and Mayor de Blasio that Geller argued indicated explicit support for the protests in defiance of the state and city's own gathering restrictions. These included Cuomo's statement that he "stand[s] behind the protesters and their message" and de Blasio's statement imploring peaceful conduct because "[i]t is too important and the message must be heard."[50]

Yet the court found such developments insufficient to render the gathering restrictions tacitly viewpoint discriminatory. It did so for two reasons: Geller overstated the degree of "encouragement" represented by the statements of public officials, and public officials must have significant latitude to decide how, exactly, to enforce mandates like the gathering restrictions. Regarding the first point, the court found that the statements by Cuomo and de Blasio were more properly characterized as "acquiescing to the inevitability of the protests, rather than actively 'encouraging' protests."[51] Regarding the behavior of police and other officials at the protests, the court likewise accepted the defendants' argument that "if robust efforts were made to enforce the gathering restrictions in response to the Floyd demonstrations, an already fraught and combustible situation would have been made worse." And to justify the underlying deference to officials on this matter, unsurprisingly, the court referred to the *South Bay* decision's discouragement of "second-guessing . . . by an unelected federal judiciary."[52]

While Geller's arguments ultimately failed, the contrasting case of *Ramsek v. Beshear* illustrates how the nuances of different local situations—in terms of the text of the gathering restrictions and behavior of local officials—have proven critical in assessments of their neutrality. *Ramsek* also involved multiple rounds of consideration at the trial and appellate level, and the results changed the second time through the cycle once the Floyd protests had commenced.

The initial lawsuit asked the District Court for the Eastern District of Kentucky to enjoin the state's blanket ban on "any event or convening that brings together groups of individuals" (which was soon revised to only apply to gatherings of more than 10 people) after Governor Andy Beshear suggested to the press that those protesting the gathering restrictions in person at the state capital might be met with punishment (pursuant, of course, to those very restrictions).[53] Although the district court initially denied the motion for lack of standing, the Sixth Circuit reversed on the notion that Ramsek in fact had standing and demonstrated likelihood of succeeding on the merits because the orders, which singled out social gatherings but permitted commercial gatherings, were content-based. Yet given the intensely factual nature of determining whether there was some particularly sound reason to distinguish large social gatherings like protests from permitted gatherings of similar size, the Sixth Circuit remanded to the district court for more intensive consideration.

In the interim, the Floyd protests began, and Governor Beshear made several affirmative statements of approval for the protests and addressed protesters supportively in person. When the District Court reconsidered the injunction against the order banning protests, it in fact found it to be content-neutral, but also deemed its tailoring insufficiently narrow. Upon Governor Beshear's appeal, the Sixth Circuit unequivocally condemned Beshear's disparate rhetoric regarding each of the groups of protesters, asserting that "[t]hreatening sanctions based upon the content of a group's political speech is a quintessential violation of the rights of free speech and assembly."[54] Yet because Beshear had rescinded the order while the case was being considered, the Sixth Circuit determined the challenge to be moot, as "[w]ith the lifting of the Order, Ramsek has achieved the relief he sought through this litigation."[55]

Overall, then, the contrasting conclusions reached in these two cases demonstrate how the line between impermissible speech restriction and reasonable discretion in enforcing the law depends on the factual minutiae of the situation in question. We can unequivocally conclude neither that the enforcement of the gathering restrictions reveals the biased abuse of legal authority by liberal officials (as right-wing media has contended) *nor* that there is no reason to suspect that the application of such restrictions in particular situations could pose constitutional problems (as perhaps defenders of local officials' support of the BLM protests might be inclined to think). Given this ambiguity, proponents of each side therefore have a basis for the feeling that the law vindicates them in their convictions—perhaps ultimately perpetuating rather than resolving the partisan impasse around coronavirus restrictions.

MASKS AND THE FREEDOM OF SPEECH

The freedom of religion and assembly issues covered to this point arguably represent the most central First Amendment issues precipitated by the pandemic; however, alongside these was a minor yet important First Amendment issue, the wearing of masks, which this section addresses. Specifically, this section shows that masks, on their face, do not seem to restrict one's freedom of speech, but they do uncover a number of free speech issues related to their symbolic expressive nature.

Masks played two roles in the pandemic. First, they were a means of mitigating the transmission of the virus. Masks served as a barrier to prevent the virus from passing from person to person, but this characterization was contested by those who questioned the efficacy of masks or the pandemic's severity. The Center for Disease Control (CDC) and Dr. Anthony Fauci, the Director of the National Institute of Allergy and Infectious Diseases, both of which initially said that masks were not needed, changed course and recommended that the public wear masks to stop the spread of the disease as the virus spread virulently. Some states soon followed this advice and mandated the wearing of masks.

Second, masks became a political issue. Shortly after the CDC and Fauci released their recommendations to wear masks, President Donald Trump highlighted that the recommendations were just that. Trump said, "With the masks, it is going to be a voluntary thing. . . . You can do it. You don't have to do it. I am choosing not to do it. It may be good. It is only a recommendation, voluntary."[56] President Trump later criticized and mocked his democratic opponent in the 2020 presidential campaign, Joe Biden, who regularly wore a mask. Similar sentiments echoed throughout parts of the public, revealing wearing masks to be a political issue.[57]

Furthermore, some believed that masks had no health benefits but were a form of social control.⁵⁸ In this regard, masks were seen as a form of punishment and censorship. Memes of punishment masks circulated on social media. These memes depicted prisoners, slaves, and women throughout history wearing leather and metal masks that physically prevented them from talking. But the cloth and medical masks that were recommended and mandated to wear do not prevent a person from speaking. Certainly, we can imagine any number of ways they might. For example, masks cover a person's mouth, which, as nonverbal communication scholars would tell us, communicates via smiles, frowns, etc. Or, it might be hard to hear someone else talk when they are wearing a mask.

But let us assume that masks do somehow prevent one from physically speaking. Would that be valid regulation of one's freedom of speech? The answer would be no for two reasons. First, masks do not discriminate against ideas. This means that the mandating of wearing is not aimed at the content of speech, but would be a regulation based on time, place, or manner, namely place and manner (e.g., indoors and/or by oral communication). Time, place, and manner restrictions on speech are valid in part if they allow the speaker alternative channels to express themselves. If masks prevented oral speech, an alternative channel could be the mask itself. One could, for example, simply write a message on their mask to express themselves.

THE COURTS ON MASKS AS A FREE SPEECH ISSUE

The Supreme Court has not addressed the relationship between the First Amendment and masks, but the circuit courts have. These cases can be broadly categorized into two categories.⁵⁹ The first addresses mask-wearing regulations to interfere with another's civil rights, and the second focuses on relegations in which masks are used to conceal the wearer's identity.

A case that exemplifies the first category involves a man known in the community for protesting corruption and air quality issues in the county courts. The man was later involved in a trial at the courthouse, which days earlier was shut down because of air quality issues. The man entered the building wearing "a paper air-filtration mask" over his mouth and nose.⁶⁰ The guards prevented him from entering because of a long-established rule that masks were not allowed to be worn in the courthouse because masked individuals could intimidate participants in trials, thereby corrupting the judicial process and individual's rights to a fair trial. After being denied entry, the man left and returned shortly afterward with his mask in a briefcase so that he could attend his trial. Once he had passed security, he donned the mask. A deputy later confronted the man and told him to remove it. The man refused and was arrested.

The man sued, and the Seventh Circuit ruled that this was not a violation of his First Amendment rights. The reasons for this conclusion were, first, that the rule was based on preventing intimidation. The opinion read:

> Imagine what a witness in a criminal case would think, or a juror, if either saw masked people sitting in the spectator section of the courtroom. Considering that courts nowadays, especially state courts hearing criminal and domestic relations cases [. . .] it would be the height of irresponsibility to allow masked people into courthouses. The very courthouse involved in this case has, the record shows, been the scene of a crime committed by a masked man.[61]

The second reason for the court's conclusion was based on the facts of the case. While the man had previously protested air quality issues, which had closed the courthouse days earlier, he was wearing the mask to protect himself from the poor quality of air within the courthouse, not as a form of protest. It is worth noting that the court did say that if the deputy's motive was to arrest the man in an effort to punish past speech or censor any protest at the moment, that could trigger First Amendment issues, but there was no record of the deputy mentioning anything in regard to a protest.

An example of the second category, cases about relegations in which masks are used to conceal the wearer's identity, involves the Church of the American Knights of the Ku Klux Klan (KKK).[62] The group applied for a permit for a parade in lower Manhattan and indicated that they would be wearing their robes and hoods, which included masks that would cover their faces but had holes to see through. Their application was rejected because the masks violated a state law banning the wearing of masks in public unless it was done in the context of entertainment or a masquerade party.

The KKK sued, saying that their freedom of speech was violated. The Second Circuit Court found that the law dated back to 1845 and was intended to prevent insurrectionists from wearing masks to disguise their identities when they attacked local police. The law was not aimed at restricting any particular viewpoint but aimed to facilitate the arrest of those who commit violence. The court also held that wearing masks (alongside the robes and hoods) was a form of symbolic expression that communicated a message. That message was that the wearer was part of a group that held certain beliefs and ideologies. However, the court said that wearing a robe and hood was sufficient to identify the wearer as part of the group. In other words, the mask communicated a message, but that message, in context, carried very little expressive weight compared to the other parts of the KKK's regalia. The court also rejected the KKK's argument that wearing masks was a form of anonymous speech. While the First Amendment protects some forms of anonymous speech, the court found no established right to anonymous speech in public demonstrations. Further, the court held:

> While the First Amendment protects the rights of citizens to express their viewpoints, however unpopular, it does not guarantee ideal conditions for doing so, since the individual's right to speech must always be balanced against the state's interest in safety and its right to regulate conduct that it legitimately considers potentially dangerous.[63]

As such, the law regulated conduct (i.e., wearing the mask) for an important state interest that outweighed the incidental infringement of speech.

A federal district court case provides a variation on this theme of masks being used to conceal one's identity.[64] In 1978, Iranian students at Texas Tech University (TTU) wanted to protest the Shah and the United States government that supported him. They applied to the university for a permit to protest, stating that they would be wearing masks. TTU denied the request because the university feared that the protesters would be more likely to become violent due to the anonymity provided by the masks. The variation comes into play in that the students feared that if they were identified, they would be retaliated against in part because the Shah's son lived nearby at the time. The facts of this particular case differed from the KKK case, and, as such, the district court came to a different conclusion.

The district court made two noteworthy observations. First, they held that masks "have become a symbol of opposition to a regime which is of such a character that its detractors believe they must disguise their identity to protect themselves."[65] Second, and most critical to the outcome of the case, the court found that while the TTU had a strong interest in preventing violence, the university had not persuasively demonstrated that violence was likely. The court found that other similar protests were relatively peaceful and, therefore, speculations of violence did not warrant suppression of speech by masked protesters.

CASE LAW APPLIED TO COVID MASKS

At the heart of each of these cases is the government attempting to proscribe the wearing of a mask by people who claim that wearing one is protected by the First Amendment. But COVID-19 allows us to examine the opposite situation. The question now becomes, what does the First Amendment say about being forced (e.g., via mandates, executive orders, etc.) to wear masks? The preceding discussion provides a number of points to consider.

First, the issue or reason surrounding the wearing of a mask in each case is related to a matter of public concern (e.g., quality of government buildings, espousing one's views about society, and advocating against a regime they oppose). Without a doubt, the COVID-19 pandemic is a matter of public concern. This goes for the virus itself as well as society's and the government's response to it, including masks.

Second, the courts in each case agreed that wearing a mask communicates to some degree or has the potential to communicate a message (e.g., the mask could be a protest about the air quality in the courthouse, masks could mark the wearer as a member of a group, and masks are a sign of opposition). The same could be said of wearing masks during the pandemic. When individuals wear a mask, they are suggesting a variety of messages (e.g., "I take this situation seriously," "I care about my health and yours," etc.).[66] Likewise, the absence of a mask can communicate other ideas (e.g., "I choose not to mask," "I don't believe masks are effective," "I'm skeptical about the seriousness of COVID," "I stand with President Trump and choose not to mask," etc.).[67] And while some may believe that masks are ineffective but wear them given the mandates, others might take the health of others seriously and thus *not* wear a mask because they feel that masks are ineffective.

The point, ultimately, is that masks function as "symbolic speech" that can communicate a range of ideas depending on the context and the individuals involved. And even though the wearing of masks has been compelled during the pandemic for a practical reason (as a form of PPE) rather than to compel a message, those forced to wear masks might feel they are being compelled to express support for particular ideas nonetheless. The compulsion of expression is an issue the Supreme Court has addressed in great detail in contexts ranging from the pledge of allegiance, license plates, unions, and parades.[68] Chief Justice John Roberts has said, "Some of this Court's leading First Amendment precedents have established the principle that freedom of speech prohibits the government from telling people what they must say."[69] If we hold, as the circuit courts have, the masks communicate, being forced to wear a mask can be seen as compelling people to express views they do not agree with.

This is an imaginative argument to be sure. But the reality of the coronavirus holds that masks are a practical matter. The reason for the masks was that they are viewed by the State as a means of mitigating the transmission of the coronavirus. And while masks carried social and political messages, those messages were secondary to their primary purpose and, as such, carried very little expressive weight in this context. This leads to our final point.

Third, in each of the circuit court cases, there was a regulation affecting the wearing of a mask regardless of the message the mask conveyed. The courts upheld the regulations due to a significant government interest (e.g., maintaining the judicial system's integrity, preventing the real threat of violence, and identifying those who cause violence). The case about Iranian students protesting clarifies that the government can regulate the wearing of masks when there is a real, credible threat of violence and not simply speculations about perceived violence. Assuming that the coronavirus is a real and serious threat to people's health and life, the government has a compelling interest in taking any reasonable steps to stop the spread of the disease. And when the government has a credible compelling interest (e.g., preserving national security, preventing the production and distribution of child obscenity, thwarting calls for lawlessness etc.) the courts have upheld regulations that might incidentally restrict speech as long as the primary purpose of the regulation is unrelated to suppressing speech (and readers will recall that this was part of the standard for evaluating "content-neutral" restrictions discussed in the earlier sections on gatherings). In our reading, therefore, the compelling interest of combating a global health crisis is of far greater importance than any incidental affliction of speech associated with wearing masks regardless of their symbolic nature.

IMPLICATIONS FOR TEACHING AND RESEARCH

In this chapter we have examined the freedom of expression conflicts that emerged during the pandemic through the lens of jurisprudence, and in this final section we provide a few suggestions for how different subfields of communication might draw on the analysis provided in the chapter both in the classroom and in scholarship. In doing so, it is informed by previous work that has demonstrated how freedom of expression issues can be integrated into different areas of the communication curriculum.[70]

Given the nature of any pandemic, there is stress, and one way to deal with that stress is to blow off steam. This is certainly true of the COVID-19 pandemic. The rancor surrounding the gathering restrictions implicates the concept of the "safety valve" in free speech theory. The seminal articulation of the safety valve idea comes from Justice Louis Brandeis, who wrote in his landmark Whitney v. California (1927) concurrence that "the path of safety lies in the opportunity to discuss freely supposed grievances."[71] In other words, liberal speech protections help to actually avert more violent clashes or bitterly held resentments by allowing citizens to "blow off steam." Burnette, Dewberry, Fox, and Arneson connect the importance of the safety valve theory with the core concept of "fair fighting" in relational communication generally and the counseling context specifically. This approach "provides people with the means to address discord and reduce stress in relationships before matters boil out of control," and it thus resonates with the logic of the safety valve theory of free speech.[72]

Connections such as these, therefore, show how the pandemic has offered a window on the ways in which free speech conflicts can be useful for elucidating concepts in adjacent but conceptually related areas of the discipline. Although the perception of double standards in the enforcement of gathering restrictions may have been the overt complaint during the pandemic, the situation also seems to generally highlight the kind of bitterness and desperation that can take root when segments of the populace feel as if they do not have meaningful ways of airing their grievances. Exploring this kind of dynamic seems like it could be just as useful for pondering the impact of the pandemic on interpersonal communication as it is in a law and policy context.

Likewise, the fixation on outdoor expressive gathering that is on display in these cases seems to conflict with the routine contention in the judicial opinions that social media platforms constituted adequate alternative venues for expression while physical gathering was deemed too dangerous. The fact that the litigants in these cases were so insistent on the importance of physical gathering reminds us of how different expressive mediums are often felt to have unique affordances and cannot simply be reduced to fungible "channels of communication." This tension raises a number of questions for communication scholars in subfields such as digital media and rhetoric, public address, interpersonal communication, and others to explore: what are the symbolic values associated with protest in physical space? Are different kinds of persuasion possible in digital and physical settings? Do digital interactions and physical gatherings of people who share common grievances each perform different social functions?

Finally, on a perhaps more universally applicable note, the acrimony over speech restrictions that has played out during the pandemic offers us an opportunity to reaffirm the importance of some core principles of argument in our classrooms. The pandemic free speech cases exemplify how intelligent people can reach different conclusions—sometimes dramatically so—about how to evaluate the significance of a particular set of facts and resolve a dispute. At the same time, they also reinforce the importance of establishing shared intellectual terrain on which these arguments are based. We must strive to take seriously the contentions of those who disagree with us while remaining committed to a collectively agreed upon set of norms and standards according to which we conduct our debates.

CONCLUSION

In each area of dispute covered in this chapter, we have seen how the circumstance of the pandemic gave rise to expressive situations that required creative adaptation of existing legal frameworks. Overall, while the pandemic has provided an opportunity to clarify some doctrinal parameters in existing First Amendment law, much of the case law has reinforced that the government has broad authority to craft regulations to address public health crises even if these regulations might have some effect on speech.

At the same time, there has been enough variability in legal outcomes to suggest that it is perhaps unwise to expect the law to unambiguously vindicate one side or another when expressive rights become laden with political significance in a particular cultural climate. As we saw in each case regarding religious gatherings, protests, and mask-wearing, it is difficult to pinpoint an exact cutoff for the government's ability to restrict expression in the name of public health—or at least one that will not be perceived to unduly burden some form of expression by its proponents.

NOTES

1. Lawrence Gostin, "Jacobson v Massachusetts at 100 Years: Police Power and Civil Liberties in Tension," *American Journal of Public Health* 95, no. 4 (2004), 576–581, https://ajph.aphapublications.org/doi/full/10.2105/AJPH.2004.055152

2. Gostin, "Jacobson," 579

3. Gostin, "Jacobson," 579.

4. Gostin, "Jacobson," 578 [Table 1].

5. Christopher Dunn, "Pandemic Bans on Public Gatherings and the First Amendment," *Law*, June 3, 2020, https://www.law.com/newyorklawjournal/2020/06/03/pandemic-bans-on-public-gatherings-and-the-first-amendment/?slreturn=20210421172040

6. Dunn, "Pandemic Bans."

7. South Bay United Pentecostal Church et. al. v. Newsom, 140 S.Ct. 1613 (2020), 1613.

8. Givens v. Newsom, 459 F. Supp. 3d 1302 (Dist. Court, ED California 2020), 1312.

9. *Givens*, 1313.

10. See e.g., the explanation here: Catherine E. Shoichet, "They Can't March in the Streets. So, They're Protesting in their Cars Instead," *CNN*, April 14, 2020, https://www.cnn.com/2020/04/14/us/coronavirus-car-protests/index.html

11. *Givens*, 1311.

12. Bayley's Campground Inc. v. Mills, 463 F. Supp. 3d 22 (Dist. Court, D. Maine, 2020), 32.

13. County of Butler v. Wolf, 486 F. Supp. 3d 883 (Dist. Court, WD Pennsylvania, 2020), 908.
14. Roman Catholic Diocese of Brooklyn v. Cuomo, 141 S.Ct. 63 (2020), 71.
15. *Diocese v. Cuomo*, 70.
16. LET THEM PLAY MN v. Walz, Civil No. 20–2505 (JRT/HB), Dist. Court Minnesota, 2020
17. Forbes v. County of San Diego, Case No. 20-cv-00998-BAS-JLB, Dist. Court, SD California, 2021
18. Quoted in Kevin Brueninger and Noah Higgins-Dunn, "Trump Slams Governors, Demands They Open Houses of Worship 'Right Now,'" *CNBC*, May 22, 2020, https://www.cnbc.com/2020/05/22/trump-slams-governors-demands-they-open-houses-of-worship-right-now.html
19. Quoted in Keith Eldridge, "Lewis Co. Sheriff Pushes Back on the Governor's Mask Mandate," *KOMO News, June 24, 2020, https://komonews.com/news/coronavirus/lewis-co-sheriff-pushes-back-on-the-governors-mask-mandate*
20. Quoted in David Crary, "More US Churches Sue to Challenge COVID-19 Restrictions," *AP*, August 13, 2020, https://www.usnews.com/news/us/articles/2020-08-13/more-us-churches-sue-to-challenge-covid-19-restrictions
21. John Whitehead, "The Rutherford Institute's Statement on the Right to Religious Freedom during COVID-19," *The Rutherford Institute*, April 9, 2020, https://www.rutherford.org/publications_resources/on_the_front_lines/statement_on_the_right_to_religious_freedom_during_covid_19
22. Chris Buice, "Churches Should Show Love for Neighbors by Closing During Coronavirus Pandemic," *Knox News*, March 20, 2020. https://www.knoxnews.com/story/opinion/2020/03/13/churches-should-show-love-neighbors-closing-during-coronavirus-pandemic/5041951002/
23. Quoted in Devon Link, "Fact Check: Pope Francis' New Book Criticizes Those Who Refuse to Wear Masks to Fight the Spread of COVID-19," *USA Today*, December 1, 2020, https://www.usatoday.com/story/news/factcheck/2020/11/30/fact-check-pope-francis-criticizes-those-who-refuse-wear-masks/6465181002/
24. Eugene Volokh, "Liberty of Movement and Assembly," *San Francisco Attorney Magazine,* October 28, 2020, https://www.sfbar.org/blog/liberty-of-movement-and-assembly/
25. John Vile, "Coronavirus and the First Amendment," The First Amendment Encyclopedia, March 31, 2020, https://161.45.158.116/first-amendment/article/1777/coronavirus-and-the-first-amendment
26. Volokh, "Liberty of Movement and Assembly."
27. Richard Read, "A Choir Decided To Go Ahead with Rehearsal. Now Dozens of Members Have COVID-19 and Two Are Dead," *Los Angeles Times*, March 29, 2020, https://www.latimes.com/world-nation/story/2020-03-29/coronavirus-choir-outbreak
28. Quoted in Read, "A Choir Decided to Go Ahead with Rehearsal"
29. Ted Slowik, "As Churches Close but Liquor Stores Remain Open, Some Ponder the Meaning of 'Essential,'" *Chicago Tribune*, March 25, 2020, https://www.chicagotribune.com/suburbs/daily-southtown/opinion/ct-sta-slowik-essential-businesses-st-0326-20200325-p23fiwranjc5tcxecvrzynrcky-story.html

30. Massey, "Mayor Berke, Chattanooga Face More Lawsuits Alleging First Amendment Violations in Response to Coronavirus," *Chattanooga Times Free Press*, April 22, 2020, https://www.timesfreepress.com/news/local/story/2020/apr/22/mayor-berke-chattanooga-face-more-lawsuits-alleging-first-amendment-violations-response-coronavirus/521268/

31. Quoted in Massey, "Mayor Berke, Chattanooga Face More Lawsuits Alleging First Amendment Violations in Response to Coronavirus."

32. Matthew Glowicki, "Rand Paul, Thomas Massie Slam Beshear Over Quarantine Plan for Easter Churchgoers," *Louisville Courier Journal*, April 10, 2020, journal.com/story/news/2020/04/10/coronavirus-paul-massie-slam-beshear-over-quarantine-plan-easter/5135624002/

33. Quoted in Glowicki, "Rand Paul, Thomas Massie Slam Beshear Over Quarantine Plan for Easter Churchgoers."

34. Glowicki, "Rand Paul, Thomas Massie Slam Beshear."

35. Calvary Chapel Dayton Valley v. Steve Sisolak, Governor of Nevada, et. al., 141 S.Ct. 1285 (2021)

36. Calvary Chapel v. Sisolak

37. *Diocese of Brooklyn v. Cuomo*, 68.

38. *Diocese of Brooklyn v. Cuomo*, 70.

39. South Bay Pentecostal Church, et. al., v. Gavin Newsom, Governor of California, et. al. [II], 141 S.Ct. 716 (2021), 720.

40. *South Bay v. Newsom [II]*, 719.

41. *South Bay v. Newsom [II]*, 721.

42. Ritesh Tandon, et. al. v. Gavin Newsom, Governor of California, et. al, 141 S.Ct. 1294 (2021).

43. Newsmax, "TRUMP TELLS ALL on riots, race relations, Biden, China." https://www.youtube.com/watch?v=mDrYocda9wA&t=920s

44. Penny Starr, "Thousands Dismiss Social Distancing in Brooklyn for Pro-Black Transgender Rally," *Breitbart*, June 15, 2020, https://www.breitbart.com/politics/2020/06/15/thousands-dismiss-social-distancing-in-brooklyn-for-pro-black-transgender-rally/

45. Fox News, "Tucker: There are two versions of the law." https://www.youtube.com/watch?v=XoI6e60-87I

46. Geller is known for staging protests in New York City relating to issues like the so-called "ground zero mosque" and immigration generally. See https://www.splcenter.org/hatewatch/2017/05/26/anti-muslim-activists-white-nationalists-and-anti-government-figures-join-pam-geller-nyc

47. Pamela Geller v. Andrew Cuomo et. al. [II], 476 F.Supp.3d 1 (SD NY, 2020), 6.

48. *Geller II*, 7.

49. *Geller II*, 10.

50. *Geller II*, 8.

51. *Geller II*, 17.

52. *Geller II*, 17.

53. Ramsek v. Beshear, No. 20–5749 (6th Cir. 2021), 4, https://law.justia.com/cases/federal/appellate-courts/ca6/20-5749/20-5749-2021-03-03.html

54. *Ramsek*, 7.
55. *Ramsek*, 8.
56. Ryan Lizza and Daniel Lippman, "Wearing a Mask Is for Smug Liberals. Refusing to Is for Reckless Republicans," *Politico*, May 1, 2020, https://www.politico.com/news/2020/05/01/masks-politics-coronavirus-227765
57. Leo H. Kahane, "Politicizing the Mask: Political, Economic and Demographic Factors Affecting Mask Wearing Behavior in the USA," *Eastern Economic Journal*, January 5, 2020, https://www.ncbi.nlm.nih.gov/pmc/articles/PMC7783295/pdf/41302_2020_Article_186.pdf.
58. Molly McCann, "Mandatory Masks Aren't About Safety, They're About Social Control," *The Federalist*, May 27, 2020, https://thefederalist.com/2020/05/27/mandatory-masks-arent-about-safety-theyre-about-social-control/
59. Hernandez v. Superintendent, 800 F. Supp. 1344 (E.D. Va. 1992)
60. Ryan v. County of DuPage, 45 F.3d 1090 (7th Cir. 1995), 1091.
61. *Ryan v. DuPage,* 1092.
62. Church of the Am. Knights of the KKK v. Kerik, 356 F.3d 197 (2nd Cir. 2004).
63. *KKK v. Kerik*, 209
64. Aryan v. Mackey, 462 F. Supp. 90 (N.D. Tex. October 19, 1978).
65. *Aryan v. Mackey*, 92.
66. Lizza and Lippman, "Wearing a Mask."
67. Alyssa Rosenberg, "The Mask Wars Are Getting Crazier. It's Time to Take a Deep Breath," *Washington Post*, May 6, 2021, https://www.washingtonpost.com/opinions/2021/05/06/mask-wars-are-getting-crazier-its-time-take-deep-breath
68. West Virginia State Board of Education v. Barnette, 319 U.S. 624 (1943); Wooley v. Maynard, 430 U.S. 705 (1977); Abood v. Detroit Bd. of Educ., 431 U.S. 209 (1977), Hurley v. Irish-American Gay, Lesbian and Bisexual Group of Boston 515 U.S. 557 (1995).
69. Rumsfeld v. Forum for Academic and Institutional Rights, Inc., 547 U.S. 47 (2006)
70. David R. Dewberry, Ann Burnette, Rebekah Fox & Pat Arneson, "Teaching Free Speech Across the Communication Studies Curriculum," *First Amendment Studies* 52, no. 1 (2018), 80–95.
71. Whitney v. California, 274 U.S. 357 (1927).
72. Dewberry et al., 82.

Chapter 4

Confronting the Coronavirus
How Public Relations Can Foster Trust during Crisis

Nneka Logan and Chelsea Woods

Most definitions of public relations position it as a strategic management function focused on building and maintaining mutually beneficial relationships. For instance, the Public Relations Society of America (PRSA) defined public relations as "a strategic communication process that builds mutually beneficial relationships between organizations and their publics."[1] Similarly, Scott Cutlip, Allen Center, and Glen Broom's widely-cited definition positioned public relations as "the management function that establishes and maintains mutually beneficial relationships between an organization and the various publics on whom its success or failure depends."[2] Others, including Robert Heath and Timothy Coombs, incorporated both relational and task elements in their definition:

> Public relations is the management function that entails planning, research, publicity, promotion, and collaborative decision making to help any organization's ability to listen to, appreciate and respond appropriately to those persons and groups whose mutually beneficial relationships the organization needs to foster as it strives to achieve its mission and vision.[3]

Carried out through a variety of strategies and tactics, public relations work largely consists of creating and disseminating strategic communication campaigns, news releases, press conferences, statements, social media posts, and other communication messages and materials. Although the mission of public relations also encompasses other vital elements, such as protecting an organization's reputation and contributing to its economic prosperity,[4] scholars contend that well-managed relationships are also vital to organizational success.[5] Embedded in public relations' relationship-centric mission is the notion that public relations serves as a liaison function and should offer value not only to organizations and publics, but also serve broader society.[6] During times of heightened uncertainty and anxiety, such as those brought about by the 2019 novel coronavirus known as COVID-19, public relations becomes even more important in helping stakeholders such as employees, customers, and communities make sense of what is happening, why it is happening, how it will affect them, and when they will emerge from troubling times.

At the time of this writing, 229,373,963 people globally have contracted the 2019 novel coronavirus known as COVID-19, with 4,705,111 succumbing to the disease.[7] In the U.S., a total of 42,034,347 people contracted COVID-19, with the virus claiming 671,728 lives so far. More than 70 percent of the adult population has received at least one vaccine dose,[8] but varying vaccination rates and increasing COVID-19 variants prolong the precariousness of the pandemic and the crises that ensue from it.

The negative economic impact of COVID-19 is unprecedented,[9] costing the global economy somewhere between an estimated $5.8 to $8.8 trillion and causing it to contract by 3.5 percent.[10] The pandemic has been an existential crisis for businesses, with many unable to survive. In the U.S. alone, the economy contracted by 19.2 percent,[11] and one economist claimed COVID-19 is "the greatest threat to prosperity and well-being the U.S. has encountered since the Great Depression."[12] The full impact of COVID-19 on American business remains unknown. What is clear, however, is that the pandemic is likely the most significant challenge most businesses have faced, leaving many in a state of ongoing crisis management,[13] and creating an unprecedented challenge for the communicators charged with making sense of the pandemic for internal and external stakeholders. COVID-19's momentous impact clearly called for the public relations community to confront the challenges inherent in the situation, including engaging in effective risk and crisis communication practices and determining businesses' responsibilities to stakeholders.

As the virus swept across the United States in spring 2020, government officials and agencies struggled to communicate about COVID-19 effectively.[14] Information seemed to change daily, prompting inconsistent claims about transmission methods and treatment options. These confusing messages were accompanied by unclear and evolving safety protocols, including mixed perspectives on the efficacy of masks, social distancing, and lockdowns.[15] The lack of clear, consistent governmental guidance on how to handle this public health crisis meant U.S. businesses had to quickly determine what their responsibilities were, to whom they were responsible, and how they should demonstrate as well as communicate their responsibilities to key constituents.

With this in mind, we examine how a pandemic response attuned to corporate social responsibility (CSR) and grounded in relationship management theory (RMT) positions corporations to act and communicate in ways that foster trust and allows those organizations to better manage the complexities of doing business during COVID-19.

Connecting CSR to RMT provides a novel theoretical framework to explore how American businesses experienced the pandemic and communicated to foster trust in their organizations among internal and external stakeholders, such as employees, customers, and communities. We apply this theoretical framework to the three stages of crisis—precrisis, crisis, and postcrisis—as well as incorporate examples from various corporations to show how uniting CSR with a relationship management approach to public relations can foster trust in organizations through crisis communications. Our perspective also has pedagogical implications for teaching communication that suggest incorporating CSR alongside relationship management provides a theoretical foundation for students that can guide them once they become practitioners in managing communications in times of both crisis and calm. We proceed, then, in four main sections: first, we review CSR; second, we review RMT; third, we use these theoretical approaches to explore business and public relations practices within the context of crisis communication; finally, we conclude with suggestions for using CSR and RMT in communication teaching, research, and practice.

CORPORATE SOCIAL RESPONSIBILITY

In 1855, when yellow fever gripped Norfolk and Portsmouth, Virginia, claiming the lives of 3,200 of the 26,000 townspeople, local newspapers told stories of how Virginia's railroad companies volunteered to help.[16] For example, the September 14, 1855, issue of the Richmond-based *Daily Dispatch* read, "We are requested to say that any thing intended for the people of Norfolk and Portsmouth will be transported free of charge over the Central Railroad. We have no doubt that the Orange and Alexandria Road will do the same. Any kind of provisions and any live animals, sheep, chickens, &c., will be transported and forwarded free of cost."[17] These early displays of CSR demonstrated its importance during a crisis. Over the years, CSR has become commonplace business practice, embedded into the operations of most leading corporations as a means to generate trust with stakeholders, enhance reputations, and advance any number of organizational objectives.

Although CSR began as a business discourse, it has evolved into an important part of public relations theory and practice,[18] with scholars defining it in a variety of ways. For example, Damion Waymer captured the essentials of the concept, defining CSR as "the notion that organizations are responsible for addressing matters—whether they be employee, consumer, community, or economic related—that are important to the communities in which they operate."[19] Timothy Coombs and Sherry Holladay defined CSR as, "the voluntary actions that a corporation implements as it pursues its mission and fulfills its perceived obligations to stakeholders including employees, communities, the environment, and society as a whole."[20] Introducing his fully functioning society theory, Robert Heath maintained corporate responsibility endeavors should "make society better through policy positions, products/services that add value to people's lives, and other activities that clearly favor the public interest over (or at least equal to) personal (partisan) interest."[21] As Young Park and Melissa Dodd explained, "CSR is generally understood as voluntary organizational actions that serve to benefit society."[22] They argued that CSR messaging that emphasizes the corporation's desire to improve society but downplays the organization's enlightened self-interested reasons for engaging in CSR should be eschewed in favor of more balanced messaging that also acknowledges the organization's desire to benefit from CSR. Similarly, survey results from public relations firm, Porter Novelli, found that "Americans want to know what companies are doing to support coronavirus relief efforts—but companies must be cautious not to seem self-promotional or self-congratulatory."[23]

Scholars are beginning to explore the connection between CSR and COVID-19. This work recognizes that the pandemic has offered organizations an avenue to "demonstrate their commitment to SR [social responsibility] through effective crisis communication that is truthful, ethical, and demonstrates an understanding of all stakeholders' concerns, and how the message will affect them."[24] Scholars exploring the relationship between COVID-19 and CSR also suggest ways for corporations to prioritize stakeholders. As Andrew Crane and Dirk Matten indicate:

> COVID-19 has clearly illustrated who should be regarded as the most "essential" stakeholders of business. Frontline workers in healthcare, food service, delivery, and public transportation, for example, have been widely recognized as critical for delivering healthcare and keeping the economy going during the pandemic. Despite being widely applauded, however, such workers have also often been exposed to infection without necessary protections . . . and remain poorly paid and economically vulnerable.[25]

The perspective provided by Crane and Dirk helps to explain why the pandemic was particularly hard on African American, Latinx, Hispanic, indigenous, and immigrant communities, who suffered higher infection and death rates.[26] Members of these communities are often disproportionately concentrated in low-paying service jobs that cannot be performed from home and that do not easily lend themselves to social distancing, which increases their exposure to COVID-19.[27] Similarly, women in the workforce were also disproportionately affected by the pandemic. Many had to balance job responsibilities with what became a perpetual second shift, in managing family responsibilities, when schools and daycares were closed. These and other pandemic-related challenges led millions of women to leave the workforce.[28] Although few people were spared the negative effects of the pandemic—regardless of race or gender—understanding the racial and gendered implications of the pandemic can help employers avoid treating employees like a monolithic group, and help communicators tailor messages to the unique needs of employee audiences, which positions them to build trust.

Trust is an important factor in an organization's relations with external constituencies as the CSR literature indicates.[29] For example, Sora Kim found that CSR communication was conducive to building trust among consumer publics.[30] Similarly, Hanna Kim, Won-Moo Hur, and Junsang Yeo found that consumers' perceptions of CSR functioned as a prerequisite for building trust in a corporate brand, with consumer brand trust serving a mitigating function in consumers' perceptions of hypocrisy, which helped to sustain organizational reputation.[31] COVID-19 compels business organizations to respond responsibly, in ways that build trust with internal and external stakeholders, as means to maintain mutually beneficial relationships.

RELATIONSHIP MANAGEMENT THEORY

RMT situates relationships as the central focus of public relations research, theory, and practice. Unlike previous approaches to public relations, which tended to focus on how messages influenced public opinion, the relational perspective directed attention to the importance of establishing and nurturing mutually beneficial relationships between organizations and publics.[32] The significance of relationships to public relations is evidenced in the concept's inclusion in this classic definition of public relations as: "The management function that establishes and maintains mutually beneficial relationships between an organization and the publics on whom its success or failure depends."[33]

A common definition of relationship management is, "the process of managing organization-public relationships in such a way as to benefit organizations and publics alike."[34] The organization-public relationships that are at the center of the relational approach to public relations are defined by John Ledingham and Stephen Bruning as "the state which exists between an organization and its key publics in which the actions of either entity impact the economic, social, political and/or cultural well-being of the other entity."[35] They also found that the quality of the relationship between employees and organizations influenced whether employees would remain with the organization or leave it: "An organization-public relationship centered around building trust, demonstrating involvement, investment, and commitment, and maintaining open, frank communication between the organization and its key public does have value in that it impacts the stay-leave decision in a competitive environment."[36] These findings arguably have relevance in crises scenarios. For example, in the emotionally charged, deeply uncertain context of a global pandemic, self-introspection, dissatisfaction with one's employer or job may lead employees to consider a career change.[37] Thus, how a company engages the relational components may influence employees' decision to stay or leave the company. How it enacts relational components may also influence customers' intent to purchase products as well as community members' decisions to engage in activist activities or support the organization amidst criticism—all of which highlight the significance of organization-public relationships during crisis.

RMT and Trust

Essentially, a relationship management approach to public relations "implies that the research and practice of the discipline should focus on an organization's relationships with its key publics, concern itself with the dimensions upon which that relationship is built, and determine the impact that the organization-public relationship has on the organization and its key publics."[38] These "key publics" may include employees, customers, community members, or other groups of individuals who share a common interest.[39] As the relational approach to public relations grew in popularity, trust became an increasingly important factor and focus of research.[40] Scholars found that trust is enhanced through relationship-building efforts.[41] Although trust may not be considered the most important variable in a relationship, it is undeniably important as the public relations literature demonstrates.

Ledingham and Bruning defined trust as "a feeling that those in the relationship can rely on each other," and "dependability, forthrightness and trustworthiness" were considered key components of trust.[42] Linda Hon and James Grunig elaborated the meaning of trust in their *PR Relationship Measurement Scale,* defining it as: "One party's level of confidence in and willingness to open oneself to the other party."[43] Trust was proposed to include additional dimensions: "integrity: the belief that an organization is fair and just . . . dependability: the belief that an organization will do what it says it will do . . . and, competence: the belief that an organization has the ability to do what it says it will do."[44] Relationship management literature also holds that organizations can inspire trust when they enact transparent internal communication, which is defined as "an organization's communication to make available all legally releasable information to employees whether positive or negative in nature—in a manner that is accurate, timely, balanced and unequivocal, for the purpose of enhancing the reasoning ability of employees, and holding organizations accountable for their actions, policies, and practices."[45] Thus, trust plays a vital role in nurturing relationships with employees through internal communication.[46]

Trust also functions as a conduit for sustaining successful relationships with external stakeholders such as customers and communities. As Eric Liguori and Stephen Pittz offered, "Maintaining current customer relationships is critical, and communicating effectively with existing customers is key to building trust."[47] According to Moronke Oshin-Martin, "trustworthiness is the hallmark of an organization's goodwill toward its stakeholders."[48]

This brief overview of the significance of trust in public relations' relationship management literature suggests that business organizations would benefit from viewing trust as a prerequisite for establishing and maintaining the quality of relationships that organizations need to sustain them in times of crisis. However, creating trust in the organization is something that should happen before the crisis, not during the crisis, because trust accrues over time, through day-to-day interactions between organizations and their stakeholders. Trust, therefore, cannot be instantaneously established as a way to mitigate crisis, but it can lessen the negative effects of crisis on organizations and publics.

UNDERSTANDING THE PANDEMIC THROUGH CRISIS

During times of heightened risk and entrenched crisis, trust is both a foundation and key objective of public relations activities.[49] Crises—especially ones concerning matters of public health and safety—are characterized by high levels of uncertainty that require transparent, honest, and easy to understand communication. These events disrupt the "normal" and hinder the ability to predict and anticipate, generating psychological discomfort and stress.[50] High amounts of uncertainty and confusion, which Karl Weick labeled "cosmology episodes," can temporarily hinder organizational and individual abilities to process and respond. These situations feel like *vu jàdé*, the opposite of *déjà vu*: "I've never been here before, I have no idea where I am, and I have no idea who can help me."[51] Health pandemics, including SARS and Ebola, have affected organizational operations in recent history.[52] However, the magnitude of COVID-19 and its impacts on society at multiple levels was more complicated than "traditional crises," which can have detrimental effects but are often location and time-bound (e.g., natural disasters) or relatively isolated, such as organizational accidents or scandals.[53] Regardless of the crisis situation, organizational leaders must help stakeholders make sense of the crisis situation and adapt.[54]

The coronavirus pandemic presented a crisis that required business organizations to engage their stakeholders thoughtfully and meaningfully in order to, "Restore their faith and trust, thereby providing a sense of stability to them."[55] Although the magnitude, type, and consequences of crises may differ, all crises share some commonalities, which are reflected in the different ways crisis has been defined in crisis literature emanating from public relations and business. One of the most general, straightforward definitions of crisis was offered by Ronald Perry, who defined it as "a system failure that creates shared stress."[56] Although this definition could apply to various crises and disasters, definitions crafted by public relations scholars and practitioners tend to focus on organizational crises and their potential impacts. For instance, Otto Lerbinger defined crisis as "An event that brings, or has the potential for bringing an organization into disrepute and imperils its future profitability, growth, and possibly, its very survival,"[57] and Coombs claimed, "A crisis is a perceived violation of salient stakeholder expectations that can create negative outcomes for stakeholders and/or the organization."[58] Healthcare organization Cassling, highlighting the sudden and unexpected nature, defined a crisis as "an event [that] demands a quick response and, if mismanaged, can result in loss of profits, increased litigation, job loss, decreased employee morale, reputation damage, decreased competitive strength, increased government intervention, increased consumer activism and decreased trust in management."[59] What these and other crisis definitions have in common is the understanding that crises fall within the realm of unexpected occurrences that threaten the credibility, stability, or existence of an organization, potentially harming stakeholders, and requiring an immediate and effective response.

In this chapter, we employ a simple but effective crisis framework that conceptualizes crises in three phases: precrisis, crisis event, and postcrisis. Understanding these stages as "discrete, but interdependent events (points of analysis)" and knowing what each requires "can advance the theory, research, and practice."[60] In each phase communicators focus on managing information and managing meaning.[61] Managing information consists of "collecting, analyzing, and disseminating information" while managing meaning "involves efforts to influence how people perceive the crisis—for instance, by attributing its cause, the character of the organization involved in the crisis, and the quality of its response."[62] In what follows, we will define each crisis stage, draw connections to CSR and relationship management imperatives, and incorporate examples of internal and external corporate communications that

Precrisis

Precrisis describes the period that precedes the acute crisis event and includes the actions that should be undertaken before a crisis ensues to help ensure minimal impact on the organization and its stakeholders, emphasizing mitigation and preparation.[63] During the precrisis phase, public relations professionals and others responsible for crisis communications are essentially searching for red flags that alert the organization to potential problems. Appropriate precrisis management requires a proactive approach to "take all possible actions to prevent crisis."[64] The precrisis stage of the crisis life cycle consists of three components: signal detection, prevention, and preparation.

The signal detection phase can be thought of in terms of the public relations activity known as environmental scanning.[65] Environmental scanning "is an ongoing method of gathering information from the environment for use by an organization in strategic decision making and issues management."[66] In other words, we can understand environmental scanning as an "early warning system for changes, issues and reputation of the organization—a type of radar to monitor trends in order to help top management plan for the future."[67] Signal detection therefore allows for communicators to spot issues as they emerge, diffuse them, and potentially avert crisis, or at least ensure that the organization is prepared to manage the crisis effectively for stakeholders and for the enterprise itself. Because most crises, including the COVID-19 pandemic, emit early warning signs that can enhance their potential to be mitigated, signal detection is crucial.

The prevention, or mitigation, stage includes issue management, risk management, and reputation management. Issue management entails "taking steps to prevent the problem from maturing into a crisis," risk management aims to lower or eliminate the level of risk, and reputation management "seeks to resolve problems in the stakeholder-organization relationship that could escalate and damage the company's reputation."[68] While effective issues management benefits an organization by allowing it to proactively address potential threats and safeguard its reputation, it can also serve stakeholder and societal interests by positioning organizations as responsible communicators and proponents of issues, risks, and public concerns.[69]

During the precrisis phase of the coronavirus pandemic, clear guidance from government officials and agencies at many levels was lacking, arguably compelling a heightened business response.[70] The federal government was criticized for downplaying the virus,[71] and issuing contradictory guidance on masks—on the one hand advising people to wear masks while on the other, the president of the United States mocked those who did.[72] The administration even violated its own social distancing guidelines.[73] Trust in public health agencies such as the Centers for Disease Control and Prevention (CDC) also declined because the organization issued incomplete information and confusing messages.[74] These missteps contributed to public mistrust of the institutions charged with caring for public health and led to an increased reliance on employers who were viewed as being more credible than the government.[75] Therefore, business organizations found themselves confronting a public health, economic, and leadership crisis that left them scrambling for ideas on how to appropriately respond to COVID-19.

One example of an organization that earned praise for its prevention efforts is the National Basketball Association (NBA). On March 11, 2020, while the federal government was minimizing the severity of COVID-19 and well before many state governments limited public gatherings, commissioner Adam Silver suspended the remainder of the basketball season.[76] This controversial action likely cost the NBA billions of dollars, but it allowed the organization to help protect more than a million basketball fans, as well as players, coaches, referees, and local communities, including people working in arenas, as well as other NBA partners from exposure to the virus through NBA-sponsored activities. Although this move did not prevent the virus from causing a full-blown crisis, it likely lessened the risk of spreading the virus through NBA-sponsored events. Suspending the season demonstrated to the public that the NBA could be trusted to do its part to protect public health, positioning it as a socially responsible organization and enhancing the organization's reputation among key stakeholders. The NBA's leadership also influenced the National Association of Collegiate Athletics, the National Hockey League, and Major League Baseball (MLB) to pause competition, which also helped them to help protect their own internal and external stakeholders.[77] Beyond sports, many other organizations also took steps to demonstrate CSR through their planning efforts as the threat of COVID-19 loomed.

Along with adopting preventative measures to mitigate a crisis's toll on an organization and its stakeholders, managers must also engage in preparation, part of the precrisis stage that includes identifying an organization's vulnerabilities. Timothy Coombs and Rebecca Costantini posited, "The core tenant of crisis management is that no organization is immune to a crisis; all organizations should prepare for crises."[78] Along with scanning for risks, managers must also be able to analyze a potential red flag, including the likelihood of it manifesting into a crisis and its potential impacts on the organization and stakeholders. Often, organizations identify multiple risks but due to resource constraints, they must prioritize select risks based on analysis before developing response plans.[79]

When COVID-19 arrived in the United States, some organizations were better prepared to confront it than others. For instance, some organizations with international or multinational operations had already experienced the virus's effects on operations.[80] However, many business organizations were unprepared for the pandemic's impact, perhaps because of the virus's novelty and ambiguity, or because more recent health crises (e.g., H1N1, Ebola, SARS) had little impact on their operations. For instance, a study conducted in early March 2020 found that only 12 percent of respondents were highly prepared while 26 percent believed the virus would have little to no impact on their business.[81] Another study published in mid-March reported that 44 percent of surveyed companies did not include infectious disease outbreaks in their crisis plans.[82] When the virus hit the United States and Europe, many companies scrambled to adapt and mobilize resources.[83] Assisting organizations that were not prepared to respond to the pandemic, California-based cryptocurrency company Coinbase open-sourced its response plan in February 2020 to help other businesses "navigate this situation and to encourage a calm, rational approach."[84] COVID-19 has essentially revealed a collective vulnerability for all organizations to consider: that now we may be entering what some scholars call "the pandemic era," characterized by a record number of highly transmissible and potentially deadly viruses such as H1N1 flu, Ebola, Zika, and of course COVID-19.[85] Thus, precrisis preparation work may now need to routinely consider the potential of pandemics.

In addition to assessing organizational vulnerabilities, the building of crisis teams, creating crisis plans, reviewing the plans, practicing the plan's actions, and holding spokesperson or media training for those who may need to speak on behalf of the organization are all important tasks during the precrisis preparation stage that can make a difference in how an organization manages crises. Previous research demonstrates how organizations that adequately plan for crises are better-positioned to adapt to unanticipated circumstances, protect their stakeholders, and safeguard their reputations,[86] fostering trust among stakeholders and publics.

It is also important to note that precrisis is the time for organizations to embed CSR into their activities, communicate about their good deeds to build trust, and establish or strengthen relationships before the crisis hits. Precrisis organization-public relationships largely dictate how stakeholders and publics perceive and act toward an organization postcrisis. Generally, organizations with high levels of social capital or goodwill with internal and external stakeholders are better equipped to manage and withstand crises.[87]

Crisis Event

Every crisis event may not be able to be handled perfectly, but every crisis event can potentially be managed appropriately because of all the literature and resources available to guide organizations on how to manage crises. Crisis management represents a set of actions "designed to combat crises and to lessen the actual damage" inflicted on the organization, stakeholders, and the industry,[88] and crisis communication is an integral part of the crisis management process. Crisis communication can be defined as, "The dialog between the organization and its public(s) prior to, during, and after the negative occurrence. The dialog details strategies and tactics designed to minimize damage to the image of the organization"[89] and entails "the collection, processing, and dissemination of information required to address a crisis situation"[90] with the goal of lessening the impact of the crisis on the organization and its stakeholders.

Although communication is certainly vital in all crisis stages, it is acutely crucial during the crisis event stage. A crisis event is a triggering event that initiates the onset of a crisis.[91] The focus of this stage is crisis recognition and crisis containment, with crisis recognition an obvious prerequisite for crisis containment. A barrier to effective crisis management and containment includes inadequate signal detection and risk management, which allow preventable issues to mature into crises. Another barrier is the inability or unwillingness to recognize something as a crisis. As Coombs advised, "People in an organization must realize that a crisis exists and respond to the event as a crisis."[92] Ignoring or downplaying crisis will not make it vanish. Such behaviors only make the crisis that much harder to contain, lengthen its duration, and increase negative consequences for the organization and its stakeholders.

During a crisis, communicators are constantly collecting, analyzing, and sharing information to enable stakeholders to make meaning of what they are experiencing. Crisis communicators accomplish their goals by providing an ethical base of instructing information and adjusting information. Instructing information tells stakeholders what to do to protect themselves in a crisis (e.g., boil water, shelter in place, evacuate, return a defective product, etc.). The emphasis of this kind of communication is on safety.[93] By the end of March 2020, many individuals believed that businesses had a responsibility to regularly communicate about protocols for protecting both employees and customers to foster trust.[94] Many businesses heeded these concerns, clearly articulating their safety protocols for patrons. For example, Walmart emphasized alternative shopping options (curbside delivery) and introduced new protective measures (plexiglass, cleaning protocols, special shopping hours for high-risk customers, store traffic limits).[95]

Adjusting information positions stakeholders to psychologically cope with the stresses and strains brought on by the crisis.[96] Adjusting information reduces uncertainty, provides reassurance, promotes emotional well-being, and shows care, compassion, and empathy. For example, in a memo to all employees, co-founder of technology company Slack said, "Don't stress about work,"[97] and he further reassured them, "We got this. Take care of yourselves, take care of your families, be a good partner. It is fine to work irregular or reduced hours. It is fine to take time out when you need it."[98] Similarly, as part of its larger COVID-19 response, Walmart offered adjusting information by advising, "We're doing everything we can to help strengthen our community of families, friends, and associates. We're taking preventative measures to keep our stores clean and maintain a healthy environment. Together, we'll get through this."[99] Collectively, instructing and adjusting information allow stakeholders to derive meaning from the chaos caused by the crisis and more effectively cope with its effects.[100]

Crisis Communication in External Contexts: Community and Customer

As communicators provide instructing and adjusting information during a crisis, it is also often important for them to target their communications to external and internal audiences. Communicating to external audiences often focuses on meeting the informational needs of customers and communities. How an organization practices CSR demonstrates its commitment to the community and customers as well as offers insights into its values and principles. Maintaining CSR practices during a crisis also provides a trust-building opportunity for an organization to strengthen its relationship with external constituents. Communication to external audiences is important during times of crisis as a report from public relations firm Porter Novelli noted: "During this time, the majority of Americans believe companies need to take a community-first, not shareholder-first approach. More than three-quarters of individuals say companies must make decisions that are in the broader interest of the community. After all, we're all in this together."[101] Many individuals also believed that the country's ability to make it through the pandemic depended on companies playing a critical role in helping address challenges.[102]

Corporations demonstrate a commitment to community in a variety of ways—from making philanthropic cash and in-kind donations, to adapting products, services, and operations to better meet the public's needs. For example, Smithfield Foods, a food processing company, donated $3 million in cash and in-kind donations to help combat hunger caused by the pandemic.[103] Starbucks gave away free coffee to people who identified themselves as essential workers,[104] and the company also has a continuously updated web page to advise customers on how to engage with the organization during the pandemic.[105] Hilton and Marriott provided free hotel rooms for frontline healthcare workers in virus hot spots.[106] Wireless carriers donated thousands of phone chargers to hospitals for employees and COVID-19 patients to help them stay in contact with loved ones.[107] As unemployment rates spiked nationwide, financial institutions such as Bank of America introduced accommodations for customers with financial struggles.[108] All of these voluntary CSR activities helped to establish or strengthen relationships with customer and community stakeholders as well as gain positive media coverage that enhanced the reputation of these organizations.

Other companies adapted their operations to help meet supply shortages created by COVID-19, helping those brands earn consumer trust.[109] Some amped up their production outputs. 3M, for example, doubled its global output of N95 respirator masks, which help protect healthcare workers from the virus.[110] Other businesses reallocated resources. For example, General Motors shifted attention from vehicle production to help produce ventilators as part of the "Stop the Spread" campaign that united public and private sector actors to fight the pandemic.[111] Hundreds of distilleries, including more than 800 craft distilleries, stopped or reduced alcohol production to make hand sanitizer, which was scarce during the initial wave of the pandemic.[112] Because apparel manufacturer Fanatics no longer needed to prioritize producing jerseys and other gear for the MLB after its season was delayed, the company teamed up with the league and produced masks and gowns to donate to health professionals.[113]

It is also important to recognize that crisis communication is riddled with paradox as communicators "are expected to communicate with certainty in highly uncertain times."[114] Although public relations practitioners and crisis communicators were not always able to communicate with certainty during the pandemic, that did not lessen the expectation to communicate credibly and with transparency.[115] To build trust, crisis communicators focus on the facts and avoid sugar coating difficult information.[116] It is also important to listen to stakeholders as there is a direct correlation between listening to stakeholders and fostering trust, particularly during times of crisis.[117] Even though external stakeholders have often been prioritized in crisis communication research, public relations scholars are increasingly recognizing that meeting the communication needs of employees is a CSR and must also be a primary focus of their crisis efforts.[118]

Crisis Communication in Internal Contexts: Employees

In addition to recalibrating communications to meet the needs of external stakeholders during the pandemic, COVID-19 also led organizations to reevaluate their communication to employees. Crises are particularly demanding of employees, who are often required to adjust to new conditions in an instant.[119] The pandemic altered work conditions as employees adopted social distancing measures or worked from home. Some organizations had to change basic business operations, including how employees were to interact with and meet customer needs. Communicating about pay cuts, furloughs, and layoffs was another challenging factor. For many organizations and employees, the cosmology episode sparked by the pandemic incited high levels of anxiety and spurred sense-making processes as "organizations had to find new ways of leading, organizing, and communicating."[120] Employees expected businesses to recognize and address certain responsibilities at the onset of the pandemic, including protecting employees and communities from the virus, adapting operations (e.g., offering remote work options, reducing direct contact), and altering HR policies (e.g., offering more sick leave to encourage symptomatic employees to say home).[121]

Employees and human resource leaders both reported a meaningful step companies took to support employees during the first months of the pandemic was instituting high-quality, transparent communication.[122] Employers' transparent internal communication[123] about the pandemic and its effects on the organization and employees' work situations helped employees manage their uncertainty, understand, and accept organizational decisions and ultimately built trust with the organization.[124] Explaining how decisions were reached and how leaders considered employees in the process is a trust-building mechanism. For some employees, employers became a "mainstay" of trust.[125]

Providing clear information about safety measures to protect employees and maintain business continuity was a hallmark of CSR that could foster trust during the pandemic. For example, several companies, including Campbell Soup Company, issued organizational policies for employees who needed to be in the workplace, including: restricted business travel, quarantine measures following any international travel, mandatory health screenings, and mask use, social distancing, and enhanced cleaning procedures.[126] Relatedly, Walmart issued its 6–20–100 Guidance, which presented key information to keep employees safe in an easy-to-understand framework: Employees were asked to stay 6 feet from other people, wash their hands with soap and water for 20 seconds, and stay home if their temperature was over 100 degrees.[127] To employees, safety regulations signaled integrity,[128] a dimension of trust that indicates the organization employs sound principles to guide its behavior.[129]

Emotional resources that help individuals manage their physiological strain are also vital for employees; they facilitate sense-making and foster the employee-organization relationship, including employee morale, engagement, and productivity.[130] Other emotional resources included an increased focus on wellness programming. For example, CVS Heath offered extra paid sick leave for employees while its Employee Assistance Program offered 24/7 access to mental health counselors for employees and their families.[131] Starbucks provided its U.S. employees with 20 free therapy sessions.[132]

Although information and emotional resources are essential, establishing and maintaining trust within the employee-organization relationship also involves employee participation. Research conducted during the pandemic on internal crisis communication highlighted the need for organizations to engage in more symmetrical forms of communication that encourage dialogue.[133] Employees are too often treated as passive information receivers as organizations prioritize top-down communication rather than horizontal (coworker-coworker) or bottom-up communication (worker to manager), even during the pandemic.[134] Rather, to fully engage employees, organizations must cultivate an environment where employees feel comfortable voicing their concerns and believe their concerns have been heard, considered, and addressed.[135]

Illustrating the complexities corporations faced during the pandemic, an organization could be praised for how it handled operations for external stakeholders on the one hand, but criticized for its treatment of employees on the other. For example, Amazon's actions to protect and support customers, communities, government, and public health agencies during early stages of the pandemic were celebrated.[136] The corporation also emphasized its employee-based efforts, highlighting its hiring plans and raising its starting wage by $2 an hour. But conflicting news reports surfaced detailing labor issues, low compensation rates, unsafe working conditions, and high infection levels,[137] and employees began circulating petitions and orchestrating protests.[138] Both Amazon and Walmart were criticized for their lack of generosity to their frontline employees as the companies reported record profits during the early months of the pandemic.[139] A common perception was that these corporations worked to satisfy surging consumer demands but failed in their foremost responsibility to protect their most vulnerable stakeholders—employees.

Situational constraints can force organizations to prioritize stakeholder obligations during a crisis,[140] and stakeholder needs and organizational priorities may evolve as the crisis situation changes.[141] However, when possible, organizations should balance the needs of internal and external stakeholders in their crisis response.[142] Crane and Matten argued that frontline and essential workers (i.e., individuals who work in healthcare settings or provide other critical services) should have been regarded as the most salient stakeholders because of their roles in sustaining society, the economy, and providing healthcare services.[143] Yet, despite being placed at a greater, involuntary risk for contracting the virus, many of these employees continued to be poorly compensated and often underprotected. Integrity is the dimension of trust that involves treating stakeholders fairly,[144] but exploiting those most at-risk jeopardized organization-public relationships as a majority of people claimed they were less likely to trust businesses that fail to protect employees.[145] Moving forward, businesses must recognize that stakeholder expectations regarding CSR are not limited to external contexts but should extend to internal stakeholders, also, especially during times of crisis.

Postcrisis

The postcrisis stage "begins when the harm, drama, confusion and uncertainty of the crisis dissipate and some sense of order is re-established."[146] Practitioners shift from managing the crisis to focusing on its effects.[147] At the time of this writing, it seems premature to suggest that we have entered into the postcrisis phase. Because identifying the specific endpoint of the crisis stage is challenging, Coombs offered that postcrisis communication is "largely an extension of crisis response communication coupled with learning from the crisis."[148] As the pandemic is not resolved, we use this section as a reflection, gleaning implications from what we have learned thus far and offering recommendations for moving forward.

Although crises often produce negative outcomes for organizations and their stakeholders, they can also generate positive impacts, including the chance to improve an organization.[149] Crises offer an opportunity for reflection by evaluating the precrisis and crisis stages to determine what went wrong and why. A central element of the postcrisis stage is organizational learning, which involves identifying these errors and charting a route forward to communicate and correct shortcomings.[150] Through learning, an organization can build resilience, enabling it to rapidly adapt in response to adversity, establishing a new sense of normalcy quickly. The seismic impacts of COVID-19 underscored the need for organizations to reflect and adjust certain policies and actions to develop this resiliency and strengthen relationships with internal and external stakeholders. For example, the pandemic transformed some workplace cultures as corporations, such as Clorox, implemented or enhanced internal communication efforts and employee wellness resources based on employee needs, thereby underscoring their commitment to employees while simultaneously building a more respected organization.[151]

At the present time, U.S. organizations are adapting to the "new normal." Some offices are gradually reopening, but others are delaying their reopening plans. Vaccine hesitancy among some individuals and new variants lead some employees to voice concerns about safety in the workplace.[152] The situation's fluidity requires ongoing, increased levels of flexibility and improvisation from business leaders and communicators,[153] as they must continue supporting and engaging employees while meeting organizational goals. At a minimum, organizations should seek to maintain employee, customer, and community trust gained during the pandemic by continuing to offer an ethical base of instructing and adjusting information, extending crisis communication tenets into the postcrisis stage as Coombs suggested.[154] Business leaders and communicators must also remember that trust-building extends beyond transparency. In the post-COVID-19 world, more employees will likely expect to have a voice in their organizations, and increasingly consumers expect brands to "do the right thing" for society not only for the bottom line.[155]

CONCLUSION

COVID-19 is testing trust in media, government, NGOs, businesses, and all of society's institutions.[156] As government officials and health agencies struggle with COVID-19 responses, individuals continue to turn to the private sector for leadership and guidance. As we look to the future, it is possible the pandemic's effects may force more businesses and communicators to wade deeper into what has become a tangled web of politics and public health. For example, organizations are having to make decisions about implementing and enforcing their own mask policies.[157] For some of their stakeholders, the core of the mask issue is safety. But for others, it is about choice and liberty, which the mask is believed to inhibit. Similarly, some see vaccines as a symbol of freedom and the route to returning to normal. Others see them as an unreasonable infringement on their personal freedoms. In either case, the public health issues of masks and vaccines have become political hot buttons that divide Americans and place businesses and their communicators in the challenging position of having to make public health decisions to protect employees, customers, and communities.

The pandemic also underscored the critical role of crisis communication by elucidating the importance of engaging in ongoing environmental scanning, preparing, and planning for crises, and cultivating a resilient organizational culture. Organizations and educators should take steps to ensure current and future public relations practitioners are equipped to address these challenges. Prior to the pandemic, one study found that among the top skills deemed important by current public relations practitioners for future practitioners were the ability to communicate effectively in today's environment of disinformation and develop a crisis communication plan.[158] The surge in mis- and disinformation circulating during the pandemic increased the need to manage multiple relationships via effective crisis communication and has intensified the need to ensure these skills are incorporated into the public relations curricula of higher education.

An examination of the effects of COVID-19 on the practice of public relations suggests that, as we embark upon the future, communicators—both scholars and practitioners—need to expand their conceptualizations of CSR to consider how politics and public health issues can intersect to shape communication and organization-public relationships in crisis contexts. Another consideration to keep in mind concerns extending conceptualization of crisis communication research. More specifically, crisis communication research has historically taken a functionalist perspective that aimed to achieve organizational objectives, such as protecting corporate profit and reputations, and satisfying external publics who could impact both. However, the public health crisis created by COVID-19 exemplified the importance of studying crises and CSR within a broader context that includes attention to traditionally less powerful actors such as employees and local communities who are often left vulnerable from the crisis and with fewer resources to confront it. Relatedly, the pandemic elucidated the need to better understand and theorize the complex and intertwined nature of contemporary crises that can affect multiple organizations, industries, publics, and geographic areas[159] including disasters, injustice, globalization, and pandemics.[160]

Attention to CSR and relationship management will help both public relations scholars and practitioners to fulfill their responsibilities to stakeholders by exercising compassion, engaging dialogically, and constantly reevaluating the role of business in a changing society. Connecting CSR to relationship management contributes a productive new way to enhance understanding of how American businesses experienced the pandemic and communicated to foster trust in their organizations as it also provides a strong foundation upon which to build future crisis research.

NOTES

1. "About Public Relations," Public Relations Society of America (PRSA), accessed August 11, 2021, https://www.prsa.org/about/all-about-pr.

2. Scott Cutlip, Allen Center, and Glen Broom. *Effective Public Relations*, 9th ed. (Upper Saddle Ridge, NJ: Pearson Education, 2006) 5.

3. Robert Heath and Timothy Coombs, *Today's Public Relations: An Introduction* (Thousand Oaks, CA: SAGE, 2006), 7.

4. PRSA, "About Public Relations."

5. Stephen Bruning, "Relationship Building as a Retention Strategy: Linking Relationship Attitudes and Satisfaction Evaluation to Behavioral Outcomes," *Public Relations Review* 28, no. 1 (2002): 39–40.

6. Donalynn Pompper, *Corporate Social Responsibility, Sustainability and Public Relations* (London: Routledge, 2015), 6; James Grunig, "Foreword," in *Public Relations as Relationship Management: A Relational Approach to the Study and Practice of Public Relations,* ed. Eyun-Jung Ki, Jeong-Nam Kim, and John Ledingham. (New York: Routledge, 2015), xxii - xxvii.

7. "WHO Coronavirus (COVID-19) Dashboard," World Health Organization, accessed September 22, 2021, https://covid19.who.int/.

8. "COVID Data Tracker," Centers for Disease Control and Prevention, accessed July 28, 2021, https://covid.cdc.gov/covid-data-tracker/#datatracker-home.

9. Eduardo Levy Yeyati and Federico Filippini, "Social and Economic Impact Of COVID-19," *Brookings,* June 2021, https://www.brookings.edu/wp-content/uploads/2021/06/Social-and-economic-impact-COVID.pdf.

10. Margeurite Dennis, "The Impact of COVID-19 on the World Economy and Higher Education," *Enrollment Management Report* 23, no. 4 (2020): 9, https://onlinelibrary.wiley.com/doi/full/10.1002/emt.30720.

11. Lucia Mutikani, "U.S. Economy Contracted 19.2% During COVID-19 Pandemic Recession," *Reuters,* July 29, 2021, https://www.reuters.com/business/us-economy-contracted-192-during-covid-19-pandemic-recession-2021-07-29/.

12. Alvin Powell, "What Might COVID Cost the U.S.? Try $16 Trillion," *The Harvard Gazette,* November 10, 2020, https://news.harvard.edu/gazette/story/2020/11/what-might-covid-cost-the-u-s-experts-eye-16-trillion/#:~:text=A%20pair%20of%20Harvard%20economists,and%20contact%20tracing%20that%20would.

13. Ligouri and Pittz, "Strategies for Small Business: Surviving and Thriving in the Era of COVID-19," 2.

14. Jill Castellano, "San Diego County Officials Give Inconsistent, Confusing COVID-19 Statements," *inewsource*, April 15, 2020, https://inewsource.org/2020/04/15/san-diego-officials-give-inconsistent-confusing-covid-19-statements; J. David Goodman, "How Delays and Unheeded Warnings Hindered New York's Virus Fight," *The New York Times,* April 8, 2020, https://www.nytimes.com/2020/04/08/nyregion/new-york-coronavirus-response-delays.html.

15. Huo Jingnan, "Why There Are So Many Different Guidelines for Face Masks for the Public," *NPR*, April 10, 2020, https://www.npr.org/sections/goatsandsoda/2020/04/10/829890635/why-there-so-many-different-guidelines-for-face-masks-for-the-public; Anthony Zurcher, "Coronavirus: Things the US Has Got Wrong—and Got Right," *BBC*, April 1, 2020, https://www.bbc.com/news/world-us-canada-52125039.

16. Nneka Logan, "The Rise of The Railroad in Virginia: A Historical Analysis of The Emergence of Corporate Public Relations in The United States," *Public Relations Inquiry* 7, no. 1 (2018): 6, https://doi.org/10.1177/2046147X17743299.

17. "The Yellow Fever Norfolk and Portsmouth Virginia in 1855," *Daily Dispatch,* Daily Accessed July 28, 2021. http://www.usgwarchives.net/va/yellow-fever/yfin5.html

18. Young Park and Melissa Dodd, "The Historical Development of Corporate Social Responsibility as a Strategic Management Function of Public Relations," in *The Moral Compass of Public Relations*, ed. Brigitta Brunner (New York: Routledge, 2017), 15–27.

19. Damion Waymer, "Does Public Relations Scholarship Have a Place in Race?," in *The SAGE Handbook of Public Relations*, ed. Robert Heath (Los Angeles: SAGE, 2010), 237–260.

20. Timothy Coombs and Sherry Holladay, *Managing Corporate Social Responsibility: A Communication Approach* (Malden, MA: Wiley-Blackwell, 2012), 8.

21. Robert Heath, "Onward into More Fog: Thoughts on Public Relations' Research Directions," *Journal of Public Relations Research* 18, vol. 2 (2006): 103. https://doi.org/10.1207/s1532754xjprr1802_2.

22. Park and Dodd, "The Historical Development of Corporate Social Responsibility as a Strategic Management Function of Public Relations," 15.

23. "Porter Novelli COVID-19 Insights for a Time of Crisis," Porter Novelli, published April 2020, https://www.porternovelli.com/wp-content/uploads/2020/04/Porter-Novelli-COVID-19-Tracker.pdf.

24. Moronke Oshin-Martin, "Ethical Public Relations, Communities of Color, and COVID-19 Crises in Summer 2020," in *Public Relations for Social Responsibility: Affirming DEI Commitment with Action*, ed. Donnalyn Pompper (Bingley, UK: Emerald Publishing Limited, 2021):19–31.

25. Andrew Crane and Dirk Matten, "Covid-19 and the Future of CSR Research," *Journal of Management Studies* 58, no. 1 (2021): 1. https://doi.org/10.1111/joms.12642; The Lancet, "The plight of essential workers during the COVID-19 pandemic," *Lancet 395* (2020): 1587. 2020;395:1587. https://doi.org/10.1016/S0140-6736(20)31200-9

26. *Ibid,* 1; "Health Equity Considerations and Racial Ethnic Minority Groups" Centers for Disease Control and Prevention, published April 21, 2021, https://www.cdc.gov/coronavirus/2019-ncov/community/health-equity/race-ethnicity.html.

27. Jennifer Liu, "More Than Half of Black, Latino, Native American Workers Hold Jobs That Require In-Person Contact," *CNBC,* December 2, 2020, https://www.cnbc.com/2020/12/02/black-latino-native-american-workers-face-higher-covid-19-exposure.html; Moronke Oshin-Martin, "Ethical Public Relations, Communities of Color, and COVID-19 Crises in Summer 2020," 22.

28. Megan Cassella, "The Pandemic Drove Women Out of the Workforce. Will They Come Back?," *Politico,* July 22, 2021, https://www.politico.com/news/2021/07/22/coronavirus-pandemic-women-workforce-500329.

29. Mobin Fatma, Zillur Rahman, and Imran Khan, "Building Company Reputation and Brand Equity Through CSR: The Mediating Role of Trust," *International Journal of Bank Marketing* 33, no. 6 (2015): 840–856. https://doi.org/10.1108/IJBM-11-2014-0166; Patricia Martínez and Ignacio Del Bosque, "CSR And Customer Loyalty: The Roles of Trust, Customer Identification with the Company and Satisfaction," *International Journal of Hospitality Management* 35 (2013): 90. https://doi.org/10.1016/j.ijhm.2013.05.009.

30. Sora Kim, "The Process Model of Corporate Social Responsibility (CSR) Communication: CSR Communication and Its Relationship with Consumers' CSR Knowledge, Trust, And Corporate Reputation Perception," *Journal of Business Ethics* 154, no. 4 (2019): 1156. https://doi.org/10.1007/s10551-017-3433-6.

31. Hanna Kim, Won-Moo Hur, and Junsang Yeo, "Corporate Brand Trust as A Mediator in the Relationship Between Consumer Perception of CSR, Corporate Hypocrisy, And Corporate Reputation," *Sustainability* 7, no. 4 (2015): 3690. https://doi.org/10.3390/su7043683.

32. Mary Ann Ferguson, "Building Theory in Public Relations: Interorganizational Relationships as a Public Relations Paradigm," *Journal of Public Relations Research* 30, no. 4 (2018): 171. https://doi.org/10.1080/1062726X.2018.1514810.

33. John Ledingham and Stephen Bruning. *Public Relations as Relationship Management: A Relational Approach to the Study and Practice of Public Relations* (New York: Routledge, 2000), xiii.

34. John Ledingham, "Relationship Management Theory," in *Encyclopedia of Public Relations,* 2nd ed., ed. Robert Heath (Thousand Oaks, CA, 2013), 781.

35. John Ledingham and Stephen Bruning, "Relationship Management in Public Relations: Dimensions of an Organization-Public Relationship," *Public Relations Review* 24, no. 1 (1998): 62, https://doi.org/10.1016/S0363-8111(98)80020-9

36. *Ibid,* 61.

37. Jennifer Levitz, "Covid-19 Was a Wake-Up Call, Leading Many to Make Lifestyle and Career Changes," *The Wall Street Journal,* April 11, 2021, https://www.wsj.com/articles/covid-19-was-a-wake-up-call-leading-many-to-make-lifestyle-and-career-changes-11618133400.

38. John Ledingham, "Relationship Management in Public Relations: Dimensions of an Organization-Public Relationship," *Public Relations Review* 24, no. 1 (1998): 56, https://doi.org/10.1016/S0363-8111(98)80020-9.

39. Shannon Bowen, Brad Rawlins, and Thomas Martin, *An Overview of the Public Relations Function,* 2nd ed. (New York: Business Expert Press, 2019), 10.

40. Eyun-Jung Ki, Jeong-Nam Kim, and John Ledingham. *Public Relations as Relationship Management: A Relational Approach to the Study and Practice of Public Relations* (New York: Routledge, 2015), 6; John Ledingham and Stephen Bruning, "Relationship Management in Public Relations: Dimensions of an Organization-Public Relationship," 58.

41. Neill and Bowen, "Ethical Listening to Employees During a Pandemic: New Approaches, Barriers and Lessons," 290.

42. John Ledingham and Stephen Bruning, "Relationship Management in Public Relations: Dimensions of an Organization-Public Relationship," 58.

43. Linda Hon and James Grunig, "Guidelines for Measuring Relationships in Public Relations," *Institute for Public Relations.* Published November 1999. http://painepublishing.com/wp-content/uploads/2013/10/Guidelines_Measuring_Relationships.pdf.

44. *Ibid,* 6.

45. Linjuan Men, "Internal Reputation Management: The Impact of Authentic Leadership and Transparent Communication," *Corporate Reputation Review* 17 (2014): 260, https://doi.org/10.1057/crr.2014.14.

46. Jo-Yun Li, Ruoyu Sun, Weiting Tao, and Yeunjae Lee. "Employee Coping with Organizational Change in the Face of a Pandemic: The Role of Transparent Internal Communication," *Public Relations Review* 47, no. 1 (March 2021): 2, https://doi.org/10.1016/j.pubrev.2020.101984; Neill and Bowen, "Ethical Listening to Employees During a Pandemic: New Approaches, Barriers and Lessons," 290.

47. Ligouri and Pittz, "Strategies for Small Business: Surviving and Thriving in the Era of COVID-19," 108.

48. Oshin-Martin, "Ethical Public Relations, Communities of Color, and COVID-19 Crises in Summer 2020," 22.

49. Truls Strand Offerdal, Sine Nørholm Just, and Oyvind Ihlen. "Public Ethos in the Pandemic Rhetorical Situation: Strategies for Building Trust in Authorities' Risk Communication," *Journal of International Crisis and Risk Communication Research* 4, no. 2 (2021): 4.

50. Timothy Sellnow and Matthew Seeger, *Theorizing Crisis Communication* (Malden, MA: Wiley-Blackwell, 2013), 6–7.

51. Karl Weick, "The Collapse of Sensemaking in Organizations: The Mann Gulch Disaster," *Administrative Science Quarterly* 38, no. 4 (1993): 633–634. https://doi.org/10.2307/2393339.

52. Roberto Cortez and Wesley Johnson, "The Coronavirus Crisis in B2B Settings: Crisis Uniqueness and Managerial Implications Based on Social Exchange Theory," *Industrial Marketing Management* 88 (2020):126, https://doi.org/10.1016/j.indmarman.2020.05.004; Brennan Day, Ruth McKay, Michael Ishman, and Ed Chung, "'It Will Happen Again.' What SARS Taught Business About Crisis Management," *Management Decision* 42, no. 7 (2004): 833, https://doi.org/10.1108/00251740410550907.

53. Fasth, Elliot, and Styhre, "Crisis Management as Practice in Small-and Medium-Sized Enterprises During the First Period of COVID-19," 2.

54. Ana Mendy, Mary Lass Stewart, and Kate VanAkin, "A Leader's Guide: Communicating with Stakeholders, And Communities During COVID-19," McKinsey & Company, published April 17, 2020, https://www.mckinsey.com/business-functions/organization/our-insights/a-leaders-guide-communicating-with-teams-stakeholders-and-communities-during-covid-19.

55. Mark Camilleri, "Strategic Dialogic Communication Through Digital Media During COVID-19 Crisis," in *Strategic Corporate Communication in the Digital Age*, ed. Mark Camilleri (Bingley, UK: Emerald Publishing Limited, 2021), 1–18.

56. Ronald Perry, "What Is a Crisis?," in *Handbook of Disaster Research*, ed. Havidan Rodriguez, Enrico Quarantelli, and Russell Dynes (New York: Springer, 2007), 1–15.

57. Otto Lerbinger, *The Crisis Manager: Facing Risk and Responsibility*. (New York: Lawrence Erlbaum, 1997), 4.

58. Timothy Coombs, *Ongoing Crisis Communication: Planning, Managing, and Responding*. (Thousand Oaks, CA: SAGE, 2019), 3.

59. "Six Elements of a Crisis Communication Plan," Cassling, accessed July 28, 2021, https://www.cassling.com/knowledge-center/six-elements-of-a-crisis-communication-plan.

60. Robert Heath, "Introduction," in *Handbook of Crisis Communication*, ed. Timothy Coombs and Sherry Holladay (Malden, MA: Wiley-Blackwell, 2010), 1–14.

61. Timothy Coombs, "Crisis Communication," in *Encyclopedia of Public Relations*, 2nd ed., ed. Robert Heath (Thousand Oaks, CA: SAGE, 2013), 221–224; Coombs, *Ongoing Crisis Communication: Planning, Managing, and Responding*, 53.

62. *Ibid*, 222.

63. Coombs, *Ongoing Crisis Communication: Planning, Managing, and Responding*, 9.

64. *Ibid*, 10.

65. *Ibid*, 34.

66. Phyllis Larsen, "Environmental Scanning," in *Encyclopedia of Public Relations*, 2nd ed., ed. Robert Heath, (Thousand Oaks, CA: SAGE, 2013), 302–303.

67. *Ibid*, 302.

68. Coombs, *Ongoing Crisis Communication: Planning, Managing, and Responding*, 11.

69. Shannon Bowen, "Ethical Responsibility and Guidelines for Managing Issues of Risk and Risk Communication," in *Handbook of Risk and Crisis Communication*, ed. Robert Heath and Dan O'Hair (New York: Francis, 2010), 343–363.

70. Dan Diamond, "Feuds, fibs and finger-pointing: Trump officials say coronavirus response was worse than known," *The Washington Post*, March 29, 2021, https://www.washingtonpost.com/health/2021/03/29/trump-officials-tell-all-coronavirus-response/; Goodman, "How Delays and Unheeded Warnings Hindered New York's Virus Fight"; Andy Slavitt, *Preventable: The Inside Story of How Leadership Failures, Politics, and Selfishness Doomed the U.S. Coronavirus Response* (New York: St. Martin's Press, 2021), 1.

71. Jessie Hellmann, "Trump Downplaying Sparks New Criticism Of COVID-19 Response," *The Hill*, July 6, 2020, https://thehill.com/policy/healthcare/506075-trump-downplaying-sparks-new-criticism-of-covid-19-response.

72. Ashley Collman, "2 Days Before His Coronavirus Diagnosis, Trump Mocked Biden for Wearing a Face Mask," *Business Insider*, October 2, 2020, https://www.businessinsider.com/trump-coronavirus-mocked-biden-face-mask-presidential-debate-2020-10.

73. Tim Rostan, "No More Social Distancing for Media in the Rose Garden as White House Decides It 'Looks Better' When Reporters Bunch Together," *Market Watch*, June 7, 2020, https://www.marketwatch.com/story/no-more-social-distancing-for-media-in-rose-garden-as-white-house-decides-it-looks-better-when-reporters-bunch-together-2020-06-05; Brooke Seipel, "Trump Draws Cheers After Defending Crowd at Club as 'Peaceful Protest,'" *The Hill*, August 7, 2020, https://thehill.com/homenews/news/511140-trump-draws-cheers-after-defending-supporters-lack-of-masks-at-briefing-as.

74. Selena Simmons-Duffin, "Poll Finds Public Health Has a Trust Problem," *NPR*, May 13, 2021, https://www.npr.org/2021/05/13/996331692/poll-finds-public-health-has-a-trust-problem.

75. "Edelman Trust Barometer 2021," Edelman, accessed July 28, 2021, https://www.edelman.com/trust/2021-trust-barometer; Mendy, Stewart, and VanAkin, "A Leader's Guide: Communicating with Stakeholders, And Communities During COVID-19."

76. Michaela Kerrissey and Amy Edmonson, "What Good Leadership Looks Like During This Pandemic," *Harvard Business Review*, April 13, 2020, https://hbr.org/2020/04/what-good-leadership-looks-like-during-this-pandemic.

77. Kerrissey and Edmonson, "What Good Leadership Looks Like During This Pandemic."

78. Timothy Coombs and Rebecca Costantini, "Crisis Management." In *Public Relations: Competencies and Practice*, ed. Carolyn Mae Kim (New York: Taylor and Francis, 2019), 129.

79. Coombs, *Ongoing Crisis Communication: Planning, Managing, and Responding*, 57; Robert Heath and Michael Palenchar, *Strategic Issues Management: Organizations and Public Policy Changes* (Thousand Oaks, CA: SAGE, 2009), 31.

80. Lydia Coutré, "How Businesses Should Prepare for COVID-19," *Crain's Cleveland Business*, March 8, 2020, https://www.crainscleveland.com/health-care/how-businesses-should-prepare-covid-19.

81. "Gartner Business Continuity Survey Shows Just 12 Percent of Organizations Are Highly Prepared for Coronavirus," Gartner Newsroom, published March 10, 2020, https://www.gartner.com/en/newsroom/press-releases/2020-03-10-gartner-business-continuity-survey-shows-just-twelve-percernt-of-organizations-are-highly-prepared-for-coronavirsu.

82. "Top-Line Findings From 'Covid-19: How Businesses Are Handling the Crisis' Study," Institute for Public Relations, published March 17, 2020, https://instituteforpr.org/wp-content/uploads/Topline-COVID-findings-3.16.2020.pdf.

83. Martin Reeves, Nikolaus Lang, and Philipp Carlsson-Szlezak, "Lead Your Business Through the Coronavirus Crisis," *Harvard Business Review*, February 27, 2020, https://hbr.org/2020/02/lead-your-business-through-the-coronavirus-crisis.

84. Lars Schmidt, "How HR Leaders Are Preparing for the Coronavirus," *Fast Company*, February 28, 2020, https://www.fastcompany.com/90469161/how-hr-leaders-are-preparing-for-the-coronavirus.

85. Harsha Gangadharbatla, "Covid-19 and Advertising: The Case for a Paradigm Shift," *Journal of Current Issues & Research in Advertising* 42, no. 1 (2021): 1, https://doi.org/10.1080/10641734.2021.1876797.

86. Chelsea Woods, "When More Than Reputation is at Risk: How Two Hospitals Responded to Ebola," *Public Relations Review* 42 (2016): 896, https://doi.org/10.1016/j.pubrev.2016.10.002.

87. Sarah Kovoor-Misra, *Crisis Management: Resilience & Change* (Thousand Oaks, CA: SAGE, 2020), 136–137.

88. Coombs, *Ongoing Crisis Communication: Planning, Managing, and Responding*, 6.

89. "Crisis Communication," Public Relations Ethics, The Arthur W. Page Center, accessed July 28, 2021, https://www.pagecentertraining.psu.edu/public-relations-ethics/ethics-in-crisis-management/lesson-1-prominent-ethical-issues-in-crisis-situations/crisis-communication/

90. Timothy Coombs, "Parameters for Crisis Communication," in *Handbook of Crisis Communication*, ed. Timothy Coombs and Sherry Holladay (Malden, MA: Wiley-Blackwell, 2010), 17-53.

91. Coombs, *Ongoing Crisis Communication: Planning, Managing, and Responding*, 8.

92. *Ibid*, 11.

93. *Ibid*, 140.

94. "Special Report: Brand Trust and the Coronavirus Pandemic," Edelman, published March 30, 2020, https://www.edelman.com/research/covid-19-brand-trust-report.

95. "Walmart Continues Focus on Health and Safety," Walmart Corporate Newsroom, published March 24, 2020, https://corporate.walmart.com/newsroom/2020/03/24/walmart-continues-focus-on-health-and-safety.

96. Coombs, *Ongoing Crisis Communication: Planning, Managing, and Responding*, 144.

97. Catherine Clifford, "CEO of Multibillion-Dollar Company Slack to Employees Amid Coronavirus: 'Don't Stress Out About Work,'" *CNBC*, March 26, 2020, https://www.cnbc.com/2020/03/26/slack-ceo-to-employees-amid-covid-19-dont-stress-about-work.html.

98. *Ibid*, para. 3.

99. "Additional Steps We're Taking for The Health and Safety of Our Associates," Walmart, published March 31, 2020, https://corporate.walmart.com/newsroom/2020/03/31/additional-steps-were-taking-for-the-health-and-safety-of-our-associates.

100. Mendy, Stewart, and VanAkin, "A Leader's Guide: Communicating with Stakeholders, And Communities During COVID-19."

101. Porter Novelli, "Porter Novelli COVID-19 Insights for a Time of Crisis."

102. Edelman, "Special Report: Brand Trust and the Coronavirus Pandemic."

103. "Smithfield Foods Supports Communities During COVID-19 Response with More Than $3 Million in Donations and Launch of 'Good Food Challenge,'" Smithfield Foods Press Room, published March 26, 2020, https://www.smithfieldfoods.com/press-room/2020-03-26-Smithfield-Foods-Supports-Communities-During-COVID-19-Response-with-More-Than-3-Million-in-Donations-and-Launch-of-Good-Food-Challenge.

104. Kelly Tyko, "Starbucks Offers Free Coffee to Health Care Workers, First Responders as Coronavirus Cases Rise," *USA Today*, December 1, 2020, https://www.usatoday.com/story/money/food/2020/12/01/starbucks-freebie-healthcare-workers-first-responders-december-coronavirus/6431086002/.

105. "At a Glance: What Customers Need to Know About Starbucks Response to COVID-19," Starbucks Press Center, updated June 29, 2021, https://stories.starbucks.com/press/2020/what-customers-need-to-know-about-starbucks-response-to-covid-19/.

106. Curtis Tate, "Hilton, Marriott Donate Free Hotel Rooms for Medical Workers Responding to Coronavirus Crisis," *USA Today,* April 12, 2020, https://www.usatoday.com/story/travel/2020/04/12/coronavirus-hilton-marriott-give-free-hotel-rooms-medical-workers/2978567001/.

107. Jay Peters, "US Wireless Carriers Are Delivering Phone Charters to Hospitals For COVID-19 Patients," *The Verge,* April 29, 2020, https://www.theverge.com/2020/4/29/21242130/att-t-mobile-verizon-iheartmedia-phone-chargers-hospitals-covid-19.

108. Laura Grace Tarpley, "In Response to COVID-19, Bank of America Is Offering Deferrals on Home Loans, Auto Loans, and Credit Cards," *Business Insider,* April 7, 2020, https://www.businessinsider.com/personal-finance/bank-of-america-covid-19-2020-4.

109. Edelman, "Special Report: Brand Trust and the Coronavirus Pandemic."

110. Dee DePass. "3M Doubles Global Production of Respiratory Masks; Warns of Counterfeits," *StarTribune,* March 20, 2020, https://www.startribune.com/3m-has-doubled-global-production-of-respiratory-masks-warns-of-counterfeits/568967952.

111. "Boost Production of Ventilators." *GMC Life,* accessed July 30, 2021, https://www.gmc.com/gmc-life/news/ventilator-production.

112. Kellen Browning, "Distilleries Raced to Make Hand Sanitizer for the Pandemic. No More," *New York Times,* August 4, 2010, https://www.nytimes.com/2020/08/04/business/distilleries-hand-sanitizer-pandemic.html.

113. Jessica Golden, "Fanatics Shifts Production from MLB Jerseys to Masks and Gowns to Fight Coronavirus," *CNBC,* March 26, 2020, https://www.cnbc.com/2020/03/26/fanatics-makes-mlb-masks-and-gowns-to-fight-coronavirus.html.

114. Timothy Sellnow, "Reflecting on Dialectical Tensions in Risk and Crisis Communication: Lessons Learned and Future Opportunities," in *Risk and Crisis Communication: Navigating the Tensions Between Organizations and the Public,* ed. Robert Littlefield and Timothy Sellnow (Lanham, MD: Lexington Books, 2015), 139–148.

115. Camilleri, "Strategic Dialogic Communication Through Digital Media During COVID-19 Crisis," 15.

116. Mendy, Stewart, and VanAkin, "A Leader's Guide: Communicating with Stakeholders, And Communities During COVID-19."

117. Neill and Bowen, "Ethical Listening to Employees During a Pandemic: New Approaches, Barriers and Lessons," 280.

118. Finn Frandsen and Winni Johansen, "The Study of Internal Crisis Communication: Toward an Integrative Framework," *Corporate Communications: An International Journal* 16, no. 4(2011): 348, https://doi.org/10.1108/13563281111186977

119. Mats Heide and Charlotte Simonsson, 2020, "Internal Crisis Communication: On Current and Future Research," in *Crisis Communication,* ed. Finn Frandsen and Winni Johansen (Berlin: De Gruyter Mouton, 2020), 259–278.

120. Kevin Ruck and Linjuan Rita Men, "Guest Editorial: Internal Communication During the COVID-19 Pandemic," *Journal of Communication Management 25,* no. 3 (2021): 185. https://doi.org/10.1108/JCOM-08-2021-163.

121. "Special Report: Trust and the Coronavirus," Edelman, published March 18, 2020, retrieved from https://www.edelman.com/research/2020-edelman-trust-barometer-special-report-coronavirus-and-trust.

122. Donald Sull and Charles Sull, "How Companies Are Winning on Culture During COVID-19," *MIT SMR,* October 28, 2020, https://sloanreview.mit.edu/article/how-companies-are-winning-on-culture-during-covid-19/.

123. Men, "Internal Reputation Management: The Impact of Authentic Leadership and Transparent Communication," 259.

124. Sabine Einwiller, Christopher Ruppel, and Julia Stranzl, "Achieving Employee Support During the COVID-19 Pandemic—the Role of Relational and Informational Crisis Communication in Austrian Organizations," *Journal of Communication Management* 25, no. 3 (2021): 248, https://doi.org/10.1108/JCOM-10-2020-0107/full/html; Li et al., "Employee Coping with Organizational Change in the Face of a Pandemic: The Role of Transparent Internal Communication," 8.

125. Edelman, "Edelman Trust Barometer 2021."

126. "Campbell's COVID-19 Response," Campbell Newsroom. Posted October 22, 2020. https://www.campbellsoupcompany.com/newsroom/news/campbells-covid-19-response.

127. Walmart, "Additional Steps We're Taking for The Health and Safety of Our Associates."

128. Sull and Sull, "How Companies Are Winning on Culture During COVID-19."

129. Linda Hon and James Grunig, "Guidelines for Measuring Relationships in Public Relations," 3.

130. Einwiller, Ruppel, and Stranzl, "Achieving Employee Support During the COVID-19 Pandemic—the Role of Relational and Informational Crisis Communication in Austrian Organizations," 235; Maria Watkins, Run Ren, Elizabeth Umphress, Wendy Boswell, Maria Triana, and Ashar Zardhoohi, "Compassion Organizing: Employees' Satisfaction with Corporate Philanthropic Disaster Response and Reduced Job Strain," *Journal of Occupational and Organizational Psychology* 88, no. 2 (2015): 449, https://doi.org/10.1111/joop.12088.

131. "COVID-19 Update: Workplace Policies and Practices," CVS Health News and Insights. Published March 18, 2020. https://cvshealth.com/news-and-insights/press-releases/covid-19-update-workplace-policies-and-practices-lisa-bisaccia-evp.

132. Stephanie Mehta, "U.S. Starbucks Employees Can Now Get Up to 20 Free Therapy Sessions," *Fast Company,* March 16, 2020, retrieved from https://www.fastcompany.com/90476917/starbucks-employees-in-the-u-s-can-get-up-to-20-therapy-sessions.

133. James Grunig, "What Is Excellence in Management," in *Excellence in Public Relations and Communication Management,* ed. James Grunig, (New York: Routledge, 1992), 219–250; Linjuan Men and Don Stacks, "The Effects of Authentic Leadership on Strategic Internal Communication and Employee-Organization Relationships," *Journal of Public Relations Research* 26, no. 4 (2014): 315, https://doi.org/10.1080/1062726X.2014.908720.

134. Mats Heide and Charlotte Simonsson, "What Was That All About? On Internal Crisis Communication and Communicative Coworkership During a Pandemic,"

Journal of Communication Management 25, no. 3 (2021): 268, https://doi.org/10.1108/JCOM-09-2020-0105.

135. Einwiller, Ruppel, and Stranzl, "Achieving Employee Support During the COVID-19 Pandemic—the Role of Relational and Informational Crisis Communication in Austrian Organizations," 234; Li et al., "Employee Coping with Organizational Change in the Face of a Pandemic: The Role of Transparent Internal Communication," 4; Neill and Bowen, "Ethical Listening to Employees During a Pandemic: New Approaches, Barriers and Lessons," 290.

136. "Amazon's COVID-19 Vaccination and Testing Blog," About Amazon, last modified July 6, 2021, https://www.aboutamazon.com/news/company-news/amazons-covid-19-blog-updates-on-how-were-responding-to-the-crisis.

137. Shirin Ghaffary and Jason Del Ray, "The Real Cost of Amazon," *Vox*, June 29, 2020, https://www.vox.com/recode/2020/6/29/21303643/amazon-coronavirus-warehouse-workers-protest-jeff-bezos-chris-smalls-boycott-pandemic; Annie Palmer, "Amazon Says More Than 19,000 Workers Got Covid-19," *CNBC*, October 1, 2020, https://www.cnbc.com/2020/10/01/amazon-says-more-than-19000-workers-got-covid-19.html.

138. Erika Hayasaki, "Amazon's Great Labor Awakening," *The New York Times Magazine*, February 18, 2021, https://www.nytimes.com/2021/02/18/magazine/amazon-workers-employees-covid-19.html.

139. Molly Kinder and Laura Stateler, "Amazon and Walmart Have Raked in Billions in Additional Profits During the Pandemic, and Shared Almost None of It with Their Workers," *Brookings*, December 22, 2020, https://www.brookings.edu/blog/the-avenue/2020/12/22/amazon-and-walmart-have-raked-in-billions-in-additional-profits-during-the-pandemic-and-shared-almost-none-of-it-with-their-workers/.

140. Chelsea Woods and Shari Veil, "Balancing Transparency and Privacy in a University Sexual Misconduct Case: A Legal Public Relations Perspective," *Journal of International Crisis and Risk Communication Research* 3, no. 1 (2020): 120, https://doi.org/10.30658/jicrcr.2.1.1.

141. Kaibin Xu and Wenqing Li, "An Ethical Stakeholder Approach to Crisis Communication: A Case Study of Foxconn's 2010 Employee Suicide Crisis," *Journal of Business Ethics* 117 (2013): 382, https://doi.org/10.1007/s10551-012-1522-0.

142. Robert Ulmer and Timothy Sellnow, "Consistent Questions of Ambiguity in Organizational Crisis Communication: Jack in the Box as A Case Study," *Journal of Business Ethics* 25 (2000): 146, https://doi.org/10.1023/A:1006183805499.

143. Crane and Matten, "Covid-19 and the Future of CSR Research," 1.

144. Hon and Grunig, "Guidelines for Measuring Relationships in Public Relations," 3.

145. Edelman, "Special Report: Brand Trust and the Coronavirus Pandemic."

146. Sellnow and Seeger, *Theorizing Crisis Communication*, 32.

147. Coombs, "Parameters for Crisis Communication," 45.

148. Coombs, "Parameters for Crisis Communication," 45.

149. Kovoor-Misra, *Crisis Management: Resilience & Change*, 53.

150. Ian Mitroff, *Why Some Companies Emerge Stronger and Better from a Crisis: 7 Essential Lessons for Surviving Disaster.* (New York, NY: AMACOM, 2005), 206.

151. Susan Caminiti, "The Most Surprising Lessons Companies Learned from Coronavirus," Nasdaq, published November 17, 2020, https://www.nasdaq.com/articles/the-most-surprising-lessons-companies-learned-from-coronavirus-2020-11-17; Kathy Gurchiek, "Workplace Lessons Learned During the Pandemic," *SHRM*, published March 29, 2021, https://www.shrm.org/hr-today/news/hr-news/pages/workplace-lessons-learned-during-covid19.aspx.

152. Lauren Hirsch and Kellen Browning, "Delays, More Masks and Mandatory Shots: Virus Surge Disrupts Office-Return Plans," *The New York Times*, July 23, 2021, https://www.nytimes.com/2021/07/23/business/return-to-office-vaccine-mandates-delta-variant.html; Ray Smith and Patrick Thomas, "As Delta Variant Rages, More Workers Are on Edge About Return to the Office," *The Wall Street Journal*, August 2, 2021, https://www.wsj.com/articles/as-delta-variant-rages-more-workers-are-on-edge-about-return-to-the-office-11627909200.

153. Heide and Simonsson, "What Was That All About? On Internal Crisis Communication and Communicative Coworkership During a Pandemic," 272.

154. Coombs, "Parameters for Crisis Communication," 45.

155. Aaron Chatterji and Michael Toffel, "The New CEO Activists," *Harvard Business Review Magazine*, January-February 2018, https://hbr.org/2018/01/the-new-ceo-activists; Edelman, "Edelman Trust Barometer 2021."

156. Edelman, "Edelman Trust Barometer 2021."

157. Andrea Hsu, "As Mask Mandates Disappear, Business Owners Make and Enforce Their Own Rules," *NPR*, May 18, 2021, https://www.npr.org/2021/05/18/997638745/as-mask-mandates-disappear-business-owners-left-to-make-and-enforce-their-own-ru

158. Arunima Krishna, Donald Wright, and Raymond Kotcher, "Curriculum Rebuilding in Public Relations: Understanding What Early Career, Mid-Career, and Senior PR/Communications Professionals Expect from Graduates," *Journal of Public Relations Education* 6, no. 1, 45. https://aejmc.us/jpre/2020/01/.

159. Yan Jin, Sung In Choi, and Audra Diers-Lawson, "Special Issue Editor's Essay: Advancing Public Health Crisis and Risk Theory and Practice via Innovative and Inclusive Research on COVID-19 Communication," *Journal of International Crisis and Risk Communication Research*, 4, no. 2 (2021): 179, https://doi.org/10.30658/jicrcr.4.2.0

160. Audra Diers-Lawson and Florian Meißner, "Editor's Essay: Moving Beyond Western Corporate Perspectives: On the Need to Increase the Diversity of Risk and Crisis Communication Research," *Journal of International Crisis and Risk Communication Research*, 4, no. 1 (2021): 169, https://doi.org/10.30658/jicrcr.4.1.5

Chapter 5

This Just Got Real

Implications of the COVID-19 Pandemic on Sport Communication

Brandi Watkins

> Right or wrong, sports have an ability to spark national conversation in ways that some other institutions no longer can or maybe never have. We look to sports for something, sometimes it's distraction, sometimes it's passion, but sometimes it's leadership.—Jody Avrigan[1]

For me, and I suspect for most people, Wednesday, March 11, 2020, started innocuously enough. I was off for spring break and went to Cincinnati to visit my parents. My mom and I went to the mall earlier in the day to exchange some shoes, we went out to lunch, then stopped by the grocery store to get food for dinner. A perfectly normal spring break afternoon. After dinner, we settled in the living room to watch television, a nightly family ritual dating back to my childhood. We debated what we should watch knowing that there were limited options that would appease all of our television watching proclivities (another important part of the nightly family ritual). The debate concluded where it often did—we would watch sports—one of the few things that we could all consistently agree on.

Like many others, I come from a sport loving family. Weekend activities were planned around various sporting events. Saturdays in the fall was for watching college football and Sunday was reserved for my dad's favorite team, the Dallas Cowboys (consequently, the Cowboys were much more fun to watch in the 1990s). Early in the year, the time reserved for the National Football League (NFL) would fade into NASCAR season at our house. I spent many Sunday afternoons napping to the almost ASMR-like roar of stock car engines whirring around a track on the television. My brother and I played sports. He played football. I played basketball. As a child of the 1990s, my love of basketball was formed by one indelible figure, Michael Jordan. Many of my favorite summer memories involve watching Jordan and the Chicago Bulls make their way through the National Basketball Association (NBA) playoffs. I would spend hours during the day in our driveway practicing free throws and post-up moves, then as the sun started to set, I would go inside to watch Jordan put on a show. All of this to say, sports always have been and always will be an important part of my life, and I know I am not the only one.

Back to that fateful Wednesday night. The Oklahoma City Thunder were hosting the Utah Jazz in a late-season NBA game that had playoff implications. We tuned to ESPN to watch the game, catching the last few minutes of the pregame show. There were reports that Utah center Rudy Gobert would be unavailable that night due to illness, but this was not unusual for this stage of the NBA season. Both teams were warmed up, the referees were on the floor, and it would be a matter of moments before the game tipped off. But then, something strange happened. A guy in a suit ran across the court. Players moved back to their respective benches, visibly confused as to what was happening. The ESPN television crew were seemingly just as confused, grappling on air to make sense of what we all were watching. I asked my dad what happened, as if he had some special inside knowledge that I did not have at the time. I turned to Twitter, which for better or for worse is always a fount of information, but tonight the tweets were as confused and uninformed as we were. Eventually, the news came down. Rudy Gobert of the Utah Jazz tested positive for COVID-19. He was the first athlete from a major American sport league to test positive for the virus. Shortly after the news of Gobert's diagnosis, the game was cancelled, and then came an avalanche of game and league suspensions and cancellations from all corners of the sport world. The next day the *Los Angeles Times* published a column titled "The Day Sports Stopped."

WHAT IS SPORT COMMUNICATION?

In the grand scheme of pedagogy and academic pursuits, sport communication is still a relatively young field. The study of sport has a multidisciplinary heritage that includes history, management, sociology, marketing, organizational behavior, and law.[2] Sports communication, in an academic sense, is a broad term that frequently encompasses a number of sub-disciplines including sport management, public relations, marketing, journalism, media studies, and history, among others. Scholars have attempted to narrow the focus of sport communication by defining the field. For example, Pedersen et al. proffered one definition of sport communication, "a process by which people in sport, in a sport setting, or through sport endeavor, share symbols as they create meaning through interaction"[3] and the authors go on to explain that "sport communication involves the sport communication process, its components, and the communication between sport industry practitioners, organizations, and internal and external stakeholders and the interrelationships between them."[4] A decade later, Robert L. Krizek proposed the following definition:

> Sport communication is the process of creating and sharing meanings by individuals participating in the embodied (combining physical and mental exertion) activity of sport. Sport communication also includes the meaning making of individuals observing that activity; governing, directing or commenting on that activity; and/or discussing the influence of sport on individuals and society.[5]

The central thesis of these two definitions is the same—sport communication is a process of creating shared meaning using sport as a lens or backdrop. Sport communication, then, requires that people engage with all the facets of sport to create a shared meaning related to the experience. Sports communication looks at the theoretical and practical implications of sport and the various organizational structures surrounding sport. It provides a lens for viewing the world and world events, including the global COVID-19 pandemic, in a way that is accessible and relevant to people's day-to-day lives.

Sport communication is a multifaceted field that encompasses the study of sport media, sport organizations, sport production, sport fandom, and the cultural and social structures that surround sport. Pertinent to this chapter, sports have been used as a lens to view and interpret world events and to critically analyze the systems in which sport operate. Sport has been used to help us better understand social issues related to identity, racism, sexism, and politics. Andrew Billings put it this way: "Sports have power; therefore, we need to teach sports. Not how to play them, I think we have that covered, but how to consume them and how to understand them . . . how to talk about them. Because when we teach sports, we often teach those larger issues as well—gender, domestic violence, religion, identity."[6] In this talk, Billings implored those in sport communication to teach how to consume and understand sport. This moves beyond looking at sports as merely an athletic competition, but instead encourages people to use sport as a lens for how we observe the world around us.

The purpose of this chapter is to examine the implications of the COVID-19 pandemic on sports and the sport communication discipline. In addition to the COVID-19 pandemic, the year 2020 in particular will also be remembered for the protests and outrage that followed the death of George Floyd, a Black man killed at the hands of a police officer. Floyd's death sparked a call for racial justice in the United States that reverberated throughout the sports world. As such, it is prudent to also consider the events related to the racial justice reckoning in conjunction with the COVID-19 pandemic in the context of sports. With this in mind, the remainder of this chapter will investigate the sports industry's reaction to the COVID-19 pandemic followed by a section recounting the events of the summer of 2020 after the death of George Floyd. The chapter concludes with a discussion related to the implications of the COVID-19 pandemic for sports communication pedagogy and scholarship.

SPORTS REACT TO THE COVID-19 PANDEMIC

The earliest reports of the novel coronavirus (COVID-19) were in December of 2019[7] and the first confirmed case in the U.S. was reported in January 2021.[8] Countries in Asia were hit particularly hard by the highly transmissible virus in early 2020, and shortly after the virus spread throughout the rest of the world causing the World Health Organization to declare the virus a global emergency on January 30[9] and then upgraded the virus to a pandemic on March 11.[10] On March 13, the U.S. was put under a state of emergency and states across the nation had to make difficult decisions regarding shelter-in-place orders and lockdowns.[11] As mentioned in the introduction to this chapter, March 11 was a pivotal day in sports as it relates to the COVID-19 pandemic; however, in order to appreciate the breadth of the COVID-19 pandemic's impact on the sporting world, it is necessary to look at the timeline of events starting in March 2020 (see Table 5.1).[12]

December 7, 2020, the U.S. Food and Drug Administration granted emergency use authorization of the Pfizer-BioNTech COVID-19 vaccine and the Moderna vaccine on December 18.[13] By March 2021, the vaccines were made available to everyone 16 years and older in the U.S.[14] Many sport franchises allowed officials to use their facilities to host mass vaccination sites in the spring. With increased vaccination rates across the country, fans were welcomed back to sporting events. Notably, by the time the NBA playoffs started in June of 2021, most of the playoff team arenas hosted fans to full or near full capacity.[15] For the MLB, whose season began in April 2021, stadiums are expected to operate at full capacity by the July 4th holiday.[16]

Table 5.1 Timeline of Sports Reactions to the COVID-19 Pandemic

2020

March 3	The NBA issues a league memo encouraging players to use fist bumps in lieu of high fives. Similarly, on March 5 the United European Football Association (UEFA) Premier League banned the traditional pregame fair-play handshake.
March 7	The NBA issues a league memo informing teams to prepare to play without fans.
March 9	Sports leagues, including the NBA, NHL, and Major League Baseball (MLB) ban reporters from locker rooms. U.S. Major League Soccer (MLS) followed suit a day later.
March 10	The Ivy League cancelled its basketball tournament, the first sport league to cancel an event because of the virus.
March 11	The NBA was the first major U.S. sports league to postpone its season. The National Collegiate Athletic Association (NCAA) announced the men's and women's basketball tournaments will be held without fans.
March 12	Major sports leagues all postponed their seasons including the MLS, MLB, NHL, Association of Tennis Professionals, Professional Golfer's Association (PGA), Ladies Professional Golf Association, and Minor League Baseball (MiLB). The NCAA cancels the men's and women's basketball tournaments for the first time since the tournament's inception in 1939. They also suspend all remaining winter and spring events. The UEFA Champions League cancelled its first game.
March 13	The English Premier League and National Association for Stock Car Racing (NASCAR) also postponed their season. The Boston Marathon was cancelled.
March 16	The NFL suspended its off-season activities.
March 17	The Kentucky Derby was cancelled.
March 20	The Scripps National Spelling Bee was cancelled.
March 24	The 2020 Olympics and Paralympics Games were postponed until 2021. This marked the first disruption to the Olympics since World War II led to the cancellation of the 1940 and 1944 Summer Olympics.
April 3	The Women's National Basketball Association (WNBA) delays the start of its season.
May 9	The Ultimate Fighting Championship (UFC) holds UFC 249 in Jacksonville, Florida. This is the first major sporting event to resume without fans during the pandemic.
May 17	NASCAR resumes its season at Darlington Speedway in South Carolina.
June 4	The NBA announces it will restart its season with 22 teams playing in what came to be known as the "NBA Bubble."
June 11	The PGA returns with the Charles Schwab Challenge in Ft. Worth, Texas.

2020	
June 15	The WNBA announced it will resume its season playing in a bubble, similar to the NBA.
June 22	MLB announced it would play a modified 60-game season starting in late July.
June 27	The National Women's Soccer League played the Challenge Cup tournament marking the return of women's sports in the pandemic.
July 8	MLS returns with a "MLS is Back" tournament.
July 23	The New York Yankees and Washington Nationals play in the first MLB game since the start of the pandemic. Dr. Anthony Fauci throws out the ceremonial first pitch.
July 24	The WNBA resumed its season in a bubble.
July 30	The NBA resumed its season in a bubble.
August 1	The NHL resumed its season with 24 teams.
August 11	In college football, the Power Five conferences announce plans for the upcoming college football season. The Southeastern Conference (SEC), Big 12, and Atlantic Coast Conference decide to play the season as scheduled. The PAC 12 and Big Ten conferences vote to postpone the season; however, both conferences will later decide to play the season.
August 26	Jacob Blake, a Black man, was left partially paralyzed after being shot by a police officer in Kenosha, Wisconsin. Players from the NBA, WNBA, MLS, and MLB refuse to play in protest.
September 3	College football season starts. Some games are postponed or cancelled due to COVID-19 protocols. The season ends in January 2021 when the University of Alabama defeated Ohio State University for the College Football Playoff National Championship with limited fan attendance.
September 10	NFL seasons starts with limited fan attendance.
September/ October	NHL, WNBA, NBA, MLB hold championship events.
December 22	NBA starts the 2020–2021 season with an abbreviated 72 game schedule. Teams play in home arenas with no or limited fan attendance.
2021	
February 7	The Tampa Bay Buccaneers played the Kansas City Chiefs in Super Bowl 55 with limited fan attendance. The NFL was able to complete its season on time with all scheduled games played.

The availability of vaccines is an important component of the COVID-19 timeline because they allow life to go back to a semblance of prepandemic normal, which include hosting sporting events with fans. However, at the time of this writing, despite widespread availability of vaccines, a fourth wave of COVID-19 infections hit the United States because of the highly contagious delta variant of the virus. This illustrates that the pandemic is an ongoing and fluid situation and we are not yet back to our normal, prepandemic routines.

THE LEGACY OF COVID-19 AND SPORTS

According to systems theory, no organization operates in a vacuum. Instead, they consist of internal and external systems within an operating environment that can impact an organization's ability to achieve its mission. We can look at this in the context of sports. The COVID-19 pandemic prohibited large gatherings of people, thus causing the temporary stoppage of sporting events. This left sport organizations with a decision—do we continue to play and if we do, how do we do it safely? The decision of the sport organizations to not have fans at games would have a direct economic impact on the organization and the surrounding community. A decision to cancel an event or a season would have consequences for television licensing and broadcast agreements. Take the NBA and WNBA, for example, their decision to finish out the season in a bubble meant that players and coaches would have to leave their families for an extended period of time, causing families to have to make adjustments. Leaving home arenas meant that the hourly workers who run the concession stands and ticket booths were left without a job or compensation. Even still, the decision to close down bars or restaurants caused a lot of fans to sit out on sporting events because they lost the social aspect of sports.

The above examples illustrate how interconnected sports can be to the fabric of daily life. Disruptions can have long reaching effects (some more serious than others). This chapter will look at the disruptions caused by the COVID-19 pandemic through the lens of sport. Through sport we are able to see how leagues had to make important decisions that could affect any number of stakeholders. More specifically, in this section I will examine the implications of the COVID-19 pandemic in three sport-related areas: (1) the ability of sports to bring people together, (2) increased discussion related to the health and well-being of athletes, and (3) the role of athletes in promoting public health.

Sports Bring People Together?

Sports grew in significance and stature, particularly in the U.S., during the Industrial Revolution. The Industrial Revolution brought sweeping changes to society and ushered in the modern era we live in today. For the first time, people left their homes and family farm to work in the new factories in larger cities, which spurred urbanization. With more individuals leaving behind families, isolation and loneliness was rampant among those who migrated to the city and to cope, many of them turned to sports. Local sport leagues developed in cities that provided new urbanites an outlet to escape from their current situation.[17] Through sports, people found companionship and belonging in a strange, new place.

The ability of sports to bring people together has been echoed throughout history. Take 9/11, for example, another event that brought life to a halt. After the terrorist attacks on the World Trade Center and the Pentagon, Americans were left wondering what to do next. When would it be ok to resume our normal lives again? What would our normal lives look like? Sports played a big role in helping us reclaim our lives again after the attacks. The 9/11 Memorial Museum hosted a special exhibit called "Comeback Season" that shows how sports helped Americans unite and heal after 9/11. The museum's website put it this way:

> In the months that followed, sports set an emotional cadence for a grieving nation. Ballparks, racetracks, and arenas offered fans a place to come together and cheer. The rituals of sport were extended to commemorate those killed on 9/11 and honor those who protect us. In stadiums around the country, millions found a path forward, combining reverence for the fallen with devotion to the games.[18]

In both of these examples, people sought out connection and escape through sport. Similar to the Industrial Revolution, many people were experiencing similar feelings of loneliness brought on by months of quarantine and isolation. Even now, many of us are wondering when or if we will ever be able to resume our normal lives again?

The parallels between the pandemic and these examples are there, but this time, it does not appear that the sports mojo is working with this significant world event. SportsPro reported that television ratings across all the major U.S. sport leagues were down significantly in 2020.[19] According to the article, NASCAR was one of the first sports to come back in mid-May of 2020, and the Real Heroes 400 race saw a 38 percent increase in viewers than in 2019. However, as the summer progressed league championships for the National Hockey League (NHL), NBA, and MLB were all lower than in 2019. The NBA Finals, which were played in October (instead of its regularly scheduled time of June) viewership dropped 49 percent from 2019, and for the MLB, the 2020 World Series was the least watched on record.[20] There was one league, however, that saw its viewership for the championship game go up and that was the WNBA. ESPN reports that ratings for Game 3 of the WNBA finals was up by as much as 15 percent.[21]

The decline in televised sport viewership during the pandemic, a time when people are spending more time at home and seeking out forms of entertainment, is interesting and has left experts and sport executives wrestling with why the magic of sport did not bring people together as it has in the past. Sports were viewed as an important part of our collective grieving and healing after the 9/11 terrorist attacks. People turned to sports, much the same way people did during the Industrial Revolution, as a way to escape and connect with others. Time and time again, people have turned to sporting events as a way to escape the doldrums of daily life or to find connection with others. Much of sport communication scholarship has focused on sport fandom and the ways that being a sport fan enriches our lives. But, as evidenced by the declining sport ratings, the COVID-19 pandemic is different than any other major, life altering event we have collectively experienced. While we have yet to unpack all the implications of the pandemic, there are some consequences that help shine light on why people did not turn to sports for comfort as they have in the past.

For starters, it is prudent to step back and take in the totality of the 2020 experience to better understand the head space of people living through a pandemic. There was a lot of uncertainty and generalized anxiety about the virus. The novelty of the virus meant that scientists and doctors did not know much about it or how to treat it. People were inundated with news stories projecting grim numbers related to infections and deaths. Lockdowns meant that some people lost their jobs or had their hours cut, which brought about more financial anxiety. Those who were fortunate enough to maintain their job had to adjust to working from home and the challenges of not being able to separate work space from living space. Parents became teachers as school closings led to virtual distance learning. Then, there was the risk of catching the virus or having a loved one catch the virus and the uncertainty that came with that. Not to mention, in the midst of this, in the U.S. and other parts of the world, there was a massive civil rights movement happening in response to police killings of unarmed Black men and women. In the U.S., there was a contentious presidential election and rampant political polarization that, frankly, soaked up a lot of the oxygen in the world.

Simply put, the pandemic and the resulting uncertainty and political upheaval, meant that people lacked the cognitive capacity to invest in something else—even sports. The Marist Center for Sports Communication surveyed sport fans in 2020 and found that sport fans were not watching as much live sports as in previous years and doing so less fervently.[22] According to Jane McManus, Director of the Marist Center for Sports Communication, "but what ratings and the results of the poll are telling us, is that fans may have other concerns at the moment."[23] Moreover, the survey found that 35 percent of sports fans cite concerns about COVID-19 as a reason why they are tuning into sports less, 20 percent of respondents indicated that the 2020 election was more important than sports, and 19 percent said they did not have free time for sports.

Another important consequence of the pandemic that warrants examination is that it took away the social aspect of sports, which is an essential component of the sport experience. In a *Washington Post* story about declining sport ratings in 2020, Mike Mulvihill, head of strategy and analytics at Fox Sports had this to say: "We just believe so strongly that the whole business of sports fuels social connection and is fueled by social connection. For obvious reasons, our whole environment of social connection is completely inside out. So, sports and the ability of sports to act as a unifying force is really undermined."[24] In 2020, people all over the world were mostly confined to their homes and not able to share in the collective watching experience that makes sports great. Fans were unable to gather in sports bars or at each other's homes to watch games. Physically attending a game was impossible. The togetherness that is inherent in the sport experience was missing from 2020 and without that, some people were not as interested or involved. It can be argued that the physical separation from others has impacted the casual sports fan more than the die-hard sports fans. Much of the drop in ratings for lives sports comes from the casual fan[25] who is more likely to watch sports for the social aspect than for the competition itself.

When analyzing the pandemic through the lens of sport, we can see just how remarkable and (hopefully) one-of-its-kind this event was. A pandemic, civil rights movement, and contentious politics left most people exhausted and anxious. While there have been other pandemics in modern history (Ebola, Zika, SARS, MERS, H1N1), none have had the impact on the global scale as the COVID-19 pandemic. Sports are not a cure-all for the ills of the world, but in the past, it has served an important role in bringing people together and inspiring hope. Children all over the world dream of being the next Simone Biles, Megan Rapinoe, Serena Williams, or LeBron James. Time after time we have turned to sports to inspire us to be better and have pride in who we are. The collective anxieties that sports brought to bear was intense and trying in so many ways. But, with the increasing availability of vaccines, we can hope that this pandemic will soon be behind us and we can once again find time and energy to devote to the things we enjoy, including sports.

Sports and Mental Health and Well-Being

Living in a global pandemic with nation-wide economic shutdowns had a tremendous effect on our lives. Anxiety and uncertainty surrounding the pandemic was rampant and presented a challenge to many around the world. Social distancing meant that people often felt lonely and isolated, which also heightened stress and anxiety. A report from the Kaiser Family Foundation found that nearly four in 10 Americans claimed that stress and worry associated to COVID-19 has had a negative impact on their mental health.[26] Health experts think the mental health effects of COVID-19 will likely linger long after the pandemic is over.[27]

Mental health among athletes has also received considerable attention in the media recently. Tennis star Naomi Osaka, who won the 2020 U.S. Open, made headlines for withdrawing from the 2021 French Open and Wimbledon in order to treat her anxiety and depression.[28] Other professional athletes have been more outspoken about their mental health including Olympic swimmer Michael Phelps and NBA player Kevin Love. Athletes for Hope, a nonprofit organization that assists athletes in making a difference in the world, reports that among elite professional athletes, 35 percent suffer from a mental health crisis.[29] Mental health concerns are not limited to professional athletes. The NCAA surveyed student-athletes who reported feeling heightened levels of mental exhaustion, anxiety, hopelessness, and depression in the last year.[30] Moreover, Black student-athletes reported additional trauma due to experiences of racism of racial trauma.[31]

The NBA seemed to outsmart COVID-19 by having players finish the season at the Walt Disney World resort in Orlando, Florida, in what came to be known as the bubble replete with strict health and safety protocols. The end result was zero positive tests for the roughly 90 days those players spent in the bubble.[32] The success of the bubble spelled good news for the league, but it took a toll on the players who were separated from friends and family for months. Paul George, forward for the Los Angeles Clippers, experienced a prolonged shooting slump while in the bubble. His explanation for the slump was candid, "I underestimated mental health. I had anxiety. A little bit of depression. Us being locked in here, I just wasn't there. I just checked out."[33] George was public about seeking help from a team psychiatrist, his coach, teammates, and family. And, to the NBA's credit, the league and NBA Players Association provided resources for players in the bubble including licensed mental health professionals on site and access to telehealth.[34]

Athletes at all levels have dealt with mental health struggles since before the pandemic. Those in sport communication should devote time to studying overall athlete well-being including mental health. Research can look at how athletes use their platform to raise awareness about mental health and providing resources for those who need help. The athlete as endorser has been studied extensively in the sports and marketing literature, and similar studies could be conducted on the athlete as an ambassador for health and wellness. Sport scholars and instructors can present case studies on athletes who are outspoken about mental health to see what is being said in relation to mental health and how athletes can affect change. The increased emphasis on mental health and wellness should also be reflected in sport communication scholarship and pedagogy.

Sports and Vaccination Campaigns

Another important area of postpandemic research is the campaign to get people vaccinated. As of this writing, nearly half (45%) of Americans are fully vaccinated against COVID-19[35] and worldwide, about 21.1% of the world's population is vaccinated.[36] Experts say that about 70–85 % of the population needs to be vaccinated to reach herd immunity.[37]

Athlete and sport response to vaccines has been mixed. NHL star David Perron was coy about announcing whether or not he was vaccinated after missing playoff games due to the COVID-19 protocols.[38] While some experts hope that celebrities and athletes will endorse getting vaccines, some are reluctant citing "misinformation and flawed public messaging from the federal government have made the vaccines controversial and something some public figures are reluctant to endorse."[39] Similarly, LeBron James, who has been outspoken on many political issues declined to speak publicly about whether or not he would get the vaccine stating a desire for privacy as the reason.[40]

Some athletes are using their public platform to educate the public and encourage people to get vaccinated. The NBA produced public service announcements featuring Bill Russell, Kareem Abdul-Jabbar, and Gregg Poppovich getting their COVID-19 vaccine and encouraging the public to do so as well.[41] In the spring of 2021, the Biden administration launched a campaign called "We Can Do This: Live" to encourage young people to get the vaccine.[42] Athletes from NASCAR, the NBA, and WNBA signed on to participate in the campaign. The Ad Council and the COVID Collaborative partnered with sports leagues including the American Horse Council, Athlete Unlimited, MLB, MLS, NASCAR, NBA, NFL, NHL, Women's Soccer League (NWSL), PGA Tour, U.S. Open Tennis Championships, WNBA, and World Wrestling Entertainment for a campaign to promote the COVID-19 vaccine.[43]

There is a notable example of a professional athlete speaking out about an important health-related topic. November 7, 1991, Earvin "Magic" Johnson announced he was retiring from basketball because he had been diagnosed with HIV, the virus that caused AIDS. By 1984, AIDS had taken the lives of 4,251 Americans.[44] Despite the stark number of lives lost to AIDS, the Reagan administration was, at first, reluctant to take it seriously. By the time Reagan gave a major address on AIDS in 1987, more than 25,000 people were dead.[45] Johnson was a five-time NBA champion and three-time league and Finals MVP, and he was a heterosexual man who announced contracting a virus was mostly viewed as a disease that only affected gay men and drug addicts.[46] Johnson spoke out about a virus that many found taboo and refused to talk about. In his announcement, Johnson said: "I'm going to be a spokesman for the HIV virus. I want young people to realize they can practice safe sex. Sometimes you're a little naïve about it and you think that something like that can never happen to you. It has happened but I'm going to deal with it. My life will go on. Life is going to go on and I'll be a happy man."[47] Since his announcement, Johnson has worked to educate the public about HIV[48] and has raised more than $10 million for HIV/AIDs research and charities.[49] Even during the COVID-19 pandemic, Johnson was outspoken on the parallels between the misconceptions about the two viruses, particularly in the Black community. During a CNN interview, Johnson said:

> African Americans are leading in terms of dying from the coronavirus and most of them in the hospital are African American. We have to do a better job as African Americans to follow social distancing, stay at home and make sure we educate our loved ones and our family members and do what we're supposed to do to keep safe and healthy. Then when you add that up, we don't have access to health care, quality health care. So many of us are uninsured. That also creates a problem, too. Just like it did with HIV and AIDS.[50]

Johnson was mostly praised for speaking out about HIV/AIDS in 1991 by public health officials, doctors, and activists,[51] but also received backlash from other NBA players.[52]

Much like Johnson's impact on discussions surrounding HIV/AIDS, today's athletes can take a similar role in promoting COVID-19 vaccines. From a pedagogical perspective, this topic brings up a great point of debate for a classroom—what is the role of athletes/public figures in speaking out about medical issues? Instructors can point to the example of Magic Johnson and his advocacy for HIV/AIDS in starting a discussion on the extent to which the public should expect athlete involvement in health messaging. Furthermore, researchers should look at the effectiveness of athletes in health messaging.

BEYOND COVID-19: THE SUMMER OF 2020 AND THE FIGHT FOR RACIAL JUSTICE

When reflecting on the events of 2020, the pandemic is obviously an important and defining aspect of the year, but another aspect that is worthy and essential for sport communication scholars and teachers to examine is the role sport and athletes played in the response and fight for racial justice. The history of sport around the world includes stories of athletes protesting and fighting for freedom and justice. Before looking at the events of 2020 and the response from the sport perspective, it is necessary to look back at how athletes have used their position in the past in the fight for civil rights.

Athletes, Activism, and Social Movements

Athletes have a rich tradition of using their platform and status to protest for social causes. In 1959, Elgin Baylor refused to play the Cincinnati Royals at a neutral site game in Charleston, West Virginia, after a hotel and restaurant refused him and two Black teammates service, and in 1961 Boston Celtics legend Bill Russell also refused to play in protest to being refused service on the basis of race.[53] In what has become one of the most iconic images in sport, U.S. sprinter Tommie Smith and John Carlos raised their hands to protest racial discrimination in America at the 1968 Olympic Games; however, after their protest, Smith and Carlos were suspended from the U.S. track and field team and were asked to leave the Olympic Games, but were able to keep their medals.[54]

One of the most notable and politically charged examples of athletes engaging in activism occurred in 2016 when Colin Kaepernick, then quarterback of the NFL's San Francisco 49ers, began kneeling during the national anthem to protest police brutality and racial injustice.[55] Kaepernick's silent protest led some to refer to him as "the face of the new civil rights movement."[56] Response to Kaepernick's protest was polarized—with some citing that he was disrespectful for not standing during the national anthem and others seeking to join him in the protest.

Athlete activism is not confined to racial discrimination or men's sports. In 1973 U.S. tennis great Billie Jean King threatened to boycott the U.S. Open until there was equal pay for the winner of the men's and women's tournaments.[57] A more recent example is the women athletes who comprise the WNBA. The players banded together to negotiate a collective bargaining agreement that gave them better pay, paid maternity leave, and improved travel conditions for away games.[58] The league has also been vocal in its support of the Black Lives Matter movement.

The Summer of 2020

The COVID-19 pandemic not only brought life to a virtual stand-still, it also highlighted inequalities in access to health care, particularly among ethnic minorities. The CDC reported that racial and ethnic minority groups were more at risk of getting sick and dying from COVID-19.[59] While COVID-19 drew attention to health inequality in the U.S., another issue was also bringing racial injustice to the forefront of the world's attention—the police killing of Black men and women in the U.S. George Floyd was murdered by police officer Derek Chauvin on May 25, 2020, in Minneapolis, Minnesota, (Chauvin was convicted of murder and manslaughter by a jury on April 20, 2021).[60] At the time of this death, Floyd was taken into custody for allegedly using a fake $20 bill at a local store. Bystanders, including 17-year-old Darnella Frazier, captured the altercation with her cell phone.[61] That footage showed Chauvin pinning Floyd to the ground with his knee on the back of his neck with Floyd repeatedly saying "I can't breathe."[62] During the trial, prosecutors said that Chauvin's knee was on Floyd's neck for nine minutes and 29 seconds.[63] The video of Floyd's death was posted to Facebook and quickly went viral. Thousands took the streets in Minneapolis to march in protest to the killing of George Floyd, and not long after, protesters took the streets in cities across the country.

George Floyd's death can, arguably, be considered the catalyst for the summer of 2020's racial unrest, but there was another killing of an unarmed Black person that also led to outrage. Two months earlier, Breonna Taylor, a 26-year-old EMT and aspiring nurse, was killed in her home while she slept as police were executing a no-knock warrant in Louisville, Kentucky.[64] Protesters chanted the refrain "say her name" in an effort to "remember black women who have not attracted the same attention as other cases."[65] The deaths of Floyd and Taylor were frequently cited in protests, but they were not the only Black people to be killed by police. CBS News reported that 164 Black men and women were killed by police between January 1 and August 31 in 2020.[66] In response to these killings, athletes from the NBA, WNBA, MLB, NFL, English Premier League, Formula One racing, PGA, and U.S. Open Tennis all continued the tradition of using their position and platform to speak out against racial injustice.[67] This exemplifies the point, when we teach sports, when we study sports, we are studying larger issues that affect our lives. The following section analyzes the ways in which, during a pandemic, athletes from across sports used their platform to speak out about racial injustice and police killing Black people in America.

Playing Sports during a Pandemic and a Time of Protest

As we know, sports did, in fact, come back after the COVID-19 hiatus. But, two leagues, the NBA and WNBA, did so under the condition that they would use their time in the bubble to continue efforts to raise awareness for racial justice and the Black Lives Matter movement.[68] The NBA Players Association and league officials announced goals such as "increasing Black representation in NBA front offices, greater inclusion of Black-owned and operated businesses, and a foundation to augment educational and economic development in the wider Black community."[69] In addition, the NBA and WNBA courts included Black Lives Matter signage and teams would often lock arms and kneel during the national anthem before games. Other leagues including the MLB, NHL, and MLS also used fundraising and social media campaigns to promote messages of unity.[70]

Athletes responded individually to the death of George Floyd. Michael Jordan, who has long been criticized for not taking a more active role in advancing racial equality, released a statement via Twitter. Lebron James took a more direct approach tweeting "Why Doesn't America Love US!!!!!????TOO [sic]."[71] Colin Kaepernick tweeted that he would provide legal assistance for protesters in Minneapolis.[72] Individually, athletes across sports and all over the world took to the streets to protest for racial equality and an end to police brutality. However, as the summer went on, another police shooting of a Black man would spur yet another round of protests.

Jacob Blake

One of the most recent and public displays of athletes using their position to speak out on civil rights occurred in August of 2020. On August 23, Jacob Blake was left paralyzed from the waist down after being shot by a white police officer seven times in Kenosha, Wisconsin.[73] Protesters once again took the streets demanding justice for Jacob Blake.

Meanwhile, in Orlando, Florida, the NBA's Milwaukee Bucks were preparing for Game 5 of their playoff series against the Orlando Magic. Milwaukee is about 40 miles from Kenosha, where Blake's shooting occurred. After a long summer of protests against police brutality, and the stress of a global pandemic, the players decided they had enough. The Bucks took a vote and decided to boycott Game 5, citing "people were discussing basketball, not discussing the issues that really mattered. They wanted to take action, not make another gesture."[74] The remaining NBA playoff teams followed suit and boycotted their playoff games, marking the first time that there was a walkout in professional sports.[75] Other NBA players took to social media to demand justice, change, and to show their support for the boycotts.[76] The WNBA and NHL followed suit by cancelling its games. The MLB cancelled some of its scheduled games while nine NFL teams called off preseason practices.[77] The NBA Players Association, the governors (what the league calls owners), and league officials met to discuss whether or not they would continue the season in the bubble. Ultimately, they decided to resume the season.

Several people spoke out in support of these demonstration efforts. John Carlos, who as previously discussed, raised his fist at the medal podium in protest at the 1968 Olympics told *TIME* magazine: "I respect the hell out of them for it. . . . Because you have to squeeze the toothpaste tube to get people to respond. And boycotting lets the powers that be, whether it's the NBA or any professional organization or corporate entity, know that they need to raise their voices. They need to get serious about the situation."[78] Similarly, sociologist Harry Edwards, who organized the Olympic Project for Human Rights, had this to say about the NBA game boycott:

> This is not a boycott against basketball any more than Kaepernick was taking a knee against the flag. . . . I just told a group of NBA players that. You're not involved in a boycott against basketball. You're involved in utilizing and leveraging the spotlight, the platform you have to make it crystal clear, not just to make a statement of protest but to send a message demanding change concerning these shootings. And what you're essentially screaming is, "Stop killing us."[79]

Former President Barack Obama took to Twitter to show his support for the players: "I commend the players on the @Bucks for standing up for what they believe in, coaches like @DocRivers, and the @NBA and @WNBA for setting an example. It's going to take all our institutions to stand up for our values."[80]

As one would expect, the sports boycott drew criticism in addition to praise. Then President Donald Trump and other unnamed White House officials criticized the athletes who refused to play in response to the Blake shooting.[81] Trump said, the NBA has become "like a political organization—and that's not a good thing I don't think that is a good thing for sports or for the country."[82] And in the same news story, presidential adviser Jared Kushner said, "I think the NBA players are very fortunate that they have the financial position where they're able to take a night off from work without having to have the consequences for themselves financially."[83]

Nearly a year later and the question still remains whether or not the stand that athletes across leagues took was effective. This largely depends on what each individual defines as effective and can take the form of whether or not there have been policy changes instituted or if the officers who shot Black men and women were brought to justice or if these actions brought about increased awareness of these issues for the general public. *New York Times* columnist Kurt Streeter put it his way:

> No longer was sports offering a gentrified protest, with league-endorsed slogans on basketball jerseys. Calm collapsed in the face of the inevitably growing power of players to make more than a statement. They took action. It shattered the bubble of normalcy that had settled upon the N.B.A. and its fans, who watched happily at home as a pandemic and protests raged.[84]

Regardless of whether these actions are ever deemed effective, these athletes who used their voice and platform to speak out against injustice are now part of the history of sports. The teams that chose not to play in support of a bigger cause will be discussed for years to come alongside names like Muhammed Ali, Billie Jean King, Kareem Abdul-Jabbar, Tommie Smith, John Carlos, and countless others who, through sport, did what they could to enact change.

IMPLICATIONS OF THE COVID-19 PANDEMIC FOR SCHOLARSHIP AND PEDAGOGY IN SPORT COMMUNICATION

The nature of the communication discipline means that those of us who teach and study it must consider, react, and respond to major events that impact the daily lives of people. Political communication scholars must consider the ever-evolving landscape of political campaigns. Public relations researchers analyze corporate crises in an effort to develop effective strategies to mitigate the negative effects of the crisis. Health communication scholars work to develop effective health campaigns. In the same way, sports communication scholars must attend to major changes and developments in sports.

COVID-19 and Sports Research

It will take several years for researchers to fully investigate the implications of the COVID-19 pandemic. Some scholars have taken up the mantle and contributed scholarship to special issues of journals across disciplines that begin to unpack the consequences of a global pandemic. For example, at the time of this writing the *International Journal of Sport Communication* published a special issue on Sport and the Coronavirus Crisis in September 2020 that includes commentaries and interviews with industry professionals spanning a number of areas related to sports including (but not limited to) implications of the pandemic on sports broadcasting,[85] effectiveness of sport organizational messaging during the pandemic,[86] and athletes and sports organization's response.[87]

Researchers studied and provided commentary on the intersection of social media and sports during the pandemic. Feder looked at the implications of the COVID-19 pandemic on the fan-athlete relationship through an examination of athletes' social media use. Feder makes the argument that during the lockdown, athletes enhanced the parasocial relationship they have with fans through publishing social media content that was focused more on their personal rather than professional lives and responding to questions from fans via Instagram Live.[88] Similarly, Yiran Su, Bradley J. Baker, Jason P. Doyle, and Meimi Yan[89] commented on athletes' use of TikTok during the pandemic and suggested that the platform can be used to "foster existing fan relationships, promote branded content, and appeal to new fan segments." Stirling Sharpe, Charles Mountifield, and Kevin Filo observed that social media was used by athletes and sport organizations to promote social and civic responsibility, fundraising, participating in physical activity challenges, and to communicate about financial contributions to the pandemic.[90]

Still others observed the implications of the pandemic for sport prominent communication industries. For example, Alexander L. Curry and Tiara Good considered what baseball reporters and fans talked about when the MLB spring training and season was postponed due to the pandemic.[91] Through a textual analysis of baseball-related ESPN headlines comparing 2019 to 2020, they found that reporters shifted focus away from the general coverage of business-oriented baseball stories (e.g., player transactions, injuries, prospects, etc.) to stories that focused more on how players are staying in shape during the hiatus and using the time away from baseball for surgeries and rehabilitations. This study shows how, while grappling with an unexpected crisis in real-time, reporters in baseball tried to maintain some of the norms of reporting baseball.

Scholars also used this issue as an opportunity to look back at some of the lessons learned from the early stages of the pandemic. Scholars have explored the impact of the pandemic on sport PR and concluded that the pandemic provided opportunities to grow the fan-athlete relationship in more meaningful ways. For example, Christie M. Kleinmann interviewed a sport PR professional who said that the lack of traditional sports moments (e.g., live sporting events) meant that practitioners and social media managers had to get creative and provide "connective content that went deeper than a sports moment" that included content that communicated "the shared experience and subsequent self-disclosure of athletes and fans, by the shedding of athletes' public persona, and by athletes and sports personnel sharing their private spaces of home and family."[92] The article concludes a challenge to readers to resume normal sports PR practices or to incorporate the lessons of the pandemic, specifically encouraging authentic connections, into the future of the practice.

This section provided an overview of the earliest perspectives on the COVID-19 pandemic and sports communication research. Most of the existing work involves commentary and essays reflecting on the pandemic in real-time. As more people get vaccinated and we start transitioning out of the pandemic and back into normal life (for lack of a better term), it is prudent for scholars to revisit the events and issues raised in these articles. Scholarship reflecting high levels of methodological rigor, critical analysis, and theory is necessary for us to start to unpack the totality of the ramifications of the COVID-19 pandemic.

COVID-19 and Teaching Sports

It was around mid-March of 2020 when teachers around the world learned that they would most likely have to convert their classes to online, distance learning. Almost like dominoes, announcements came from universities telling students to return to their homes and for instructors to learn Zoom. As anyone with experience teaching online will tell you, there are some classes that are going to be easier to teach online than others. Theory and lecture-based classes, with a little imagination, can transfer to an online setting fairly well. Applied, skills-based classes, particularly those that involve a lab, are slightly more difficult.

Generally speaking, sports classes tend to rely more on the applied, skill-based side of things. Sports courses that are more oriented to journalism and broadcast operate best in a lab setting with close contact between instructors and students. Into the fall semester of 2020, some universities offered hybrid or in-person classes that followed strict health and safety protocols. While adhering to such protocols allowed for the in-person experience, it also presented a new set of challenges. In a studio or lab setting, there was the issue of space and how many people would be allowed in the space at a time. Instructors would have to come up with plans including face masks, plexiglass, and hand sanitizer. Student learning about sports broadcasting had to wear a face mask while on camera, which made grading on-air presence a difficult endeavor.

Another difficulty in teaching sports during the pandemic was the lack of sports in general. Students in sports broadcasting courses would, in the past, have access to games or stadiums to get invaluable real-time experience. This year, they would not be allowed in a booth to call games and were not able to conduct one-on-one interviews. Instead, they did like the professionals had to do and that was pivot. If they were unable to sit in the booth to call a game, then they would call it from a monitor, much like professional sports broadcasters were doing. Similarly, interviews were conducted via Zoom and in 2020 everyone did everything on Zoom.

None of these scenarios represent ideal learning environments (I would argue not even for the courses that transitioned to online more easily), but it was reflective of the moment. It is not overstating it to say that the COVID-19 pandemic caused everyone in all industries to make the best with what they had. Bill Roth, Professor of Practice in the Sports Media and Analytics program at Virginia Tech, taught in-person sports broadcasting courses in the fall semester. He described his experience as generally being one of trial and error, saying "we learned and adjusted as the semester progressed."[93] And that, in and of itself, is a valuable lesson for students to take with them in their future careers. No matter what field you are working in, being resourceful, innovative, and able to adapt are essential life skills that hopefully students and instructors alike will take away from this pandemic experience.

NOTES

1. ESPN 30 for 30, *March 11, 2020*, podcast audio, December 21, 2020. https://www.espn.com/radio/play/_/id/30571269
2. Paul M. Pedersen, Kimberly S. Miloch, and Pamela C. Laucella. *Strategic Sport Communication.* (Champaign, IL: Human Kinetics, 2007).
3. Pedersen, Miloch, and Laucella, *Strategic Sport Communication*, 195
4. Pedersen, Miloch, and Laucella, *Strategic Sport Communication*, 205
5. Robert L. Krizek, "Sport and Ethnography: An Embodied Practice Meets and Embodied Method," in *Defining Sport Communication,* ed. Andrew C. Billings (New York: Routledge, 2017), 4.
6. TEDxTalks. "Using Sports for Social Change | Andrew Billings | TEDxBirminghamSalon." YouTube. October 09, 2014. https://www.youtube.com/watch?v=xfjZ-tWFxpA.
7. Brody J. Ruihley and Bo Li. "Sport and the Coronavirus Crisis Special Issue: An Introduction," *International Journal of Sport Communication* 13, no. 3 (2020): 289, https://doi.org/10.1123/ijsc.2020-0254
8. Derek Bryson Taylor, "A Timeline of the Coronavirus Pandemic," *New York Times,* March 17, 2021, https://www.nytimes.com/article/coronavirus-timeline.html.
9. Taylor, "Timeline."
10. Ruihley and Li, "Sports and Coronavirus," 289–290.
11. Ruihley and Li, "Sports and Coronavirus," 289–290.
12. Source material for the timeline: Ben Axelrod, "It's Been One Year Since COVID-19 Shutdown Sports: A Timeline of the Past Year," *WKYC Studios,* March 11, 2021, https://www.wkyc.com/article/sports/coronavirus-sports-year-timeline/95-ff73b8df-03dd-4a7c-8212-e8b8482b81ab; ESPN News Services, "NBA Suspends Season Until Further Notice After Player Tests Positive for Coronavirus," *ESPN,* March 11, 2020, https://www.espn.com/nba/story/_/id/28887560/nba-suspends-season-further-notice-player-tests-positive-coronavirus; Ahiza García-Hodges, Yuliya Talmazan, and Arato Yamamoto. "Tokyo 2020 Olympics Postponed Over Coronavirus Concerns," *NBC News,* March 24, 2020, https://www.nbcnews.com/news/world/tokyo-2020-olympics-postponed-over-coronavirus-concerns-n1165046; Avery Yang, "Timeline: How Coronavirus Is Upending the Sports World," *Sports Illustrated,* March 12, 2020. https://www.si.com/sports-illustrated/2020/03/12/coronavirus-timeline-sports; Joseph Zucker, "Timeline of Coronavirus' Impact on Sports," Accessed June 1, 2021. https://bleacherreport.com/articles/2880569-timeline-of-coronavirus-impact-on-sports.
13. "COVID-19 Frequently Asked Questions," U.S. Food and Drug Administration, last modified May 27, 2021, https://www.fda.gov/emergency-preparedness-and-response/coronavirus-disease-2019-covid-19/covid-19-frequently-asked-questions.

14. Jacqueline Howard, "All 50 States Now Have Expanded or Will Expand Covid Vaccine Eligibility to Everyone 16 and Up," *CNN Health,* April 5, 2021, https://www.cnn.com/2021/03/30/health/states-covid-19-vaccine-eligibility-bn/index.html.

15. "Where NBA Teams Stand on In-Arena Attendance." NBA News, May 28, 2021, https://www.nba.com/news/where-nba-teams-stand-on-in-arena-attendance.

16. Matt Traub, "How Many Fans Will Be Allowed at Major League Baseball Games This Season?" *Sports Travel*, July 5, 2021, https://www.sportstravelmagazine.com/how-many-fans-will-be-allowed-at-major-league-baseball-games-this-season-capacity/.

17. Pedersen, Miloch, and Laucella, "Strategic Sport Communication."

18. "Comeback Season: Sports After 9/11," 9/11 Memorial Museum, Accessed June 1, 2021, https://www.911memorial.org/visit/museum/exhibitions/past-exhibitions/comeback-season-sports-after-911.

19. Sam Carp, "You Can't Watch Everything at Once: Why U.S. Sports TV Ratings have been Down during the Pandemic," *SportsPro,* December 11, 2020, https://www.sportspromedia.com/analysis/us-sports-tv-ratings-decline-nfl-nba-finals-world-series-nhl-covid-19

20. Alex Reimer, "Why Sports TV Ratings Will Likely Still Suffer in 2021," *Forbes,* December 16, 2020, https://www.forbes.com/sites/alexreimer/2020/12/16/why-sports-tv-ratings-will-likely-still-suffer-in-2021/?sh=2445acad2acf.

21. Jimmy Traina "Sports Ratings have Tanked Across the Board While Cable News Thrives: TRAINA THOUGHTS," *Sports Illustrated,* October 14, 2020, https://www.si.com/extra-mustard/2020/10/14/sports-cable-news-ratings-2020.

22. "Marist Center for Sports Communication/Marist Poll Results & Analysis," Marist Poll, October 14, 2020, http://maristpoll.marist.edu/marist-center-for-sports-communication-marist-poll-results-analysis/#sthash.2BDlQWPw.EeFulQwZ.dpbs.

23. Marist Poll, "Poll Results," para 4.

24. Ben Strauss, "So Many Sports, So Few Viewers: Why TV Ratings are Way Down During the Pandemic," *The Washington Post*, October 16, 2020, https://www.washingtonpost.com/sports/2020/10/16/sports-ratings-down-pandemic-politics/.

25. Strauss, "So Many Sports."

26. Sara Berg, "As Pandemic Enters Year 2, Mental Health Burden Becomes Clearer," *AMA,* April 16, 2021, https://www.ama-assn.org/delivering-care/public-health/pandemic-enters-year-2-mental-health-burden-becomes-clearer.

27. Alvin Powell, "Pandemic Pushes Mental Health to the Breaking Point," *The Harvard Gazette,* January 27, 2021, https://news.harvard.edu/gazette/story/2021/01/pandemic-pushing-people-to-the-breaking-point-say-experts/.

28. "World No. 2 Naomi Osaka Withdraws from Wimbledon to Take 'Personal Time with Friends and Family,'" ESPN, June 17, 2021, https://www.espn.com/tennis/story/_/id/31653392/world-no-2-naomi-osaka-withdraws-wimbledon-take-personal-friends-family.

29. "Mental Health and Athletes," Athletes for Hope, Accessed June 18, 2021, https://www.athletesforhope.org/2019/05/mental-health-and-athletes/.

30. Greg Johnson, "Pandemic Continues to Impact Student-Athlete Mental Health," *NCAA,* February 16, 2021, https://www.ncaa.org/about/resources/media-center/news/pandemic-continues-impact-student-athlete-mental-health.

31. Johnson, "Pandemic Continues."

32. Kelcie Pegher, "Coronavirus Today: The NBA Bubble Worked," *Los Angeles Times*, October 12, 2020, https://www.latimes.com/science/newsletter/2020-10-12/coronavirus-today-nba-bubble-success-covid-lakers-coronavirus-today.

33. Mark Medina, "Challenges of Isolated Life in the Bubble and to NBA Players' Playoff Stress: 'I Just Checked Out,'" *USA Today*, last updated September 7, 2020, https://www.usatoday.com/story/sports/nba/2020/09/07/nba-players-grapple-with-mental-health-inside-nba-bubble/5742849002/, para 4.

34. Baxter Holmes, "Navigating the Mental Aspects of Life in the NBA Bubble," *ESPN*, July 17, 2020, https://www.espn.com/nba/story/_/id/29478260/navigating-mental-aspects-life-nba-bubble.

35. Joshua Holder, "Tracking Coronavirus Vaccinations Around the World," *The New York Times*, last updated June 19, 2021, https://www.nytimes.com/interactive/2021/world/covid-vaccinations-tracker.html.

36. Our World in Data, "Coronavirus (COVID-19) Vaccinations," *Statistics and Research*, Accessed June 19, 2021, https://ourworldindata.org/covid-vaccinations.

37. "How Much of the Population Will Need to Be Vaccinated Until the Pandemic is Over?," Cleveland Clinic, May 5, 2021, https://health.clevelandclinic.org/how-much-of-the-population-will-need-to-be-vaccinated-until-the-pandemic-is-over/.

38. Eric Berger, "What it Means When Sports Stars Stay Coy About their COVID-19 Vaccine Status," *USA Today*, June 16, 2021, https://www.usatoday.com/story/sports/2021/06/16/sports-athletes-covid-19-vaccinations/7716013002/.

39. Berger, "Sports Stars," para 6.

40. Berger, "Sports Stars."

41. Mark Medina, "Bill Russell on Receiving COVID-19 Vaccine: 'This is One Shot I Won't Block,'" *USA Today*, February 4, 2021, https://www.usatoday.com/story/sports/nba/2021/02/04/bill-russell-receives-covid-19-vaccine-part-nba-promotion/4384813001/.

42. Berkeley Lovelace Jr., "Biden Administration to Use Celebrities, Athletes in Campaign to Combat Covid Vaccine Hesitancy," *CNBC*, April 22, 2021, https://www.cnbc.com/2021/04/22/white-house-to-use-celebrities-athletes-in-ad-campaign-to-combat-covid-vaccine-hesitancy.html.

43. The Ad Council. "Willie Nelson, Thirteen Major Sports Leagues and Organizations Team Up with the Ad Council and COVID Collaborative's National 'It's Up to You' COVID-19 Vaccine Education Initiative." *Cision PR Newswire*, March 23, 2021, https://www.prnewswire.com/news-releases/willie-nelson-thirteen-major-sports-leagues-and-organizations-team-up-with-the-ad-council-and-covid-collaboratives-national-its-up-to-you-covid-19-vaccine-education-initiative-301253252.html.

44. Justin Tinsley, "Twenty-Five Years Ago Today, Magic Johnson Announced He Had HIV," *The Undefeated*, November 7, 2016, https://theundefeated.com/features/twenty-five-years-ago-today-magic-johnson-announced-he-had-hiv-los-angeles-lakers/.

45. Tinsley, "Magic Johnson."

46. Sarah Moughty, "20 Years After HIV Announcement, Magic Johnson Emphasizes: 'I Am Not Cured,'" *PBS Frontline*, November 7, 2011, https://www.pbs.org/

wgbh/frontline/article/20-years-after-hiv-announcement-magic-johnson-emphasizes-i-am-not-cured/.

47. Tinsley, "Magic Johnson," para 6.

48. Moughty, "20 Years After HIV Announcement."

49. Mark Medina, "Magic Johnson compares HIV and Coronavirus Pandemic Misconceptions and Impact on Black Community," *USA Today*, April 10, 2020, https://www.usatoday.com/story/sports/nba/2020/04/10/magic-johnson-compares-coronavirus-hiv-aids-misconceptions-black-impact/5128687002/.

50. Medina, "Magic Johnson Compares," para 6.

51. Mark Heisler, "From the Archives: Magic Johnson's Career Ended by HIV-Positive Test. Lakers Star Says: 'I Plan to go on Living for a Long Time,'" *Los Angeles Times*, November 7, 2016, https://www.latimes.com/sports/lakers/la-sp-magic-johnson-hiv-test-archives-20161107-story.html.

52. Bill Oram, "Magic Johnson's HIV Announcement was a Game-Changing Moment for Society," *Los Angeles Daily News*, last updated August 28, 2017 https://www.dailynews.com/2016/11/06/magic-johnsons-hiv-announcement-was-a-game-changing-moment-for-society/.

53. Shannon Ryan, "Timeline: A Look Back at Some of the Most Prominent Sports Protests Over the Years," *Chicago Tribune*, September 9, 2020, https://www.chicagotribune.com/sports/ct-athlete-protests-timeline-liststory-20200909-yl4x7b3hk5gkxj5wdxqwdmxfrq-list.html.

54. Ryan, "Prominent Sports Protests."

55. Steve Keating, "Athletes Bring Fight for Equality into Sporting Arena in 2020," *Reuters,* December 14, 2020, https://www.reuters.com/article/sport-yearender-protests-race/athletes-bring-fight-for-equality-into-sporting-arena-in-2020-idUSKBN28P06E.

56. Jason Reid, "How Colin Kaepernick Became a Cause for Activists, Civil Rights Groups and Others," *The Undefeated,* August 22, 2017, https://theundefeated.com/features/how-colin-kaepernick-became-a-cause-for-activists-civil-rights-groups/, para 1.

57. Ryan, "Prominent Sports Protests."

58. Brittney Oliver, "The Women of the WNBA are Leading the Way for Activism in Sports—and Have Been for Years," *Glamour,* September 3, 2020, https://www.glamour.com/story/the-women-of-the-wnba-are-leading-the-way-for-activism-in-sports-and-have-been-for-years.

59. "Health Equity Considerations and Racial and Ethnic Minority Groups." Centers for Disease Control and Prevention. Last modified April 19, 2021. https://www.cdc.gov/coronavirus/2019-ncov/community/health-equity/race-ethnicity.html.

60. Luis Andres Henao, Nomaan Merchant, Juan Lozano, and Adam Geller. "For George Floyd, a Complicated Life and Consequential Death," *AP News*, April 20, 2021, https://apnews.com/article/george-floyd-profile-66163bbd94239afa16d706bd6479c613.

61. Li Cohen. "Teen who Recorded George Floyd's Death Speaks Out: 'It made me realize how dangerous it is to be Black in America,'" *CBS News*, May 26, 2021, https://www.cbsnews.com/news/darnella-frazier-george-floyd-black-america/.

62. Meredith Deliso, "Timeline: The impact of George Floyd's Death in Minneapolis and Beyond," *ABC News,* April 21, 2021, https://abcnews.go.com/US/timeline-impact-george-floyds-death-minneapolis/story?id=70999322.

63. Amy Forliti, Steve Karnowski, and Tammy Webber. "Police Chief: Kneeling on Floyd's Neck Violated Policy," *AP News*, April 5, 2021, https://apnews.com/article/derek-chauvin-trial-live-updates-c3e3fe08773cd2f012654e782e326f6e.

64. Bridget Read, "What We Know About the Killing of Breonna Taylor," *The Cut*, last modified September 29, 2020, https://www.thecut.com/2020/09/breonna-taylor-louisville-shooting-police-what-we-know.html.

65. "Breonna Taylor: Protesters Call on People to 'Say Her Name,'" *BBC News U.S. and Canada*, June 7, 2020, https://www.bbc.com/news/world-us-canada-52956167, para 3.

66. Li Cohen, "Police in the U.S. Killed 164 Black People in the First 8 Months of 2020. These are Their Names. (Part 1: January-April)," *CBS News*, September 10, 2020, https://www.cbsnews.com/pictures/black-people-killed-by-police-in-the-u-s-in-2020/.

67. Keating, "Athletes Bring Fight."

68. Sean Gregory, "Why Jacob Blake's Shooting Sparked an Unprecedented Sports Boycott," *Time*, last modified August 27, 2020, https://time.com/5883892/boycott-nba-mlb-wnba-jacob-blake/.

69. Dain TePoel and John Nauright. "Black Lives Matter in the Sports World," *Sport in Society*, 24 no. 5 (2021): 693–696. https://doi.org/10.1080/17430437.2021.1901392., para 3.

70. TePoel and Nauright, "Black Lives Matter."

71. "Athletes React to the Death of George Floyd Ongoing Civil Unrest in Minneapolis and Other Cities," NBC Sports, May 31, 2020, https://www.nbcsports.com/washington/wizards/athletes-react-death-george-floyd-ongoing-civil-unrest-minneapolis-other-cities., para 4.

72. Jim Reineking, "Sports Figures React on Social Media to the Death of George Floyd in Minneapolis," *USA Today Sports*, last modified May 29, 2020, https://www.usatoday.com/story/sports/2020/05/29/george-floyd-sports-figures-react-situation-minneapolis/5288501002/.

73. Joe Barrett, "Jacob Blake Shooting: What We Know about the Shooting in Kenosha," *The Wall Street Journal*, January 6, 2021, https://www.wsj.com/articles/jacob-blake-shooting-11598368824.

74. Kurt Helin, "Milwaukee Bucks Boycott Game 5 of Playoff Series in Protest of Jacob Blake Shooting," *NBC Sports*, August 26, 2020, https://nba.nbcsports.com/2020/08/26/milwaukee-bucks-boycott-game-5-of-playoff-series-in-protest-of-jacob-blake-shooting/, para 1.

75. Kurt Streeter, "With Walkouts, a New High Bar for Protests in Sports is Set," *The New York Times,* August 27, 2020, https://www.nytimes.com/2020/08/27/sports/basketball/kenosha-nba-protests-players-boycott.html.

76. Helin, "Milwaukee Bucks."

77. Adam Kilgore and Ben Golliver. "Most Sports Leagues Pause with Second Day of Protests, Some more Unified than Others," *The Washington Post*, August 27, 2020, https://www.washingtonpost.com/sports/2020/08/27/sports-protests/.

78. Gregory, "Why Jacob Blake," para 5.

79. Kilgore and Golliver, "Most Sports Leagues Pause," para 6.

80. Ryan Young, "LeBron James, NBA World React after Bucks Walkout Over Jacob Blake Shooting," *Yahoo! Sports*, August 26, 2020, https://www.yahoo.com/lifestyle/lebron-james-nba-world-react-twitter-milwaukee-bucks-boycott-playoff-game-jacob-blake-shooting-kenosha-210416874.html, para 6.

81. Libby Cathey, "Trump White House Officials Criticize NBA Players Amid Jacob Blake Protests," *ABC News*, August 27, 2020, https://abcnews.go.com/Politics/trump-white-house-officials-criticize-nba-players-amid/story?id=72651348.

82. Cathey, "Trump White House," para 2.

83. Cathey, "Trump White House," para 4.

84. Streeter, "With Walkouts," para 7.

85. Roxanne Coche and Benjamin J. Lynn, "Behind the Scenes: COVID-19 Consequences on Broadcast Sports Production," *International Journal of Sport Communication* 13, no. 3 (2020): 484–493. https://doi.org/10.101123/ijsc.2020-0231. Michael M. Goldman and David P. Hedlund, "Rebooting Content: Broadcasting Sport and eSports to Homes During COVID-19," *International Journal of Sport Communication* 13, no. 3 (2020): 370–380. https://doi.org/10.1123/ijsc.2020-0227.

86. Timothy Mirabito, Robin Hardin, and Joshua R. Pate, "The Fractured Messaging of the National Collegiate Athletic Association and Its Members in Response to COVID-19," *International Journal of Sport Communication* 13, no. 3 (2020): 324–334. https://doi.org/10.1123/ijsc.2020-0249.

87. Stirling Sharpe, Charles Mountifield, and Kevin Filo, "The Social Media Response from Athletes and Sport Organizations to COVID-19: An Altruistic Tone," *International Journal of Sport Communication* 13, no. 3 (2020): 474–483. https://doi.org/10.1123/ijsc.2020-0220.

88. Lillian Feder, "From ESPN to Instagram LIVE: The Evolution of Fan-Athlete Interaction Amid the Coronavirus," *International Journal of Sport Communication* 13, no. 3 (2020): 458–464. https://doi.org/10.1123/ijsc.2020-0233.

89. Yiran Su, Bradley J. Baker, Jason P. Doyle and Meimi Yan, "Fan Engagement in 15 Seconds: Athletes' Relationship Marketing During a Pandemic on TikTok," *International Journal of Sport Communication* 13, no. 3 (2020): 436–446. https://doi.org/10.1123/ijsc.2020-0238, 436.

90. Sharpe, Mountifield, and Filo, "Social Media Response."

91. Alexander L. Curry and Tiara Good, "Talking Baseball When There is No Baseball: Reporters and Fans During the COVID-19 Pandemic," *International Journal of Sport Communication* 13, no. 3 (2020): 551–558. https://doi.org/10.1123/ijsc.2020-0246.

92. Christie M. Kleinmann, "Do We Really Want Sports Public Relations to Return to Normal?," *International Journal of Sport Communication* 13, no. 3 (2020): 586–592. https://doi.org/10.1123/ijsc.2020-0232, 589.

93. Bill Roth, Email message to Author, June 17, 2021.

Chapter 6

Public Address in a Time of Crisis

Robert C. Rowland, Justin W. Kirk, and Michael Eisenstadt

In *Federalist 10*, widely seen as one of the most important essays about American democracy, James Madison first described a number of threats to the emerging American democracy and then argued that the organizing principle that would make the new American republic function was what he called "a republican remedy for the diseases most incident to republican government."[1] That remedy was the give and take of public discourse that would both ensure that the views of all citizens were represented and that ultimately a sensible solution to the problem of the moment could be crafted. Madison was not naïve about the quality of public deliberation. In *Federalist 10* he focused on the threat posed by factions, what we now would label partisanship, to democratic decision-making, while in *Federalist 37*, he observed somewhat dryly "that public measures are rarely investigated with that spirit of moderation which is essential to a just estimate or their tendency to advance or obstruct the public good." While he was clear-eyed about threats to democracy, recognizing problems such as fear mongering and blame shifting that have plagued the American republic ever since, he still believed that free and open debate could facilitate reasonable representative governance. His faith came from a belief that public reason enacted in the give and take of debate in Congress and in public discourse would provide a check on dangerous action and lead to wise policy choice. Ultimately, Madison's "republican remedy" was based in his belief that over time the better argument would win out since as he noted in *Federalist 41*, "A bad cause seldom fails to betray itself."[2]

It is through the study of public address that scholars have tested whether Madison's faith in democratic deliberation and debate was warranted. Public address scholars have focused on all aspects of rhetorical practice in the public sphere, analyzing, for instance, presidential, legislative, and judicial rhetoric, but also the rhetoric of campaigns, social movements, and other contexts in which people use rhetoric to influence policy or culture. Scholars also have studied genres of public communication, as well as various styles, ideologies, cultural practices, ceremonial rhetoric aimed at producing the value consensus necessary to undergird reasonable public deliberation, and other dimensions of public deliberation.[3] The scope of public address scholarship is quite broad, including all those places where individuals or groups use rhetoric for some social purpose. Similarly, public address scholars have used any number of theoretical approaches to illuminate, describe, or evaluate public rhetoric. Scholars have focused on the argumentative, narrative, value-laden, and aesthetic dimensions of public rhetoric, as well as applied a host of theories, from the dramatism of Kenneth Burke, to detailed argument analysis, to a focus on affect or style as crucial dimensions of public talk.[4] Thus, while some stereotype public address scholarship as a narrow contemporary version of neo-Aristotelian criticism, in fact, public address scholarship has enormous breadth, both in the topics covered and the theoretical approaches used. For example, one of the authors of this chapter has applied narrative theory, mythic analysis, argumentative analysis, allegorical criticism, ideological analysis, Burkean theory, theories of affect, genre theory, movement theory, and psychological approaches to authoritarianism in published works of public address.[5]

At the same time that public address scholarship has great breadth, it retains a core focus on the way that rhetoric is used by the public, representatives of the public, and others in the public sphere. In approaching this discourse, public address scholars have taken a much broader approach than have scholars in related fields, such as political science. In his seminal book, *The Rhetorical Presidency*, Jeffrey K. Tulis argued that, "Since the presidencies of Theodore Roosevelt and Woodrow Wilson, popular or mass rhetoric has become a principal tool of presidential governance."[6] Tulis's narrow conception of the "rhetorical presidency" as a modern development has proved immensely influential and countless scholars have focused on how presidents use the strategy of "going public" to influence public opinion.[7] In contrast, as David Zarefsky noted in his memorable essay responding to Tulis, public address scholars have recognized that "The Presidency Has Always Been a Place for Rhetorical Leadership."[8] George Washington, Abraham Lincoln, and other early presidents may not have used the same technologies to present their messages as did later presidents, but rhetorical processes were still central to their enactment of the presidency.[9] More broadly, public address scholars recognize that rhetoric is central to the business of the public in a democratic society. It is through the give and take of public (and sometimes private) talk that the business of the public is done. When Madison's "republican remedy" works effectively, all stakeholders are represented, and pragmatic decisions are made that reflect the will of the majority, but also protect the rights of all others. When, as occurs far too often, public deliberation breaks down or key stakeholders are denied the right to participate or subjected to outright discrimination, the result is failed public policy and sometimes even state sanctioned violence against groups deemed "Other" from "real" Americans.

To this point, we argue in this chapter that democratic governance at all levels, whether of a nation such as the United States, or of a business, religious, or social organization, is defined by the principle that citizen stakeholders talk first and then the public, often through their representatives in legislative bodies, decides. Public address scholars serve the crucial role of unpacking that public talk by identifying patterns in movements, genres, ideologies, or styles of discourse, explaining how it works or why it failed, and evaluating cases where the public sphere denied access to minority groups or other stakeholders, or failed to fulfill its problem-solving function. If rhetoric is the lifeblood of democratic societies of all kinds, public address scholars are the rhetorical hematologists who study how effectively rhetoric circulates in the body politic.

Nowhere is public address more important than in a time of crisis. The global pandemic that began at the very end of 2019 provides a powerful test of that rhetorical circulation in the world's oldest democracy, the United States. Over the course of 2020, the COVID-19 pandemic created a public health crisis that in turn led to an economic crisis and exposed a crisis in American policing in which Americans of color were disproportionately threatened by police violence, often ending in tragic deaths.[10] These three intertwined crises can be seen as aspects of a larger political crisis. As David Litt observed in *Time,* "what has cost the United States so many lives and jobs during the pandemic is not, at root, a failure of public health. It's a failure of democracy."[11] The core issue at the heart of the crisis was whether American democracy continued to work in a way that both allowed all stakeholders access to the public sphere and produced sensible policies addressing the three dimensions of the overarching political crisis.

A full treatment of the three dimensions of the political crisis would require multiple essays or books. However, in order to illustrate the centrality of public address scholarship to studies that assess the role of rhetoric in American democracy, we will set aside the economic concerns and conduct case studies of two key moments in the pandemic and the battle for racial justice—a briefing on the pandemic conducted by President Donald Trump and his COVID Taskforce on April 23, 2020, and the contrasting rhetoric of protesters and President Trump prior to and following the action of the police to clear Lafayette Square and Lafayette Park of protesters before a photo op by President Trump at St. John's Church. These two incidents can be considered snapshots, what Kenneth Burke called representative anecdotes, of public deliberation concerning the three intertwining crises that constituted the political crisis facing the nation in 2020.[12]

In discussing these "snapshots" of a nation confronting intertwining public health, economic, racial justice, and political crises, the remainder of this chapter sketches the importance of public address scholarship in explaining the crises and points to failures in public debate and deliberation that limited the capacity of the nation to address the crises. In describing the two snapshots of the crises facing the nation in 2020, we draw on a series of essays that have approached public policy controversies through the lens of what Robert Rowland has labelled the "liberal public sphere." By liberal Rowland does not mean contemporary liberal political ideology, but a broader sense of liberalism that undergirds both contemporary progressive and conservative movements, although not contemporary populist movements.[13] Rowland uses this term to distinguish his approach from the analysis of the public sphere by critical and cultural critics, whose treatment of the contestation between publics and counterpublics is focused on important issues related to inclusion/exclusion in public deliberation, but much less focused on the resolution of public policy disputes.[14] Rowland, whose treatment of the liberal public sphere is largely consistent with the broad approach to the public sphere taken by Jürgen Habermas, is, unlike Habermas, focused on contemporary public policy disputes, rather than the historical description of the evolution of the public sphere.[15] In what follows, we first develop a theoretical approach to unpacking rhetoric in the liberal public sphere, then present analyses of the two case studies, next comment on future research and the pedagogy of public sphere research, and finally draw conclusions.

A THEORETICAL ORIENTATION: THE "LIBERAL PUBLIC SPHERE"

The liberal public sphere is based in a broadly liberal theory rooted in the Enlightenment that undergirds democracy itself. Liberalism as a political theory, as opposed to contemporary progressive ideology, is broad enough to include both the modern progressive movement, including transformative figures from FDR to Barack Obama, as well as advocates of small government conservatism, most notably Ronald Reagan. A broadly liberal approach to the public sphere is appropriate since, as Orlando Patterson noted, "liberalism reigns supreme as the leading, and one might even say, overwhelming doctrine in the West . . . Its central ideas seem to inform nearly all political and economic discourse."[16] Liberalism as a wide-ranging political theory, as opposed to an ideological doctrine, embraces principles of democracy including the right to vote, protections for civil liberties, freedom of the press, and so forth. At its very core, "the republican remedy" that Madison referenced is fundamentally rhetorical. Ultimately, the representatives of the public in Congress and the Courts vote, but first they talk, they argue back and forth. Moreover, the representatives of the public are selected only after elections, which again are preceded by public talk. Thus, rhetoric is at the very center of the liberal public sphere. It functions as the currency of public deliberation and in another way as the undergirding superstructure that protects democracy itself. The words in the Constitution, the Federalist Papers, the Bill of Rights, the Declaration of Independence, speeches by Lincoln, King, both Roosevelts, Reagan, and Obama, served as more than just public persuasion of the time, but as enactments of basic values in the world's oldest democracy. The United States often has not lived up to those words, most notably with slavery and segregation, but as Dr. Martin Luther King, Jr. noted in the "I Have a Dream Speech," "the magnificent words of the Constitution and the Declaration of Independence" are "a promissory note to which every American was to fall heir. This note was a promise that all men, yes, black men as well as white men, would be guaranteed the 'unalienable Rights' of 'Life, Liberty and the pursuit of Happiness.'" King then restated a faith in the power of rhetoric to make the republican remedy function" "But we refuse to believe that the bank of justice is bankrupt. We refuse to believe that there are insufficient funds in the great vaults of opportunity of this nation. And so, we've come to cash this check, a check that will give us upon demand the riches of freedom and the security of justice."[17]

It is through rhetoric that the liberal public sphere can redeem the promissory note, providing justice to all. And it is also through rhetoric that the liberal public sphere can work through practical problems of the moment. Correspondingly, it is through the study of public address that we assess the success or failure of the liberal public sphere in cashing that promissory note and in solving problems facing the nation. Thus, it is appropriate to consider how the liberal public sphere responded to the practical problems of pandemic and economic decline, as well as the moral problem of racist violence.

It is also important to recognize that while all of the democracies of the West (including nations such as Japan and South Korea in East Asia) share a commitment to a broadly liberal political theory, even as those nations shift back and forth from progressive to conservative political ideologies, there is a great contrast between these democracies and autocracies and totalitarian societies. Dictators like Hitler and Stalin used rhetoric, but for purposes of maintaining their power, not democratic deliberation. The same point applies today to autocrats such as Vladimir Putin in Russia.

The question then is how to assess public address in the liberal public sphere. Fortunately, a means of doing so has been developed that judges the degree to which the important participants in the public sphere fulfil their responsibilities. Rowland argues that in a well-functioning liberal public sphere four key actors must each fulfill a central role in order for public debate to be both inclusive and lead to sensible decisions. Representatives of the public must present authentic arguments in support of whatever their view is on a policy dispute, as opposed to inauthentic political posturing. The media fulfill the role of informing the public about the policy dispute, by accurately reporting the arguments of each side and providing background information, such as summaries of the best available expert testimony on a topic. The role of the expert community is to inform the public directly and indirectly through the media about what the best evidence reveals concerning a given policy dispute. Finally, the key function fulfilled by the public is to pay enough attention to the ongoing policy dispute that they can in turn support elected officials, the representatives of the public, who they believe have the best solution to the problem. If all four actors fulfill their roles, the public will have enough information about an issue to choose between the competing proposals. Over time, the give and take of debate will result in sensible and inclusive policy action that effectively confronts the problem of the moment. On the other hand, if any actor fails to fulfill their responsibility there is grave risk that key groups of stakeholders may be denied participation in the public sphere or suffer discriminatory treatment and the policy problem/crisis will not be resolved. Unfortunately, both of these problems were evident in the two snapshots of the public sphere that we discuss next.

Before considering the snapshots, it is important to recognize that the liberal public sphere is a means of describing and evaluating how effectively the circulation of public address functioned in American democracy on any given issue. The approach is descriptive and evaluative, but its aim is not to reform public deliberation, although conclusions drawn from case studies could inform reform efforts. In this way, the liberal public sphere can be distinguished from some approaches to deliberative democracy, which attempt to change how the public deliberates, often by infusing expert briefings with citizen discussion meetings. One example of such effort is a proposal to mandate that a national "deliberation day" in which citizens discuss issues after receiving briefing papers occurs prior to elections.[18]

TRUMP'S QUACKERY: A BLEACH INJECTION FOR THE LIBERAL PUBLIC SPHERE

After COVID-19 emerged in the U.S. in early 2020, a number of shocks to the nation's institutions occurred. According to studies in several metropolitan cities, the prevalence of COVID-19 was grossly underreported due to a combination of a lack of testing capabilities and a surge in asymptomatic infections.[19] The infection rate and death toll skyrocketed, more than doubling in a 10-day period between April 13 and April 23, 2020.[20] In retrospect, there is strong evidence that the actual death total was vastly higher than the reported death total. Statistical models have found that excess mortality from the pandemic was approximately 50% higher than the reported death total.[21] The crisis led to an economic collapse in which more than 15% of the U.S. workforce filed for unemployment, with no clear plan to continue providing unemployment benefits to sectors of the economy that had completely shut down.[22] Hospitals in several regions were overrun, strapped for cash, and closing down at an accelerated rate.[23] Combined, these shocks posed a grave danger. Robert Redfield, Director of the Center for Disease Control and Prevention, noted that even if the virus could somehow be contained, the potential for a second outbreak would put "unimaginable strain" on the U.S. healthcare system and would be even more difficult to manage than the ongoing outbreak.[24] Among the underlying factors influencing the crisis was "a gap between how academic research operates and how the public understands that research," particularly the transmission of information from public health officials to citizens via the President of the U.S. and the media.[25]

The expert community's task of reporting scientific information to the public has proven difficult in the digital age. Since the expert community is "bound by an ethical obligation to speak precisely and to hew to the facts," experts are unlikely to make concrete public claims unless there has been sufficient evidence-based deliberation.[26] A reluctance to report information quickly can complicate the situation for experts, since the public has access to information, which often consists of rumors or outright falsehoods, traveling across social media platforms at blistering speeds. Public health officials are expected to "project their message above the noise," but, "disinformation comes and goes at high speeds."[27] Given the rapid evolution of the virus and information about it, health experts were required to report to a confused and often angry public. The public, "Unsettled by months of stay-at-home orders, confused by rampant misinformation, distraught over the country's blunders, and embroiled in yet more culture wars over masks and lockdowns," lashed out at health experts for either failing to handle the virus or providing inadequate information.[28]

In order to maintain credibility and rapport with the public, the expert community must have support from the elected representatives tasked with communicating scientific findings to the media and the public. This too proved to be a difficult task for public health officials in the U.S. Dr. Anthony Fauci, the leading public health expert on pandemics in the U.S., was perhaps the most frequent victim of public attacks over the nation's response to the virus. In early March 2020, Fauci told the public that they need not wear a mask, a statement he later retracted as the CDC updated its COVID-19 guidelines to encourage mask wearing. Rather than affirming the work of public health officials and demonstrating support for them, President Trump capitalized on public backlash to distance himself from the expert community. Not only did the Trump administration restrict public health officials' access to televised press briefings on coronavirus, but Trump went as far as retweeting "a call for Fauci to be fired for telling CNN that more could have been done to stop the spread of the virus" on April 12, 2020.[29]

Even with a lack of support from the Trump Administration and with the media driven by politics and ratings, public health officials were remarkably resilient in their efforts to report information on COVID-19. Fauci, for example, found "creative ways to get his message out. He embarked on an intensive schedule of public outreach, securing interviews with National Basketball Association star Stephen Curry on Instagram, Facebook chief executive officer Mark Zuckerberg via Facebook Live, and comedian Trevor Noah in a YouTube video that has been viewed nearly 12 million times."[30] Unfortunately, no matter how valiant these efforts were, public health messaging was at a significant disadvantage, competing with a President promoting conspiracies and a media with an insatiable appetite for such quackery. Moreover, members of the scientific community advising the White House felt they had to placate the president even though they recognized that he "did not actually make decisions about the virus based on reliable data."[31]

THE APRIL 23, 2020, COVID PRESS BRIEFING

On April 23rd, 2020, President Trump addressed the nation during a press briefing on COVID-19. In previous administrations, briefings about disease outbreaks primarily had been conducted by the Centers for Disease Control and other medical professionals.[32] However, President Trump used the briefings as a substitute for campaign rallies, transforming them into a platform for his political agenda and an opportunity to spread disinformation for political gain.[33] During the briefings, Trump occasionally shared scientific updates that accurately reflected the situation on the ground, but these remarks were overshadowed by false claims, exaggerations, and dangerous suggestions.

A key moment of the April 23 briefing occurred when Trump introduced Bill Bryan, the acting head of the Directorate of Science and Technology for the Department of Homeland Security to deliver an update on the COVID-19 virus. Although Bryan lacked a medical background, he was well known for holding "an influential perch with far-reaching authority over research, development and testing at the agency as well as for first responders across the country."[34] In addition to informing the public about the half-life of the COVID-19 virus in various temperatures, environments, and humidity levels, Bryan explained that DHS had been conducting experiments to test the efficacy of disinfectants as a method to kill the virus. Specifically, he said,

> We're also testing disinfectants readily available. We've tested bleach, we've tested isopropyl alcohol on the virus, specifically in saliva or in respiratory fluids. And I can tell you that bleach will kill the virus in five minutes; isopropyl alcohol will kill the virus in 30 seconds, and that's with no manipulation, no rubbing—just spraying it on and letting it go. You rub it and it goes away even faster. We're also looking at other disinfectants, specifically looking at the COVID-19 virus in saliva.[35]

Although Bryan was careful to add that, "This is not the end of our work as we continue to characterize this virus and integrate our findings into practical applications to mitigate exposure and transmission," the claim that disinfectants could eliminate the virus piqued President Trump's attention.[36]

At the conclusion of Bryan's report, President Trump made a series of comments, about which in most cases Bryan had no chance to reply. One reply dealt specifically with disinfectants. Trump said,

> I see the disinfectant, where it knocks it out in a minute. One minute. And is there a way we can do something like that, by injection inside or almost a cleaning. Because you see it gets in the lungs and it does a tremendous number on the lungs. So it would be interesting to check that. So, that, you're going to have to use medical doctors with. But it sounds—it sounds interesting to me.[37]

Though Bryan was unable to respond to Trump directly, a member of the press posed a question about disinfectants, asking, "the President mentioned the idea of cleaners, like bleach and isopropyl alcohol you mentioned. There's no scenario that that could be injected into a person, is there?"[38] Bryan, in a clear example of disciplined reason, replied, "No, I'm here to talk about the findings that we had in the study. We won't do that within that lab and our lab."[39] At this point, Trump interrupted Bryan to clarify, "It wouldn't be through injection. We're talking about through almost a cleaning, sterilization of an area. Maybe it works, maybe it doesn't work. But it certainly has a big effect if it's on a stationary object."[40] Trump's attempt to spin findings of scientific research on the virus had dangerous effects that would become quite evident in the days that followed the briefing.

THE MEDIA AND PUBLIC RESPONDS TO TRUMP'S BLEACH INJECTION

On the day following the April 23, 2020, COVID-19 press briefing, President Trump attempted to retract his statement about using disinfectants as a cure for the COVID-19 virus. When pressed by one journalist on the issue, Trump claimed, "I was asking the question sarcastically to reporters like you just to see what would happen."[41] His prior remarks suggest otherwise, however; as only a day earlier he added to the suggestion, "I'm not a doctor. But I'm, like, a person that has a good you-know-what," referring to his brain.[42] Moreover, when *Washington Post* reporter Phillip Rucker suggested "People tuning into these briefings—they want to get information and guidance and want to know what to do. They're not looking for rumors," Trump replied, "I'm the president and you're fake news."[43] Trump's quackery was an outright rejection of reason, lacking scientific basis. He made it "abundantly clear during Thursday's briefing that he has no qualms about making huge leaps of faith to sell some hope."[44]

It was not just mainstream media outlets that castigated Trump for his remarks. He was also widely criticized by leading conservative commentators. George Will, perhaps the most influential conservative commentator since the Reagan Administration, wrote of the briefing, "Trump, heretofore a mere snake-oil salesman, was suddenly peddling death to the credulous."[45] In fairness, there were those who defended his claims even after the floundering attempt to retract them. Cristina Cuomo, *CNN* anchor Chris Cuomo's spouse who contracted COVID-19, continued pedaling the idea that she recovered from the virus by treating herself with bleach. She claimed that bleach helped to "combat the radiation and metals in my system and oxygenate it" thus overcoming COVID-19.[46] White House Press Secretary Kayleigh McEnany released a statement accusing the mass media of taking Trump's remarks out of context. She said, "Leave it to the media to irresponsibly take President Trump out of context and run with negative headlines."[47]

Fact-checking websites largely supported the conclusion that Trump had presented dangerous medical advice. For example, Adam Edelman of NBC noted, "Trump did indeed speculate that an injection of the sort could have a curative effect."[48] Even the most supportive fact check of the president, PolitiFact, concluded that Trump "did express interest in exploring whether disinfectants could be applied to the site of a coronavirus infection inside the body, such as the lungs."[49] Of course, it was that expression of "interest" that led public health experts to issue warnings to the public, warnings that later proved prescient, when poison control hotlines reported a growing problem with poisonings. President Trump did everything he could to undercut the media, even attacking the "fake" news on five occasions in the April 23, 2020, briefing, although he did not point to a specific error in any instance.[50] President Trump previously had explained to Lesley Stahl why he attacked the media so often, "You know why I do it? I do it to discredit you all and demean you all so when you write negative stories about me, no one will believe you."[51] Overall, the media, what Trump often dismissively labeled "fake news," did their job in accurately reporting what occurred at the briefing. Of course, representatives of the public including the president have every right to correct errors by the press, but there is grave danger for the liberal public sphere when a representative of the public, especially the president, attacks and demeans the media for partisan reasons.

In stark contrast to the Trump Administration, the expert community and disinfectant manufacturers rushed to warn the public about the dangers of ingesting bleach and other chemicals. Lysol, for instance, released a statement, "As a global leader in health and hygiene products, we must be clear that under no circumstance should our disinfectant products be administered into the human body."[52] Disinfectant manufacturers were joined by "the CDC, EPA, and other state emergency management agencies," with statements "that disinfectants were in no shape or form to be used inside the human body."[53] A small group of Republicans in Congress expressed concern about Trump's comments. Indiana Senator Mike Braun, typically a staunch Trump supporter, said, "Sometimes when you're not clear with how you say things, especially when you are at a high level where people watch, it's best probably not to venture into areas that you may not know a lot about."[54] Given all the warnings from the expert community and others, one would expect the public to respond accordingly. Unfortunately, this was not the case.

Within a day of the press briefing where President Trump suggested that bleach could be used to cure the COVID-19 virus, there were an alarming number of poison control cases. The Maryland Emergency Management Agency reported "more than 100 calls to its hotline," leading it to publish a warning, "This is a reminder that under no circumstances should any disinfectant product be administered into the body through injection, ingestion or any other route."[55] Data from the New York City Poison Control Center revealed "exposure to specific household cleaners and disinfectants increased more than twofold after the President's comments."[56] Dr. Ngozi Ezike, Director of Public Health for the state of Illinois, reported "a significant increase in calls to poison control" in the days following Trump's comments.[57] Even with experts moving swiftly to "assure the US population that Trump's claims were completely unfounded," there were more than one hundred "hospitalizations across the country" related to poisoning from a disinfectant and "hundreds of calls from people asking about the curative properties of disinfecting products" made to various medical services.[58] Craig Spencer, Director of Global Health in Emergency Medicine at Columbia University, summarized the situation by claiming, "My concern is that people will die. People will think this is a good idea . . . This is not willy-nilly, off-the-cuff, maybe-this-will-work advice. This is dangerous."[59] The CDC later reported alarming survey results finding "that 4% of respondents consumed or gargled diluted bleach solutions, soapy water and other disinfectants in an effort to protect themselves from the coronavirus."[60]

The April 23, 2020, press briefing on COVID-19 offered a snapshot of the hard work that the expert community conducted to combat the coronavirus pandemic, hard work that was often significantly undercut, if not completely drowned out, by a president casting doubt on science, a media ecosystem obsessed with the president's quackery, and a public that lacked access to trustworthy sources of information. While members of the public could have sought information directly from the CDC website, such reliance on expert testimony was critiqued by a president who insisted on taking the lead in pandemic briefings, rather than leaving the science and medicine to the experts. Perhaps the most prestigious public science journal, *Nature*, decried Trump's taking center stage in public health briefings, arguing, "The Trump administration must stop sidelining the CDC."[61]

When President Trump offered dangerous suggestions such as using bleach to treat the COVID-19 virus, it carved out space for "Anti-vaccination groups and those opposing the current public health measures" to vigorously amplify their messages, "using the moment and the messaging to deepen mistrust of public health authorities, accusing them of moving the goalposts and implying that we're being conned."[62] At issue was not a lack of effort from the expert community, but rather, a clear lack of consistent messaging between the expert community, the media, and elected officials. Dr. Irwin Redlener of the National Center for Disaster Preparedness at Columbia University explained, "The inconsistency of the response is what's been so frustrating . . . If we had just been disciplined about employing all these public health methods early and aggressively, we would not be in the situation we are in now."[63] Most importantly, he added, Trump simply did not "understand how many people followed his advice."[64] As a result of the public taking "Trump more seriously than they should," people were put into distressing situations, sometimes resulting in casualties.[65] With the president abandoning reason for ratings, "instead of mounting a unified front," the U.S. response to the COVID-19 virus was "disjointed, cavalier, and fatalistic."[66]

CRUSHING DISSENT AS A PHOTO-OP(PORTUNISM)

On May 25, 2020, at the height of the COVID-19 pandemic, Derek Chauvin, white Minneapolis police officer, murdered black Minneapolis resident George Floyd. Video revealed that Chauvin knelt on Floyd's neck for nearly nine-and-a-half minutes until Floyd died in police custody.[67] Chauvin was later convicted of murder and will serve substantial time in state prison.[68] On May 26, videos recorded by bystanders became public and widespread protests began around the nation.[69] In Washington, D.C., Black Lives Matter protests began in Lafayette Park on May 29.[70] On June 1, U.S. Park Police, in conjunction with local law enforcement, issued dispersal orders to the protesters and cleared the park with tear gas and anti-riot tactics.[71] Simultaneously, President Donald Trump delivered a brief speech from the Rose Garden denouncing the protesters and then walked across Lafayette Park to St. John's Episcopal Church, where a small fire during protests the previous evening had produced what Egan Millard of the Episcopal News Service called "minor damage."[72] In this case study, we examine each liberal public sphere actor in turn to explain how the events on June 1 in Lafayette Park and the surrounding political and media discourse exposed major failures in the nation's effort to build an equitable and just society.

Among the public representatives involved in the events of June 1, one essential actor was President Trump. Trump, after learning of the arson at St. John's, took several actions that revealed his disdain both for reasonable public arguments and the process of deliberation itself. The president devised a publicity stunt with the help of advisors to attend the church. He delivered a scathing and hyperbolic attack on the Black Lives Matter movement from the Rose Garden at 6:43pm, walked from there to St. John's across the now-cleared Lafayette Park at 7:01pm, and finally posed for photographs for the media while holding a Bible eight minutes later.[73] In his brief remarks from the White House, Trump called protesters "professional anarchists," "violent mobs," "arsonists, looters, rider rioters, Antifa," and "dangerous thugs."[74] He labelled the actions of the protesters "domestic terror," situating himself between the "mobs" and "law and order." In this way, President Trump enacted a form of American exceptionalism that undermined public deliberation. Combining aspects of heroic demagoguery and paternalism,[75] President Trump expressed a promise to restore America to greatness and wove a tapestry of disunion, pitting the protesters against patriots and "law-abiding Americans."[76] Trump clearly laid out the structure of this exhortation in the final section of his Rose Garden speech:

> We have one, beautiful law. And once that is restored and fully restored, we will help you, we will help your business, and we will help your family. America is

founded on the rule of law. It is the foundation of our prosperity, our freedom and our very way of life, but where there is no law, there is no opportunity. Where there is no justice, there is no liberty, where there is no safety, there is no future.[77]

In this passage, Trump drew a stark dichotomy between "law and order" and the right of peaceful protest. He did this by suggesting that Black Lives Matter protesters had threatened "rule of law" producing a situation in which "there is no liberty . . . there is no safety." In fact, the "overall levels of violence and property destruction were low, and most of the violence that did take place was, in fact, directed against the BLM protesters." The overwhelmingly peaceful nature of the protests is evident in the finding that "96.3 percent of events involved no property damage or police injuries, and in 97.7 percent of events, no injuries were reported among participants, bystanders or police."[78] There were property losses of between $1 and $2 billion according to one study, a figure far less than many natural disasters.[79] And not all of that property damage was committed by protesters. As noted, violence often was initiated by the police and in the at least one case, a white supremacist in Minneapolis helped "incite riots and looting."[80] In other words, the critique of protesters for threatening "safety" was misleading and divisive since the protests were predominantly peaceful and what violence did occur was often initiated by the police or others. Trump's attack on protesters positioned the president "as the demagogic hero" who would save the American people from violence that was happening only rarely and typically because the police initiated it.[81] This application of American exceptionalism constituted a direct attack on the liberal public sphere. By denying the legitimacy of the protest, Trump implicitly attacked the right of all Americans to participate in the political process.[82] Clearly, Trump did not uphold his responsibility to both present reasonable arguments and represent the diversity of the nation.

One might ask why Trump's attack on protesters as dangerous rioters resonated so strongly with many Americans, when it was largely untrue? The answer is that while his message was untrue, it still "rang true" for many, especially those who drew their information from a media ecosystem supportive of Trump.[83] That ecosystem sustained a sense of public knowledge for his supporters.[84] Trump used rhetoric to generate "truths and values previously unknown" in order to sustain the narrative that the nation was threatened by dangerous protesters.[85] In essence, Trump drew on his supporters' perception of a dangerous world in which rioters threatened their community. In fact, this world did not exist, except in the rhetoric of Trump and his supporters in the media.

The media, in order to uphold their responsibility to the public, must report faithfully and impartially about the policy dispute in question. In the case of the Lafayette Park protests, the media constructed a narrative that not only enabled Trump to portray himself as a strongman, but did so in a way that presumed causation without evidence. Many leading news organizations presumed that President Trump ordered Lafayette Park to be cleared of protesters so that he could have the photo op. For example, the *New York Times* implicated the president, concluding that Trump ordered police to clear the park for his photo opportunity at St. John's. The article stated that "the police used tear gas and flash grenades to clear out the crowd that had gathered across the street in Lafayette Square *so Mr. Trump could walk to St. John's Episcopal Church afterward and pose for photographs.*"[86] Similarly, NPR titled a report "Peaceful Protesters Tear-Gassed to Clear Way for Trump Church Photo-Op" based on the Facebook post of a protester in attendance.[87] *Politico* reported that "Lafayette Square should not have been cleared with tear gas and rubber bullets to accommodate President Donald Trump's visit."[88] The *New York Times* went so far as to explicitly blaming the president for the scenes in Lafayette Park, casting Trump as the architect of a "scene of mayhem."[89] The *Washington Post* led with the claim that "Donald Trump militarized the federal response to protests of racial inequality" and added that Trump was "taking the rare step of mobilizing the military to use force to quell the unrest."[90] Clearly, these representations cast Trump as the director of events on June 1, using active verbs such as mobilizing and militarizing to imply direct involvement without supporting evidence. Public officials such as Tim Scott, Senator from South Carolina, and D.C. Attorney General Racine repeated this version of events as well.[91] Broadly, the conventional wisdom was that the President himself, acting through law enforcement, directed the clearing of the park *so that* he could take a photograph for the media in front of St. Johns. However, after a year of expert analysis, it became clear that this version of events was not accurate.

The role of the expert community is to inform the public by publicizing the best available research and analysis. On June 8, 2021, the Inspector General of the U.S. Department of the Interior released findings that the initial response from media presumed far too much about Trump's role in clearing the protesters from the park. The report concluded:

> The evidence we obtained did not support a finding that the USPP cleared the park to allow the President to survey the damage and walk to St. John's Church. Instead, the evidence we reviewed showed that the USPP cleared the park to allow the contractor to safely install the antiscale fencing in response to destruction of property and injury to officers occurring on May 30 and 31. Further, the evidence showed that the USPP did not know about the President's potential movement until mid-to late afternoon on June 1—hours after it had begun developing its operational plan and the fencing contractor had arrived

in the park, [This finding led the IG to conclude] weaknesses in communication and coordination may have contributed to confusion during the operation and the use of tactics that appeared inconsistent with the incident commander's operational plan.[92]

The IG report was based on interviews with more than 20 park officials and officers involved in the actions that day, a review of radio communications and transmissions, as well as video footage of the day from the Secret Service, and examination of other forms of direct eyewitness and expert evidence. Given this information, it is clear the media leapt to an inaccurate conclusion, an occurrence that reinforces the need for the media to apply strict fact checking procedures to their reporting and resist the temptation to rush to publish stories that seem to reflect a dominant storyline, without checking to make sure that storyline is true. In this case, the expert community upheld their responsibility by producing a report that contradicted the common wisdom about the events that day.

In order to ensure equity, justice, and sensible policy action, the public must inform themselves sufficiently to ensure representatives of the public, media, and experts are held to account for their work. In that way, the Black Lives Matter movement was created to respond to the fundamental failure of public officials to protect black Americans from being killed by police officers. Black Lives Matter is a decentralized, nonviolent protest against police brutality and other forms of antiblack violence and represents a clear example of the public acting to fill a gap left by other actors. In D.C., the segment of the public that includes Black Lives Matter occupied the area in and surrounding Lafayette Park to express their right to peacefully protest in support of justice for George Floyd. Lafayette Park was occupied as part of the public's response to a failure in the liberal public sphere, the failure to protect and value black lives.

In this case, Trump and other officials failed in their responsibility to accurately and faithfully present reasoned arguments confronting the crisis in policing that led to the murder of George Floyd and many others. Rather, Trump used largely peaceful protests to label protesters as violent radicals, a claim that was both false and incredibly divisive. The media, especially the partisan media on the political right, delivered the headlines that Trump wanted. The mainstream media, in contrast, was both quite critical of Trump and accurately reported, even if belatedly, events. However, given Trump's attacks on the media, criticism of his actions by the media helped him construct an image as a powerful strongman. In this way, the media unintentionally obliged the president, casting him in the role he desired, implying that Trump controlled and directed the scene. It took over a year for the media to correct their reporting.[93] In the events and words related to the clearing of

Lafayette Park, the expert community and a portion of the public fulfilled their role within the liberal public sphere. The expert community gathered and presented the data, telling a story of what actually happened. Protesters including those associated with Black Lives Matter, fought for justice with powerful demonstrations and even more powerful arguments. Their battle was in the best traditions of American democracy.

IMPLICATIONS FOR TEACHING AND RESEARCH

Earlier, we compared the public address that circulates throughout the American political and cultural system to blood circulating in the human body and observed that, as with bodily health, problems of circulation in public rhetoric can be extremely dangerous. Public address scholars describe and diagnose those problems of rhetorical circulation.

The interlocking crises that the nation faced in 2020 and 2021 suggest that rhetorical circulation of ideas in the United States is on occasion deeply flawed. While the expert community made missteps in the response to the pandemic and related crises facing the nation, they quickly followed the data and pointed to the importance of masking and other steps needed to lessen the impact of the pandemic. Other actors in the public sphere were less consistent in fulfilling their responsibilities. In the introduction of this chapter, we mentioned Madison's description in the Federalist Papers of threats to democratic deliberation. The two case studies indicate that those threats remain potent today. In that way, the case studies demonstrate that threats to the liberal public sphere are anything but new. The case studies also demonstrate that tools for analyzing public address remain quite powerful for exposing problems in rhetorical circulation. The crises of 2020 and 2021 did not change public address, but, rather, pointed to the continuing importance of research in the area.

Two implications can be drawn for future research on and teaching about public address. First, past research in public address and the case studies conducted in this chapter both point to the importance of understanding rhetoric in the context of a particular situation. One of the great insights of public address scholarship is that rhetorical processes have to be understood in relation to the specific situation and cultural context in which they occurred. The pandemic and the BLM protests both occurred at the beginning of a divisive election campaign in which President Donald Trump was running for reelection on a nationalist populist message based on grievance and fear.[94] When the pandemic forced President Trump to halt holding rallies, it was only natural that he look for an alternative forum to grab public attention. It was that situational dynamic which led him to use pandemic briefings as a substitute for rallies. Something similar happened with the BLM protests. With much of the country shutdown, President Trump needed a new enemy to blame for problems facing the nation. He attacked BLM protesters not because they actually were violent, but because he could create fear by depicting them as dangerous. The key point is that his actions in the pandemic briefing and in his various attacks on BLM protesters only can be understood in the context of the particular political situation facing him and the nation.

Another indication of the importance of careful analysis of context for public address is to consider how different the situation could have been had a different leader been president. After the tragic death of George Floyd, former Republican nominee for President and current Republican Senator from Utah, Mitt Romney, marched with BLM protesters, rather than attacking them. Romney said, "he wanted to find 'a way to end violence and brutality, and to make sure that people understand that black lives matter.'"[95] Had he been president, such actions might have cooled tempers and led to a national reflection on the horrors of American racial history and the need for genuine reconciliation. It is easy to imagine that a pragmatic conservative such as Romney might have deferred to experts in the CDC, putting the nation on a very different path confronting the pandemic than the path followed by the Trump administration. The key point is that rhetorical processes can only be understood in the context of the particular situation. Public address scholarship is a particularly useful approach for understanding the way that rhetoric functions in a given situation and cultural context.

A second implication relates to the focus of public address scholars on the resonance or lack of resonance of works of rhetoric. Some have viewed a focus on the resonance or on the effects of rhetoric as dated, creating a situation in which "many critics no longer focus on how a work functioned for a situated audience," based on the view that a consideration of audience influence is "uninteresting and not very revealing."[96] The two case studies, as well as a host of studies of public address, demonstrate that a consideration of how and why some works of rhetoric strongly resonate, while others do not, is anything but uninteresting and often can be quite revealing. The pandemic briefing that we discussed earlier in this chapter illustrates that point. Trump's remarks about bleach were important precisely because they had resonance. If they had actually been sarcastic and recognized as such by the audience, they would have had little import. In fact, as we noted, the comments led to a rash of poisonings. The statements were also part of a systematic campaign to downplay the importance of the virus.

It is important to consider what could have happened if President Trump had deferred to the CDC and other medical authorities and used his presidential bully pulpit to support consistent mask wearing and economic shutdowns to get the pandemic under control. If he had supported those actions, the pandemic might have been treated as simply a national public health crisis calling for actions such as wearing masks and never become a national political crisis.

Public address scholarship provides an important vehicle for placing rhetoric in the context of a particular place/time/culture and explaining resonance or lack of resonance in that context. Contrary to the criticisms of the approach, careful analysis of situation and resonance does not lead to simplistic analysis, but to a rich consideration of the way that rhetorical strategies work or fail to work for particular purposes with specific audiences. Such analysis can explain, for example, why calls for racial justice achieved so little in the period from the end of Reconstruction to the Second World War, but also why those calls for inclusion and justice became much more resonant in the late 1950s and 1960s.

One concept that is particularly valuable for exploring the situatedness of public address and explaining resonance or lack of resonance is the idea of a critical puzzle. A critical puzzle is a case where rhetoric resonates in an unexpected way or where rhetoric fails to resonate when either past experience or rhetorical theory indicates that it should resonate. One obvious example of a critical puzzle is Donald Trump's rapid ascent from reality TV star to president, despite lacking any political experience. There are many such puzzles in contemporary and historical rhetorical practice. Public address theory and criticism provides a powerful means of resolving those puzzles and therefore clarifying rhetorical circulation in American democracy.

CONCLUSION

The analysis of two snapshots reflecting the three interlocking crises that formed aspects of the larger political crisis facing the United States in 2020 exposed major weakness in the public sphere. The two snapshots of that larger political crisis function as "representative anecdotes" encompassing key dimensions of failure in the public sphere. For example, the case study of the pandemic briefing reveals a heavily politicized public sphere in which Trump Republicans were largely divorced from the scientific reality of the pandemic. One obvious example is the politicization of mask wearing. After a short period in which experts balanced the available evidence on the benefits of mask wearing, the scientific consensus quickly evolved to support the value of wearing masks to prevent spread of the disease.[97] This scientific consensus confronted the "Trumpian right's treatment of masks as a symbol of tyranny," creating a situation in which Trump supporters were much less likely to wear masks than other Americans.[98] If Trump consistently had supported masks, the public health response to the pandemic might have been much more effective.

Trump used pandemic briefings to support his political agenda, rather than to inform the nation about steps needed to containing the pandemic. He even argued that personal use of a widely available, but quite dangerous household product, bleach, could potentially eradicate the disease, a comment that created an apoplectic response from public health officials. Despite a performance that devalued science in favor of what can only be called quackery, his support remained quite stable. The net result of this briefing and a host of others was to turn a public health crisis into a partisan contest, politicizing mask wearing and later vaccination. There is widespread agreement that Trump's rhetoric as well as the rhetoric and policies of his administration made the U.S. response to the pandemic much less effective than that in western nations such as Canada where sensible public health policy drove decision-making.[99] Even one of the leading members of Trump's own pandemic taskforce, Dr. Deborah Birx, who served as "coronavirus response coordinator," concluded that because of Trump's words and actions, "hundreds of thousands of Americans may have died needlessly."[100] *The Washington Post* summarized Birx's comments as indicating that "most coronavirus deaths in the United States could have been prevented if the Trump administration had acted earlier and more decisively."[101]

The analysis of the second snapshot is also revealing. Trump's attacks on the demonstrators in his Rose Garden speech and other contexts resonated with many, despite the fact that BLM protests were overwhelmingly peaceful and much of the limited violence that occurred was initiated by the police or in at least one case a white supremacist. It is instructive that Trump supporters and other Republicans continue to believe that Black Lives Matter protesters as well as Antifa commit a great deal of public violence, when in fact political violence in the United States is overwhelmingly committed by members of far right groups, most of whom are fervent Trump supporters.[102] The public sphere clearly fails when utter falsehoods are treated as scripture and when large groups of peaceful law-abiding Americans are treated as dangerous Others.

Overall, the two snapshots suggest major failings in the primary actors in the liberal public sphere, save the expert community. The expert community worked hard to get the facts right and present them to the public, the media, and to representatives of the public. When experts such as Dr. Anthony Fauci made errors, they quickly corrected them. Fauci and many others worked tirelessly to inform key stakeholders in the public sphere. Often, the good work of the expert community was disregarded or even attacked. Partisan right-wing media emphasized creating outrage rather than informing the public. Leaders such as President Trump were focused on political, rather than public health needs. Finally, while some among the public fought for social justice, a very large segment of the general public drew their information from untrustworthy social media sources, with many subscribing to conspiracy theories. In confronting the crises facing the nation in 2020 and 2021 the liberal public sphere fared quite poorly.

In these two snapshots of the political crisis facing the nation, Madison's republican remedy was undermined by President Trump's transformation of a medical briefing into a pro-Trump rally and his use of a Rose Garden speech to demonize citizens fighting for racial justice. As former George W. Bush speechwriter and conservative columnist, Michael Gerson, observed, these two snapshots "exemplified a type of politics where cruelty is the evidence of commitment, brutality is the measure of loyalty and violence is equated with power."[103]

While the conclusions drawn from the case studies of the liberal public sphere are quite concerning for what they reveal about the state of American democracy, they are reassuring in what they reveal about the state of research in public address. American democracy is constituted through the give and take of rhetoric and argument. Public address scholars are uniquely positioned to explain that process and to point toward potential solutions when it falls short.

NOTES

1. On the importance of *Federalist 10* see Lance Banning, *The Sacred Fire of Liberty: James Madison and the Founding of the Federal Republic* (Ithaca, New York: Cornell University Press, 1995), 204.

2. James Madison, *Writings* (New York: Library of America, 1999), 167, 194, 230.

3. See for example the groundbreaking study of genres of presidential rhetoric in Karlyn Kohrs Campbell and Kathleen Hall Jamieson, *Presidents Creating the Presidency: Deeds Done in Words* (Chicago: University of Chicago Press, 2008). Also see a study of the history, culture, and rhetoric of George Washington's First Inaugural in Stephen Howard Browne, *The First Inauguration: George Washington and the Invention of the Republic* (University Park, PA: Pennsylvania State University Press, 2020); as well as research on the evolution of national identity in Vanessa B. Beasley, *You, The People: American National Identity in Presidential Rhetoric* (College Station, TX: Texas A & M University Press, 2004). For a study of fantasy as a particular form of rhetoric see Ernest G. Bormann, *The Force of Fantasy: Restoring the American Dream* (Carbondale, IL: Southern Illinois University Press, 1985). For a study of the influence of a particular form of free market ideology see Robert Asen, *Invoking the Invisible Hand: Social Security and the Privatization Debates* (East Lansing, MI: Michigan State University Press, 2009). For studies of particular speeches see two books on important speeches by Ronald Reagan, Mary E. Stuckey, *Slipping the Surly*

Bonds: Reagan's Challenger Address (College Station, TX: Texas A & M University Press, 2006); Robert C. Rowland and John M. Jones, *Reagan at Westminster: Foreshadowing the End of the Cold War* (Texas A & M University Press, 2010).

4. A good example of the diversity of public address scholarship can be found in *World War II and the Cold War: The Rhetoric of Hearts and Minds: A Rhetorical History of the United States, Significant Moments in American Public Discourse, Volume VIII*, ed. Martin J. Medhurst (East Lansing, MI: Michigan State University Press, 2018), where authors take a variety of approaches to key moments in public address from the prelude to World War II through the Reagan administration. Other examples include *Twentieth-Century Roots of Rhetorical Studies*, eds. Jim A. Kyupers and Andrew King (Westport, CT: Praeger, 2001); *Landmark Essays on American Public Address*, ed. Martin J. Medhurst (New York, NY: Routledge, 1993); Stephen E. Lucas, "The renaissance of American public address: Text and context in rhetorical criticism," *Quarterly Journal of Speech* 74 (1988): 241–260.

5. See for example, Robert C. Rowland, *Donald Trump's Rhetoric and American Democracy* (Lawrence, Kansas: University Press of Kansas, 2021); Robert C. Rowland, "The Populist and Nationalist Roots of Trump's Rhetoric," *Rhetoric & Public Affairs* 22 (2019): 343–388; Robert C. Rowland and John M. Jones, "Reagan's Farewell Address: Redefining the American Dream," *Rhetoric & Public Affairs* 20 (2017): 635–665; Robert C. Rowland and John M. Jones, "Reagan's Strategy for the Cold War and the Evil Empire Address," *Rhetoric &Public Affairs* 19 (2016): 427–464; Mike Milford and Robert C. Rowland, "Situated Ideological Allegory and *Battlestar Galactica*," *Western Journal of Communication* 76 (2012): 536–551; Robert C. Rowland, "Barack Obama and the Revitalization of Public Reason," *Rhetoric and Public Affairs* 14 (2011): 693–725; Robert C. Rowland and John M. Jones, "One Dream: Barack Obama, Race, and the American Dream," *Rhetoric and Public Affairs* 14 (2011): 125–154; Robert C. Rowland and John M. Jones, "Reagan and the Evil Empire," in *World War II and the Cold War: The Rhetoric of Hearts and Minds: A Rhetorical History of the United States, Significant Moments in American Public Discourse, Volume VIII*, ed. Martin J. Medhurst (East Lansing, MI: Michigan State University Press, 2018), 415–466; Robert C. Rowland, "Donald Trump and the Rejection of the Norms of American Politics and Rhetoric," in *An Unprecedented Election: Campaign Coverage, Communication, and Citizens Divided*, ed. Benjamin R. Warner, Dianne G. Bystrom, Mitchell S. McKinney, and Mary C. Banwart (Santa Barbara, CA, ABC-CLIO, 2018), 189–205; Robert C. Rowland, "Obama's Rhetoric of Myth and Reason," in *Reconsidering Obama: Reflections on Rhetoric,* ed. Robert Terrill, (New York: Peter Lang, 2017), 51–68; Robert C. Rowland, "Purpose, Evidence, and Pedagogy in Rhetorical Criticism," in *Rhetorics and Effects: Past, Present and Future,* eds. Amos Kiewe and Davis Houck, (Columbia, SC: University of South Carolina Press, 2015), 59–81; Robert C. Rowland, "The Rhetorical Constraints Limiting President Obama's Domestic Policy Advocacy," in *The Making of Barack Obama: The Politics of Persuasion,* eds. Matthew Abraham and Erec Smith (Anderson, SC: Parlor Press, 2013), 17–51; Robert C. Rowland, "The Battle for Health Care Reform and the Liberal Public Sphere," in *Exploring Argumentative Contexts,*

eds. Frans H. van Eemeren and Bart Garssen (Amsterdam: John Benjamins, 2012), 269–288.

6. Jeffrey K. Tulis, *The Rhetorical Presidency* (Princeton: Princeton University Press, 1987), 5.

7. See for example, Samuel Kernell, *Going Public: New Strategies of Presidential Leadership,* 4th ed. (Washington: *CQ Press*, 2007).

8. David Zarefsky, "The Presidency Has Always Been a Place for Rhetorical Leadership," in *The Presidency and Rhetorical Leadership*, ed. Leroy G. Dorsey (College Station: Texas A & M University Press, 2002), 20–41.

9. Browne makes this point quite clear in his groundbreaking analysis of Washington's First Inaugural address.

10. One careful study found that Black Americans are killed by the police at more than twice the rate of white Americans. See Niall McCarthy, "U.S. Police Shootings: Blacks Disproportionately Affected," *Statista*, July 15, 2020, https://www.statista.com/chart/21857/people-killed-in-police-shootings-in-the-us/.

11. David Litt, "The Coronavirus Crisis in the U.S. Is a Failure of Democracy," *Time*, May 20, 2020, https://time.com/5839195/coronavirus-democracy-failure/.

12. Kenneth Burke, *A Grammar of Motives* (New York: Prentice Hall, 1945), 59–61; also see Barry Brumett, "The Representative Anecdote as a Burkean Method, Applied to Evangelical Rhetoric," *Southern Speech Communication Journal* 50 (1984): 1–23.

13. See for example, Robert C. Rowland, "Campaign Argument and the Liberal Public Sphere: A Case Study of the Process of Developing Messages in a Congressional Campaign," *Argumentation and Advocacy* 42 (2006), 206–215; Rowland, "The Battle for Health Care Reform,"; Robert C. Rowland, "A Liberal Theory of the Public Sphere," in *Critical Problems in Argumentation*, ed. Charles Arthur Willard, (Washington: NCA, 2005), 281–287; Robert C. Rowland, "Ebola and the Liberal Public Sphere," in *Recovering Argument*, ed. Randall A. Lake (New York: Routledge, 2018), 188–194.

14. See for example the essays in Robert Asen and Daniel C. Brouwer, eds., *Counterpublics and the State* (Albany: State University of New York Press, 2001).

15. Habermas was focused on the historical development of the public sphere. However, his focus on the importance of reasoned discourse is consistent with the methodological approach developed in liberal public sphere theory. See Jürgen Habermas, *The Structural Transformation of the Public Sphere* (T. Burger and F. Lawrence, Trans), (Cambridge, MIT Press, 1989).

16. Orlando Patterson, "The Liberal Millennium," *The New Republic*, November 8, 1999, 54.

17. Dr. Martin Luther King, Jr., "I Have a Dream," August 28, 1963, https://www.americanrhetoric.com/speeches/mlkihaveadream.htm.

18. For the "deliberation day" proposal see Bruce Ackerman and James S. Fishkin, *Deliberation Day* (New Haven, CT: Yale University Press, 2004). For research in the field of rhetoric focused on deliberative democracy see *The Public Work of Rhetoric: Citizen-Scholars and Civic Engagement (Studies in Rhetoric/Communication)*, eds. John M. Ackerman and David J. Coogan (Columbia, SC: University of

South Carolina Press, 2010); *Rhetorical Democracy: Discursive Practices of Civic Engagement*, eds. Gerard A. Hauser and Amy Grimm (New York, NY: Routledge, 2004); Martin Carcasson, Laura W. Black, and Elizabeth S. Sink, "Communication Studies and Deliberative Democracy: Current Contributions and Future Possibilities," *Journal of Public Deliberation 6* (2010), 1–42.

19. Nicole Chavez, Faith Karimi, and Eric Levenson, "Coronavirus spread 'under the radar' in US major cities since January, researchers say," *CNN*, April 23, 2020, https://www.cnn.com/2020/04/23/health/us-coronavirus-thursday/index.html.

20. Lisa Shumaker, "U.S. coronavirus death toll doubles in 10 days to more than 50,000: Reuters tally," *Reuters*, April 24, 2020, https://www.reuters.com/article/us-health-coronavirus-usa-casualties/u-s-coronavirus-death-toll-doubles-in-10-days-to-more-than-50000-reuters-tally-idUSKCN2261C9.

21. Institute for Health Metrics and Evaluation, "Estimation of excess mortality due to COVID-19," May 13, 2021, http://www.healthdata.org/special-analysis/estimation-excess-mortality-due-covid-19-and-scalars-reported-covid-19-deaths.

22. Natalie Sherman, "Coronavirus: US unemployment claims hit 26.4 million amid virus," *BBC*, April 23, 2020, https://www.bbc.com/news/business-52398837.

23. Josh Salman and Jayme Fraser, "Coronavirus strains cash-strapped hospitals, could cause up to 100 to close within a year," *USA Today*, April 25, 2020, https://www.usatoday.com/story/news/investigations/2020/04/25/coronavirus-strains-cash-strapped-hospitals-could-cause-mass-closures/2996521001/; Casey Tolan, Ashley Fantz, and Collette Richards, "Rural hospitals are facing financial ruin and furloughing staff during the coronavirus pandemic," *CNN*, April 21, 2020, https://www.cnn.com/2020/04/21/us/coronavirus-rural-hospitals-invs/index.html; Amy Brittain, Ted Mellnik, Dan Keating, and Joe Fox, "How a surge of coronavirus patients could stretch hospital resources in your area," *The Washington Post*, April 10, 2020, https://www.washingtonpost.com/graphics/2020/investigations/coronavirus-hospitals-data/; Alisa Chang, "U.S. hospitals hit by financial 'triple whammy' during coronavirus pandemic," *National Public Radio*, April 23, 2020, https://www.npr.org/sections/coronavirus-live-updates/2020/04/23/843012119/u-s-hospitals-hit-by-financial-triple-whammy-during-coronavirus-pandemic.

24. "Coronavirus: US health official warns of dangerous second wave," *BBC*, April 22, 2020, https://www.bbc.com/news/world-us-canada-52378845.

25. Zeynep Tufekci, "5 Pandemic Mistakes We Keep Repeating," *The Atlantic*, February 26, 2021, https://www.theatlantic.com/ideas/archive/2021/02/how-public-health-messaging-backfired/618147/.

26. Victoria Smith and Alicia Wanless, "Unmasking the Truth: Public Health Experts, the Coronavirus, and the Raucous Marketplace of Ideas," *Carnegie Endowment for the Humanities*, July 16, 2020, https://carnegieendowment.org/2020/07/16/unmasking-truth-public-health-experts-coronavirus-and-raucous-marketplace-of-ideas-pub-82314.

27. Smith and Wanless.

28. Ed Yong, "The Pandemic Experts Are Not Okay," *The Atlantic*, July 7, 2020, https://www.theatlantic.com/health/archive/2020/07/pandemic-experts-are-not-okay/613879/.

29. Smith and Wanless.
30. Smith and Wanless.
31. Phillip Bump, "Birx both exemplifies and blames the cherry-picking that shaped the Trump presidency," *Washington Post,* January 25, 2021, https://www.washingtonpost.com/politics/2021/01/25/birx-both-exemplifies-blames-how-cherry-picking-data-shaped-trump-presidency/.
32. Nell Greenfieldboyce, "As The Coronavirus Crisis Heats Up, Why Isn't America Hearing From The CDC?" *NPR*, March 25, 2020, https://www.npr.org/sections/health-shots/2020/03/25/821009072/as-the-coronavirus-crisis-heats-up-why-arent-we-hearing-from-the-cdc.
33. Rowland, *The Rhetoric of Donald Trump*, 102–112.
34. Paul LeBlanc, "Homeland Security official who detailed effect of temperature on coronavirus isn't a scientist but has a long military background," *CNN*, April 24, 2020, https://www.cnn.com/2020/04/23/politics/who-is-bill-bryan-dhs/index.html.
35. Bill Bryan, "Remarks by President Trump, Vice President Pence, and Members of the Coronavirus Task Force in Press Briefing," April 23, 2020, https://trumpwhitehouse.archives.gov/briefings-statements/remarks-president-trump-vice-president-pence-members-coronavirus-task-force-press-briefing-31/.
36. Bryan.
37. Donald Trump, "Remarks by President Trump, Vice President Pence, and Members of the Coronavirus Task Force in Press Briefing," April 23, 2020, https://trumpwhitehouse.archives.gov/briefings-statements/remarks-president-trump-vice-president-pence-members-coronavirus-task-force-press-briefing-31/.
38. Trump, "Remarks by President Trump."
39. Bryan.
40. Trump, "Remarks by President Trump."
41. Deb Riechmann, Kevin Freking, and Aamer Madhani, "Trump suggested studying injections of disinfectant to treat coronavirus, then said he was being sarcastic. Here's video and a transcript," *Chicago Tribune*, April 24, 2020, https://www.chicagotribune.com/coronavirus/ct-nw-trump-white-house-sunlight-heat-fight-virus-20200424-7dnhtyxltvdazkp24mybuefmou-story.html.
42. Riechmann, Freking, and Madhani.
43. Aaron Rupar, "Trump just mused about whether disinfectant injections could treat the coronavirus. Really," *Vox*, April 23, 2020, https://www.vox.com/2020/4/23/21233628/trump-disinfectant-injections-sunlight-coronavirus-briefing.
44. Rupar.
45. George Will, "Trump's disinfectant remarks were tantamount to peddling death," *Washington Post*, April 24, 2020, https://www.washingtonpost.com/opinions/trumps-idiotic-remarks-should-be-condemned-by-anyone-who-cares-about-the-nations-health/2020/04/24/1da7e53e-864a-11ea-878a-86477a724bdb_story.html. Will was not alone among conservatives in critiquing Trump. For example, Scott Gottlieb, who served as administrator of the FDA in the Trump Administration felt the need to warn the American people not to "take a disinfectant or inject a disinfectant for the treatment of anything, and certainly not the treatment of coronavirus." Gottlieb is quoted in David Smith and Kari Paul, "Debacle of Trump's coronavirus

disinfectant comments could be tipping point," *The Guardian,* April 25, 2020, https://www.theguardian.com/us-news/2020/apr/25/donald-trump-coronavirus-disinfectant-sarcastic-tipping-point.

46. Christi Carras, "Trump wonders if injecting bleach kills coronavirus, but Cristina Cuomo bathes in it," *LA Times,* April 24, 2020, https://www.latimes.com/entertainment-arts/story/2020-04-24/coronavirus-cristina-cuomo-chris-cuomo-clorox-instagram.

47. Riechmann, Freking, and Madhani.

48. Adam Edelman, "Fact check: Did Trump say people should inject bleach to fight Covid-19?" *NBC News,* October 23, 2020, https://www.nbcnews.com/politics/2020-election/live-blog/2020-10-22-trump-biden-election-n1244210/ncrd1244478#blogHeader. Also see Glenn Kessler, Salvador Rizzo and Meg Kelly, "Fact-checking the first Trump-Biden presidential debate," *Washington Post,* September 30, 2020, https://www.washingtonpost.com/politics/2020/09/30/fact-checking-first-trump-biden-presidential-debate/; Robert Farley and Eugen Kiely, "The White House Spins Trump's Disinfectant Remarks," *FactCheck.org,* April 24, 2020, https://www.factcheck.org/2020/04/the-white-house-spins-trumps-disinfectant-remarks/.

49. PolitiFact, "On COVID-19, Donald Trump said that 'maybe if you drank bleach you may be okay,'" April 24, 2020, https://www.politifact.com/factchecks/2020/jul/11/joe-biden/no-trump-didnt-tell-americans-infected-coronavirus/.

50. Trump, "Remarks by President Trump."

51. "Lesley Stahl: Trump admitted mission to 'discredit' press," *CBS News,* May 23, 2018, https://www.cbsnews.com/news/lesley-stahl-donald-trump-said-attacking-press-to-discredit-negative-stories/.

52. Riechmann, Freking, and Madhani.

53. Robert Glatter, "Calls To Poison Centers Spike After The President's Comments About Using Disinfectants To Treat Coronavirus," *Forbes,* April 25, 2020, https://www.forbes.com/sites/robertglatter/2020/04/25/calls-to-poison-centers-spike--after-the-presidents-comments-about-using-disinfectants-to-treat-coronavirus/?sh=699b717f1157.

54. Riechmann, Freking, and Madhani.

55. Riechmann, Freking, and Madhani.

56. Glatter.

57. Glatter.

58. "Coronavirus: Trump Disinfectant Claims Cause 100 Hospital Admissions," *Real Madrid,* April 25, 2020, https://en.as.com/en/2020/04/25/other_sports/1587834179_103339.html.

59. Coronavirus: Trump disinfectant claims.

60. Cecelia Smith-Schoenwalder, "CDC: Some People Did Take Bleach to Protect From Coronavirus," *U.S. News,* June 5, 2020, https://www.usnews.com/news/health-news/articles/2020-06-05/cdc-some-people-did-take-bleach-to-protect-from-coronavirus.

61. Nature, "The Trump administration must stop sidelining the CDC," July 28, 2020, https://www.nature.com/articles/d41586-020-02231-6.

62. Tufekci.

63. "Public health experts say U.S. COVID-19 response marked by grave missteps," *PBS*, October 29, 2020, https://www.pbs.org/newshour/health/public-health-experts-say-u-s-covid-19-response-marked-by-grave-missteps.
64. "Public health experts."
65. Rupar.
66. Ed Yong, "How the pandemic defeated America," *The Atlantic*, September, 2020, https://www.theatlantic.com/magazine/archive/2020/09/coronavirus-american-failure/614191/.
67. Evan Hill, Ainara Tiefenthäler, Christiaan Triebert, Drew Jordan, Haley Willis and Robin Stein, "How George Floyd Was Killed in Police Custody," *New York Times*, May 31, 2020, https://www.nytimes.com/2020/05/31/us/george-floyd-investigation.html.
68. Tim Arango, Shaila Dewan, John Eligon and Nicholas Bogel-Burroughs, "Derek Chauvin is found guilty of murdering George Floyd," *New York Times*, April 20, 2021, https://www.nytimes.com/live/2021/04/20/us/derek-chauvin-verdict-george-floyd.
69. Audra D. S. Burch and John Eligon, "Bystander Videos of George Floyd and Others Are Policing the Police," *New York Times*, May 27, 2020, A1.
70. "Review of U.S. Park Police Actions at Lafayette Park," Office of the Inspector General, U.S. Department of the Interior, June 8, 2021, https://www.doioig.gov/sites/doioig.gov/files/SpecialReview_USPPActionsAtLafayettePark_Public.pdf.
71. Katie Rogers, Jonathan Martin, and Maggie Haberman, "As Trump Calls Protesters 'Terrorists,' Tear Gas Clears a Path for His Walk to a Church," *New York Times*, June 2, 2020, A1.
72. Egan Millard, "Fire causes minor damage to St. John's, the 'church of presidents' in Washington, during night of riots," *Episcopal New Service*, June 1, 2020, https://www.episcopalnewsservice.org/2020/06/01/fire-causes-minor-damage-to-st-johns-the-church-of-presidents-in-washington-during-night-of-riots/.
73. Tom Gjelten, "Peaceful Protesters Tear-Gassed To Clear Way For Trump Church Photo-Op," *NPR*, June 1, 2020, https://www.npr.org/2020/06/01/867532070/trumps-unannounced-church-visit-angers-church-officials.
74. Donald J. Trump, "President Trump's Rose Garden speech on protests," CNN, https://www.cnn.com/2020/06/01/politics/read-trumps-rose-garden-remarks/index.html.
75. Jennifer Mercieca, *Demagogue for President: The Rhetorical Genius of Donald Trump* (College Station: Texas A&M University Press, 2020), 81.
76. Trump, "Rose Garden speech on protests."
77. Trump, "Rose Garden speech on protests."
78. Erica Chenowith and Jeremy Pressman, "This summer's Black Lives Matter protesters were overwhelmingly peaceful, our research finds," *Washington Post*, October 16, 2020, https://www.washingtonpost.com/politics/2020/10/16/this-summers-black-lives-matter-protesters-were-overwhelming-peaceful-our-research-finds/. Others found a very similar pattern. See Sanya Mansoor, "93% of Black Lives Matter Protests Have Been Peaceful, New Report Finds," *Time*, September 5, 2020, https://time.com/5886348/report-peaceful-protests/;

79. Jennifer A. Kingson, "Exclusive: $1 billion-plus riot damage is most expensive in insurance history," *Axios*, September 16, 2020, https://www.axios.com/riots-cost-property-damage-276c9bcc-a455-4067-b06a-66f9db4cea9c.html.

80. Karma Allen, "Man who helped ignite George Floyd riots identified as white supremacist: Police," *ABC News*, July 29, 2020, https://www.axios.com/riots-cost-property-damage-276c9bcc-a455-4067-b06a-66f9db4cea9c.html.

81. Mercieca, 124.

82. Mercieca, 203–213.

83. See Rowland, *The Rhetoric of Donald Trump*.

84. Lloyd F. Bitzer, "Rhetoric and Public Knowledge," in *Rhetoric, philosophy, and literature: An exploration,* ed. Don M. Burks, (West Lafayette: Purdue University Press, 1978), 83, 88–9.

85. Bitzer, 68.

86. Rogers, Martin, and Haberman, emphasis added.

87. Gjelten.

88. "Tim Scott: Lafayette Square should not have been cleared for Trump," *Politico.com*, June 2, 2020, https://advance-lexis-com.libproxy.unl.edu/api/document?collection=news&id=urn:contentItem:6035-TWB1-F118-900N-00000-00&context=1516831.

89. Peter Baker, Maggie Haberman, Katie Rogers, Zolan Kanno-Youngs, Katie Benner, Haley Willis, Christiaan Triebert and David Botti, "How Trump's Idea for a Photo-Op Led to Havoc in a Park," *The New York Times*, June 2, 2020, https://www.nytimes.com/2020/06/02/us/politics/trump-walk-lafayette-square.html.

90. Philip Rucker, Robert Costa, Josh Dawsey and Seung Min Kim, "Trump mobilizes military, threatens to use troops to quell protests across U.S.," *Washington Post*, June 1, 2020, https://www.washingtonpost.com/politics/trump-mobilizes-military-threatens-to-use-troops-to-quell-protests-across-us/2020/06/01/10212832-a416-11ea-bb20-ebf0921f3bbd_story.html.

91. "Tim Scott" and States News Service, "Statement by Ag Racine on President Trump's Unconscionable Order to Assault Peaceful protesters Around Lafayette Square," *States News Service*, June 2, 2020, https://advance-lexis-com.libproxy.unl.edu/api/document?collection=news&id=urn:contentItem:6025-HXD1-JCBF-S06V-00000-00&context=1516831.

92. "Review of U.S. Park."

93. Domenico Montanaro, "Watchdog Report Says Police Did Not Clear Protesters To Make Way For Trump Photo-Op," *National Public Radio*, June 9, 2021, https://www.npr.org/2021/06/09/1004832399/watchdog-report-says-police-did-not-clear-protesters-to-make-way-for-trump-last-; Stephanie Ebbs and Benjamin Siegel, "Police did not clear Lafayette Square so Trump could hold 'Bible' photo op: Watchdog," *ABC News*, June 10, 2021, https://abcnews.go.com/Politics/police-clear-lafayette-park-area-trump-hold-bible/story?id=78171712; Melissa Quinn, "Watchdog finds clearing of protesters from Lafayette Park wasn't for Trump photo op," *CBS News*, June 9, 2021, https://www.cbsnews.com/news/trump-photo-op-lafayette-park-protesters-report/; Dan Mangan, "Trump Bible photo op not reason cops violently cleared George Floyd protest outside White House, feds claim," *CNBC*, June 9,

2021, https://www.cnbc.com/2021/06/09/protestors-cleared-outside-white-house-for-fence-not-trump-photo-op.html; Ashraf Khalil, "Federal probe: Protest not broken up due to Trump photo op," *Associated Press*, June 9, 2021, https://apnews.com/article/donald-trump-george-floyd-government-and-politics-a9931785996ddfafcc42dcdde9f50df5.

94. Rowland develops this point in considerable detail in *The Rhetoric of Donald Trump*.

95. Michelle Boorstein and Hannah Natanson, "Mitt Romney, marching with evangelicals, becomes first GOP senator to join George Floyd protests in D.C.," *Washington Post*, June 8, 2020, https://www.washingtonpost.com/dc-md-va/2020/06/07/romney-protest-black-lives-matter/.

96. Rowland, "Purpose, Evidence, and Pedagogy in Rhetorical Criticism," 60. For a very useful discussion of the continuing relevance of considerations of resonance or effect see the essays in Amos Kiewe and Davis Houck, eds., The Effects of Rhetoric and the Rhetoric of Effects: Past, Present, Future (Studies in Rhetoric/Communication) (Columbia, South Carolina: University of South Carolina Press, 2015).

97. Caitlin McCabe, "Face Masks Really Do Matter. The Scientific Evidence Is Growing," *The Wall Street Journal*, August 13, 2020, https://www.wsj.com/articles/face-masks-really-do-matter-the-scientific-evidence-is-growing-11595083298.

98. Ari Schulman, "The Coronavirus and the Right's Scientific Counterrevolution," *The New Republic*, June 15, 2020, https://newrepublic.com/article/158058/coronavirus-conservative-experts-scientific-counterrevolution. For research indicating that Trump supporters wore masks less often than others see Eric W. Dolan, "Trump's reluctance to wear a mask appears to have rubbed off on his followers," *PsyPost*, May 2, 2021, https://www.psypost.org/2021/05/trumps-reluctance-to-wear-a-mask-appears-to-have-rubbed-off-on-his-followers-6063.

99. German Lopez, "If the US had Canada's Covid-19 death rate, 100,000 more Americans would likely be alive today," *Vox*, September 9, 2020, https://www.vox.com/future-perfect/2020/9/9/21428769/covid-19-coronavirus-deaths-statistics-us-canada-europe.

100. Sheryl Gay Stolberg, "Trump's former pandemic coordinator suggests that a restrained response may have cost hundreds of thousands of lives," *New York Times*, April 30, 2021, https://www.nytimes.com/live/2021/03/28/world/covid-vaccine-coronavirus-cases.

101. Amy B. Wang, "Birx tells CNN most U.S. covid deaths 'could have been mitigated' after first 100,000," *Washington Post*, March 27, 2021, https://www.washingtonpost.com/politics/2021/03/27/birx-tells-cnn-most-us-covid-deaths-could-have-been-mitigated-after-first-100000/.

102. Jenny Gross, "Far-Right Groups Are Behind Most U.S. Terrorist Attacks, Report Finds," *New York Times*, January 20, 2021, https://www.nytimes.com/2020/10/24/us/domestic-terrorist-groups.html.

103. Michael Gerson, "The threat of violence now infuses GOP politics. We should all be afraid," *Washington Post*, May 20, 2021, https://www.washingtonpost.com/opinions/2021/05/20/trump-republicans-violent-threats-election-2024/.

Chapter 7

Health Communication Research and Social Implications during the COVID-19 Pandemic

YoungJu Shin, Yu Lu, and Shristi Bhochhibhoya

This chapter addresses both health communication research and its social implications during the COVID-19 pandemic. First, we begin with the overview of the current situation of the COVID-19 pandemic and health consequences, and then move to a discussion of the relationship between anti-Asian discrimination and health. Next, the role of health communication in family and interpersonal relationships during the COVID-19 pandemic is discussed, followed by a short section on the practical implications for public health interventions. We conclude with suggestions for teaching and research.

CURRENT SITUATION OF THE COVID-19 PANDEMIC AND HEALTH CONSEQUENCES

The novel coronavirus disease has spread globally since it was first identified in Wuhan, China in December 2019.[1] This infectious disease is caused by severe acute respiratory syndrome coronavirus 2 (SARS=CoV-2).[2] Since then, the virus has rapidly spread and affected more than 200 countries and territories around the globe. World Health Organization subsequently declared a Public Health Emergency of International Concern on January 30, 2020, and declared it as a pandemic on March 11, 2020.[3] Although 78% of the cases were reported to be asymptomatic as presented in a report on April 1, 2020,[4] symptomatic cases have manifested various clinical symptoms including fever, cough, fatigue, headache, diarrhea, muscle soreness, and dyspnea.[5] COVD-19 affects people of all ages and characteristics but vulnerable populations including elderly populations and people with underlying medical conditions are at higher risk for severe disease and complications.[6] In the United States, approximately 80% of the deaths occurred among the elderly population (>65 years old).[7] Similarly, 90% of deaths occurred among individuals aged 70 years or above in Italy.[8] Based on a report published on July 4, 2021, the total number of cases reported globally exceeds 183 million while approximately 4 million people have succumbed to death due to COVID-19 and its complications.[9]

COVID-19 mainly transmits from person to person through the respiratory droplets and aerosol. Additionally, since the virus remains viable on inanimate objects, people can also be infected by touching contaminated surfaces, such as door handles or handrails where there are frequent human interaction,[10] and then touching their own eyes, mouth, and nose. To curb these transmissions and limit the infections, a number of preventive measures were strictly enforced around the world including quarantine, social isolation, national/state-level lockdowns, and curfews.[11] Various countries around the world enforced strict public health policies of social distancing and restriction of activity and mobility. Although these restrictions vary, in their timing and severity, government and health officials advised people to stay at home, limit gathering, and only leave their residence for an essential reasons such as buying groceries, collecting medications, and accessing or working in health care facilities.[12] In many of the countries, national-level authorities and local authorities ordered the shutdown of schools, educational institutions, public transportations (trains, national and international flights), religious/faith-based organizations, and movie theaters; hospitals and health care centers were only the exception.[13] Millions of workers lost jobs while many worked fewer hours, which resulted in increased stress related to financial instability.[14]

Due to the economic shutdown and instability triggered by extended lockdown, "stay at home" orders and isolation, there has been an increase in the prevalence of various health-related problems. The COVID-19 pandemic impacted the life of the general population as physical health, mental health, and lifestyle behaviors were affected. Due to the lack of in-person schooling, children and adolescents were found to engage in more screen time, decreased number of hours doing physical activity, sleeping irregularly, and eating less appropriate diets.[15] In a study conducted in Pakistan, 98% of patients living with chronic diseases reported that lockdown had affected their daily routine while 71% of the participants reported mental health issues since the pandemic.[16] Additionally, 53% of the patients living with chronic illness missed their routine medical checkup which can have detrimental effects on the management of chronic illness.

Social isolation is encouraged and practiced during the pandemic to avoid transmission of the disease. However, studies indicate that many people across the world experience elevated levels of mental health disorders including anxiety, depression, and loneliness due to social isolation during the pandemic.[17,18] The pandemic brought about an "epidemic of despair" as there was a rise in serious anxiety, mental health problems, eccentric behavioral patterns, anger, alcoholism, and suicidal ideation among people.[19] The magnitude of despair was noticed by a sudden increase in the Emergency Department visits for suspected suicide attempts of adolescents aged 12–27 years, especially among adolescent girls.[20] Young adults were found to engage in alcohol and marijuana use to escape from boredom and relieve feelings of distress.[21] Before COVID, youths often engaged in substance use to fit-in in social gatherings and as a form of celebration. On the contrary, youths started to use alcohol to self-medicate and to cope with depression during the pandemic.[22] A massive rise in the purchased volumes of alcohol was reported in Australia,[23] the United Kingdom, and the United States in March of 2020 alone.[24] A recent study conducted in Canada confirmed that fewer adolescents were using alcohol and marijuana, but among the adolescents who were using alcohol and marijuana, the frequency of use increased compared to pre-COVID times.[25] Similar results were also reported in the US where college students self-reported to have increased their alcohol use frequency during the pandemic.[26] While looking at a different demographic of the population, the use of alcohol was used by older population (>55 years old) as their coping strategy. Social isolation and shelter-in-place guidelines were strictly reinforced especially for older people which may trigger or worsen anxiety, substance abuse, and depression.[27] Approximately 10% of the older adults increased their weekly consumption of alcohol when compared to their usual pre-COVID-19 behavior. Older adults who reported to have some forms of mental health outcomes (depression, anxiety, and loneliness) were more likely to report increased alcohol consumption when compared to older adults who do not have any prior mental health symptomology.[28]

As the virus continues to spread around the world with its new variant, it brought multiple new stressors into the life of the people including the closure of businesses, economic vulnerability, and uncertainty.[29] Through all of that, children and their mothers were at the most vulnerable position. The incidences of family violence, especially intimate partner violence, child abuse, and elder abuse, escalated during and after the pandemic started, and this pattern was being repeated around the globe.[30] The escalated number in violence at homes increased calls to the Domestic Violence Helpline and increased traffic at abuse help websites, for example, in Spain, an increase of 20% in calls was reported to its helpline in the first few days of lockdown and in the UK, calls to the UK Domestic Violence Helpline increased by 25% within a week of the announcement of strict lockdown measures.[31] Furthermore, an increase in domestic homicide was reported in a number of affected countries.[32] The "stay at home" orders were more unraveling and problematic to people living and surviving abusive relationships. For them, home is often the place where abuse happens and repeats. Stringent restriction measures forced by governments cut off their avenues to seek help and take shelter in a safer place than their homes. These stressors from abusers in the time of uncertainty take a toll on survivors' physical and mental health.

ANTI-ASIAN DISCRIMINATION AND HEALTH DURING THE COVID-19 PANDEMIC

In addition to dealing with all the aforementioned challenges/consequences brought about by the COVID-19 pandemic that faces everyone, one group at particularly higher risk than others are Asian populations across the world, due to the surge of discrimination toward Asians since the outbreak. In this section we discuss Asian discrimination in the U.S. as a case example to first describe the incidences of discrimination toward Asian Americans and then the health consequences associated with it.

Racial/ethnic based discrimination, in particular these targeting Asian Americans is on the rise since the start of the pandemic.[33] A Pew Research Center survey of 9,654 U.S. adults conducted in June 2020 noted that 39% of U.S. adults reported it is more common for people to express racist or racially insensitive views about people who are Asian than it was before the coronavirus outbreak.[34] Examining twitter posts, Thu Nguyen and colleagues reported that the proportion of negative tweets referencing Asians increased by 68.4% (from 9.79% in November to 16.49% in March) while the proportion of negative tweets referencing other racial/ethnic minorities (e.g., Blacks and Latinx) remained relatively stable.[35] About 31% of Asian adults, in comparison to 21% of Black, 15% of Hispanics, and 8% of Whites, have been subject to slurs or jokes because of their race or ethnicity since the outbreak began, and 26% of Asian, compared to 20% of Black, 10% of Hispanics, and 9% of Whites, feared someone might threaten or physically attack them.[36] A national study conducted in March 2020 found that 42% of the 1,141 U.S. adults surveyed had been engaging in at least one discriminatory behavior toward people of Asian descent.[37] The rates of discrimination incidences toward Asians differ a lot by ethnic groups[38] with Chinese being the highest discriminated group followed by Koreans.[39] When combining all Asian groups, in a national representative internet panel of American adults, Cary Wu and colleagues reported 22% of Asian Americans and 21% of Asian immigrants experienced COVID-19-related discrimination.[40] A particularly alarming number comes from a study conducted with a sample of 543 Chinese American parents and their children[41] in which 32% of parents and 46% of youth reported experiencing and over 76% of both parents and youth witnessing at least one incident of COVID-19 related discrimination online (e.g., being said mean or rude things due to race/ethnicity) and over 50% of parents and youth experienced and 89% of parent and 92% of youth witnessed at least one incident of COVID-19 related discrimination in person (e.g., being treated unfriendly or unwelcoming due to being Chinese). Between March 19, 2020, to June 30, 2021, 9,081 anti-Asian hate incidents (including verbal harassment, shunning, physical assault, civil rights violations, and online harassment) across the U.S. were documented with 13.7% of them being physically assaulted, according to a report from the Stop AAPI Hate website established by the Asian Pacific Policy and Planning Council.[42] Due to the known underreporting issue of hate crimes[43] and the Stop AAPI Hate website being a relatively new self-report tool not well known in the Asian community, the actual number of incidences could be much higher. This trend of discrimination surge is also reflected in a national database that while consisting for 5% of the U.S. population, 13% of the texters that reached out for help from the Crisis Text Line in early 2020 were Asians[44] despite the well-known low service utilization among Asian Americans.[45]

Common incidences of anti-Asian discrimination ranged from microaggression to hate crimes, including subtle hint, verbal harassment, shunning, workplace discrimination, being barred from transportation, being turned away by businesses, physical assaults, and attempted murder and homicide (e.g., been pushed down into train track, been stabbed with a knife, been shot with a firearm, or been lit on fire), with many assaults targeting women and elderly, some even attacks children.[46] Notably, research suggests that covert discrimination (e.g., being treated with less courtesy) was more prevalent than overt discrimination (e.g., being called names or threatened) prepandemic but since COVID, more overt discrimination, including verbal and physical harassment, has been reported.[47] It is documented that among self-reported discrimination incidences, physical assault rates had increased from 10.2% in 2020 to 16.7% in 2021, marking a dangerous trend.[48] Particularly at risk of being targeted and victimized are women, youth, immigrants, international students, those less educated, those with limited English proficiency, healthcare workers, and business owners and employees.[49]

The life conditions of Asians have been severely affected by COVID-related discrimination. Minority communities are known to be at higher risk of virus exposure, due to their over-representation in the low-wage, essential workforce at the front lines as well as inability to socially distance due to housing conditions, and unequal health care access.[50] Despite the common "model minority" myth (i.e., Asian Americans are considered as healthy and wealthy), Thomas Le and colleagues pointed out that the aggregated data of good health are largely driven by healthier, affluent Asian American subgroups, neglecting underserved Asian American subgroups.[51] The surge of discrimination further exacerbates the situation. Americans of Asian descent have reported a growing fear of being in public because of the harassment they experienced or witnessed during the COVID-19 pandemic, even feared leaving home for routine tasks such as grocery shopping.[52] At the beginning of the pandemic before masks were not mandated/normalized, many Asians had to choose between the risk of being verbally or physically attacked for wearing a mask as an Asian versus the risk of contracting COVID-19 virus without a mask.[53] Worrying their Asian family, friends, spouses who are Asian to be discriminated adds additional mental toll for Asian and non-Asian people.[54] In a qualitative interview study conducted by the authors, Chinese Americans living in the U.S. shared surviving tips to protect themselves from hate crimes including avoid going out; while in public, avoid places with few people and avoid times at or after sunset, watch for surroundings (in case people quickly approach them with a weapon), stand far away from the track when waiting for the subway or train (in case someone attempts to push them down into the track). These tips may be helpful to reduce chances of being physically harmed, while being at odds with the CDC (2021) guidelines to exercise as a means to cope with stress during the pandemic. Le and colleagues argue, subgroups of Asian Americans (e.g., the undocumented, low-income, elderly, and limited-English-proficient) may be the most adversely affected during the COVID-19 pandemic in the U.S., especially due to the fears of seeking care because of the current climate of anti-Asian xenophobia.[55]

As aforementioned, a surge of anti-Asian hate crimes was recorded[56] and significant increase of mental health help seeking reported.[57] Tyler Reny and Matt Barreto found that Google searches for "Chinese virus" and "Kung Flu" increased dramatically since March 2020.[58] An analysis of Twitter and online image message boards identified a surge in the use of Sinophobic slurs beginning in late January 2020, compared to data from before the pandemic.[59] Social media and video games, due to its anonymity nature, serve as an excellent platform for discrimination. Online discrimination was among the most common form of reported racial/ethnic discrimination.[60] Not surprisingly, deterioration of mental health has been observed as a result among Asian Americans since the pandemic, contributing to enlarged gap of health disparities. For example, although COVID-19 related discrimination was associated with increased mental disorder for all Americans, Asian Americans reported fewer mental health conditions than their White American counterparts pre-pandemic, yet reported higher level of mental disorder than Whites since the onset of the pandemic.[61] The link between discrimination and poor mental health is well established among Asian Americans prior pandemic (see Gee et al., 2009 for a review).[62] Several studies examined the effect of COVID-19 related anti-Asian racism on mental health in Asian Americans and observed elevated levels of mental disorders, depressive symptoms, anxiety, and sleep difficulties associated with discrimination experiences.[63]

Although data is still lacking on the physical health consequences of COVID-19 related discrimination in Asian Americans, research has found that these who experience racial/ethnic discrimination may experiences hypervigilance, avoidance, flashbacks, and nightmares related to the racial discrimination incidences[64] and somatic expressions, including headaches, heart palpitations, dizziness, confusion, and difficulty concentrating.[65] Racial/ethnic discrimination experiences have been further linked to reduced life satisfaction and self-esteem, increased symptoms of anxiety and depression, suicidal ideation, exacerbation of a range of chronic health conditions, including cardiac disease, respiratory conditions, pain and disability, and higher all-cause mortality in Asian Americans.[66] Furthermore, discrimination can lead to reduced access to health services and help seeking in Asian Americans[67] who already report a general low rate of health care service utilization.[68]

THE ROLE OF HEALTH COMMUNICATION

In this section, we will discuss communication in family and interpersonal relationships during the COVID-19 pandemic, followed by the practical implications for public health interventions and suggestions for teaching and research. First, let us discuss the role family plays during the pandemic.

Family Communication

Since the COVID-19 outbreak, family relationships have been profoundly impacted. Changing relational interdependence, renegotiating a role in the family, and navigating work-life balance, to name a few, require a new perspective in family communication research during the pandemic.[69] Family also faces uncertainty due to the adjustment to and threat caused by the COVID-19 and health-related information. For example, parents with adolescent and college children report the practice of the coronavirus contagion control further escalates uncertainties about social interaction at various occasions at home and school.[70] When dealing with the uncertainty, parents' sense of self-efficacy plays a key role. Studies show that crisis self-efficacy and protective self-efficacy was positively related, meaning that as parents report stronger competence in their ability to manage a crisis situation like the COVID-19 pandemic, they are highly likely to hold stronger self-efficacy to protect their children from the threat caused by the crisis. Parents' knowledge about COVID-19 significantly mediated the positive association between crisis self-efficacy and protective self-efficacy, suggesting that as parents have higher levels of crisis self-efficacy, they report better understanding of the risks associated with COVID-19, which in turn, leads to higher degrees of protective self-efficacy. When it comes to the information sources for parents, television was the most popular source, followed by health care providers such as pediatrician and physician, other family members, and friends. Website and social media including Facebook and Twitter are also identified as information channels.[71] With regard to the technology usage, parent distraction with technology (i.e., the level of distraction that is caused by technology in parenting) is found to negatively affect child social competence during the pandemic. Recent research in Croatia shows that as parents are more distracted by the technology when interacting with children, children's sense of social competence decreases.[72] The same study also indicates that high levels of parents' emotional stability protect children against the negative effect of technological distraction. That is, the inverse effect of parent distraction with technology on children's social competence can be lessened as long as parents remain emotionally stable while interacting with children.

In addition to the impact of COVID-19 on parent-child relationships, the outbreak and spread of the coronavirus also severely affected family interaction and caregiving. For instance, at long-term care homes, the residents and their loved ones are encouraged to take alternative visit approaches including video and phone calls, window visits, and outdoor in-person visits during the pandemic.[73] Since social connections are essential to psychological and physical well-being of long-term care residents, health care providers and caregivers need to deal with the public health crisis and adjust to the immediate changes in their interactions. Not only does the pandemic affect the parent-child relationships, but it also influences transnational intergenerational communication in a global context. Recent study explores communication modes (i.e., face-to-face and technology-mediated communication) between migrant children in Poland and their grandparents in their homelands and highlights the importance of face-to-face communication for transgenerational relationships.[74]

Interpersonal Communication

The COVID-19 pandemic has triggered a turning point for renegotiation and reformation of interpersonal relationships, including romantic relationships. Romantic couples have to handle the COVID-19 related stress together and while coping with the unexpected crisis, romantic partners experience changes in interdependence, intimacy, and communication. Various coping strategies are identified as seeking escape from the relationship, reinforcing intimacy and connection, managing routines, engaging social networks, practicing mindfulness, purposeful use of time, setting boundaries, and planning for the future.[75] During the public health crisis, seeking and sharing health information and accessing and providing support are critical for individuals' mental and physical health.[76] Individuals tend to use different communication channels for different purpose. For example, Choi and Choung (2021) found that during the COVID-19 pandemic, people who used phone calls and video chats for social connection were less likely to report loneliness, which, in turn, led to increases in life satisfaction.[77] However, those who reported using phone calls and Facebook and Instagram for information seeking were more likely to experience loneliness, which linked to decreases in life satisfaction. Jennifer Ihm and Chul-Joo Lee revealed that among Korean adults, individuals with more social resources (i.e., social network density, the feeling of closeness, and frequency of communication via face-to-face, phone call, email, and social media) reported better well-being.[78] Specifically, frequent interaction and communication with others were positively related to cognitive well-being, whereas informational support was significantly associated with affective well-being. Moreover, it was found that feeling of closeness was a significant predictor for cognitive, affective, and physical well-being. Similarly, in Lebanon, individuals who reported self-isolation were more likely to experience depression, irritability, and loneliness.[79] The same study also indicated that social support significantly reduced the depressive symptoms and poor sleep quality. In the U.S., pregnant women reported that social support helps to lower stress and gain knowledge about pregnancy during the pandemic. These women shared their experience of receiving socially distant instrumental support while lacking medical professional support.[80] Among older adults, the internet is identified as a way to cope with the coronavirus related stress.[81] More specifically, chat software (e. g., Zoom, Skype, or WhatsApp) were used as the largest increased communication channels during the pandemic, followed by the online websites for shopping or medical appointments, online newspapers, social networking services, and websites for hobbies and interests. While older adults' stress levels were negatively related to interpersonal communication via chat software and online websites for errands, the internet use for leisure was positively associated with their well-being.

Interpersonal communication scholars have also documented the differential effects of interpersonal communication and mediated information sources about COVID-19 information (i.e., traditional media, social media, and health websites). In the U.S., Samantha Nazione, Evan Perrault, and Kristin Pace's study showed that individuals reported having conversations about COVID-19 with family the most, followed by friends, coworkers, and health care professionals.[82] Their findings also indicated that more people spent time on health websites, and they had more conversations about COVID-19 with others. Frequent use of health websites also predicted performing preventive behaviors against the coronavirus infection. In Nigeria, research indicated that interpersonal communication is imperative to create an awareness of the pandemic and promote preventive behaviors such as handwashing, social distancing, and avoiding the use of handshakes in rural communities.[83] Other studies revealed that the exposure to the traditional media coverage about COVID-19 information and the use of social media significantly related to depression, whereas the use of social media and interpersonal communication about the COVID-19 significantly associated with stress among the U.S adults.[84] In China, social media serves as the main source of the COVID-19 related information. Among Chinese social media users, individuals who spent more than an hour for seeking the information about the coronavirus reported higher levels of anxiety than those searching for the information less than an hour.[85] Chinese individuals also reported information seeking from official government sources using mobile devices, while information sharing with family members takes place via private communication channels such as private texts or the social media chatting channel, WeChat.[86] As the coronavirus continues evolving, individuals are likely to experience information fatigue and emotional burnout, which causes less information seeking behavior than information scanning. In the U.S., compared to popular social media platforms like Facebook and Twitter, mobile instant message services (e. g., WhatsApp and Telegram) are regarded as more private and intimate spaces to communicate with others.[87] Nguyen et al.'s study explored that the use of video calls, text messages, social media, and online games as a means for social connection with friends and family.[88] Age, gender, living status, and internet access all exert significant influences on individuals' increased use of digital communication during the time in which a restricted face-to-face interaction was forced. In particular, individuals who were younger, women, lived alone, and concerned about their Internet access were more likely to utilize digital communication.

Interpersonal communication plays an integral role in dealing with COVID-19 related stress. In its guidelines, the CDC suggests talking with people who one trusts, such as friends and family, as a healthy way to cope with COVID-19 related stress.[89] In Romania, the use of humorous information about COVID-19 is found to alleviate anxiety and promote social distancing from people infected with the coronavirus and further mitigate the negative effect of the COVID-19 information on negative mood caused by the pandemic.[90] Additionally, Woo and Joo found in their study while COVID-19 racial discrimination was positively associated with depressive symptoms, communications with a spouse/partner buffered the mental burden of racial discrimination.[91] Interestingly, they also found those who shared their experience in online ethnic communities displayed stronger depressive symptoms than who did not, further highlighting the importance of in-person communication with someone the individual trusts. Suyeon Lee and Sara Waters also found that social support buffered the effect of discrimination on depressive symptoms among Asians in the U.S.[92]

With regard to health information seeking behaviors, Crowley and colleagues found that as individuals reported higher desires to learn about the coronavirus (uncertainty discrepancy), they were likely to experience higher levels of anxiety as well as lower levels of their ability to cope with information about COVID-19.[93] It was also discovered that the greater individuals reported their ability to find credible information about COVID-19, the greater they reported cognitive reappraisal (i.e., actively re-evaluating fears associated with the coronavirus) and direct information seeking (i.e., searching for news about the coronavirus). Indirect information seeking (i.e., reliance on others sharing information about the coronavirus) significantly predicted preparations such as buying extra foods, medicine, and household supplies, whereas the same behavior was inversely related to prevention behaviors including avoiding traveling and social gathering, as well as staying 6 feet apart.

The COVID-19 pandemic generates more challenges for patient-provider relationships. Health care professionals report excessive burden and psychological distress due to high demands of care and under the circumstances, they are required to adapt to the online communication when offering a telehealth service.[94] Barriers of patient-provider communication are identified as reduced communication channels and absence of family.[95] Offering support for health care providers and providing resources for strategic communication for culturally sensitive telehealth interactions are recommended to mitigate emotional distress and results in better quality of patient care.[96]

While a majority of research has paid close attention to the importance of verbal communication and different channels of communication, few scholars highlight the role that nonverbal communication plays in human interaction. In particular, the use of facial expression is essential to deliver communicative messages along with other verbal and nonverbal cues. In this regard, mask wearing causes more difficulty in communicating with others and creating interpersonal connection.[97] People need to practice a new skill set that helps navigate interpersonal communication in an absence of facial expression due to face covering.

PRACTICAL IMPLICATIONS FOR PUBLIC HEALTH INTERVENTIONS

As Nurit Guttman and Eimi Lev claim, health interventionists should be mindful of ethical concerns communicating uncertainty about the coronavirus and unintended consequences such as increases in health inequities and stigmatization during the pandemic.[98] When promoting proactive practices including wearing face masks, social distancing, and hand sanitizing, health practitioners must offer resources to encourage and sustain protective behaviors and provide alternatives to replace the limited interactions with others. What is more, emphasis on the severity of the virus infection and the efficacy of engaging in protective health behaviors offers more effective strategies than stressing individuals' vulnerability to the disease.[99] Based on the research findings showing that health consequences of specific behavioral beliefs (i.e., mask wearing beliefs and social distancing beliefs) served as significant predictors for adopting protective practices,[100] it is suggested that health interventions should be designed to highlight the benefits of desirable health practices. When attempting to reduce the spread of misinformation, health communication researchers should take account of the different usage of communication channels in interpersonal relationships and develop the intervention messages based on the target audience.[101] Because digital communication and/or mediated communication becomes more prevalent during the pandemic, health communication researchers and practitioners are recommended to take account of digital inequality.[102] Another way of effectively disseminating public health interventions is to employ entertainment-education, which conveys educational messages in a form of entertainment. Entertainment-education enables to strategically target the local context, and effectively tailor and disseminate health messages, through existing infrastructure. In this way, it is easier to build the trust and acquire support from the local communities than starting from the beginning.[103] Furthermore, recent research highlights the importance of cultural contexts because some COVID-19 prevention interventions failed to address the community voices at the margin and further exacerbated the marginalization of communities at the margins.[104] Marginalized communities (e. g., racial and ethnic background, religious practice, immigration status, age, and certain health conditions) are severely affected by COVID-19 related health disparities and placed at higher risks of negative health consequences including increase in anxiety and lack of confidence in dealing with the pandemic.[105] More global efforts are needed to reduce the health disparities resulting from the lack of cultural sensitivity and neglect on the voice of the minorities.

SUGGESTIONS FOR TEACHING AND RESEARCH

The COVID-19 pandemic has influenced so many different levels of our lives and introduced the notion of so-called *new normal* life which inevitably shapes personal, social, and professional lives. Here we propose practical suggestions for teaching and research in the field of communication. In terms of teaching pedagogy, instructors should recognize that students are severely affected by the long lasting pandemic. Students have struggled a great deal with their emotional distress due to the social isolation, which consequently leads to poor physical health outcomes. Thus, instructors should be mindful of the ongoing stressors that cause harmful effects on students' well-being as well as their academic performance. Instructors should show their understanding of many challenges that students are currently facing and further provide emotional support and encouragement by sharing their sympathy and empathy with students. When designing the course, instructors also need to provide a room for flexibility for the class assignment due date or even consider reducing workloads, in comparison to the prepandemic course design. Utilizing technology for the class (e.g., using Zoom while offering the live lecture and discussion in face-to-face class) is another way for students who are not able to attend the class in person. As discussed previously, validating students' emotions is very helpful to build a rapport with students and create a sense of belonging and support community to the entire class. Most importantly, the critical role that instructors can play is to ensure that students can successfully move forward with their academic advancement and professional development while dealing with high level of uncertainties on individual, social, and global levels.

With regard to research in the age of the COVID-19 pandemic, communication scholars should put continuous efforts to discover the new findings of human interaction and quality of life, as well as to investigate the longitudinal effects of the pandemic on individuals from a wide range of communicative contexts from family and interpersonal relationships, work relationships, to health implications. The practice of the "new normal" life may have profound effects on human communication and interaction and more investigation is required to better understand its social and cultural implications in our society. For example, communication researchers can revalidate the existing theories in the context of the pandemic (e.g., communication privacy management theory, communication theory of identity, health belief model, theory of motivated information management, uncertainty management theory, theory of planned behavior), to name a few, in order to demonstrate how people communicate their private information, negotiate identities, process the coronavirus related health information, and change their behaviors toward social distancing, wearing masks, and getting vaccinated utilizing qualitative and/or quantitative research methodology. Furthermore, communication scholars and practitioners can also collaborate with interdisciplinary research teams to develop a health intervention that helps mitigate the deleterious effects on individuals and to reduce health disparities in the marginalized populations during the pandemic. Lastly, communication research can also make impacts on social movement that raises an awareness of anti-Asian racism and hate speech and creates a safe space for people to engage in public discourses about this social problem. One might think that the pandemic will eventually be under control but the unintended consequences and residuals may make longer impacts than expected and leave a scare in my peoples' hearts and their memory.

In conclusion, rather than feeling overwhelmingly helpless and hopeless, accepting the fact that it is inevitable to live our lives with the coronavirus is the first step to move forward. Communication instructors and researchers can make substantial contributions to the scholarship by paying close attention to the global impacts on human communication, in the age of the COVID-19 pandemic.

NOTES

1. Hongzhou Lu, Charles W. Stratton, and Yi-Wei Tang, "Outbreak of Pneumonia of Unknown Etiology in Wuhan, China: The Mystery and the Miracle," *Journal of Medical Virology* 92, no. 4 (2020): 401.

2. Zunyou Wu and Jennifer M McGoogan, "Characteristics of and Important Lessons from the Coronavirus Disease 2019 (Covid-19) Outbreak in China: Summary of a Report of 72 314 Cases from the Chinese Center for Disease Control and Prevention," *JAMA* 323, no. 13 (2020): 1239.

3. Tedros Adhanom Ghebreyesus, "WHO Director-General's Opening Remarks at the Media Briefing on Covid-19–11 March 2020," *World Health Organization* 11 (2020).

4. Michael Day, "Covid-19: Four Fifths of Cases Are Asymptomatic, China Figures Indicate," *BMJ* 369 (2020): 369.

5. Xiaobo Yang et al., "Clinical Course and Outcomes of Critically Ill Patients with Sars-Cov-2 Pneumonia in Wuhan, China: A Single-Centered, Retrospective, Observational Study," *The Lancet Respiratory Medicine* 8, no. 5 (2020): 475.

6. Jeremy AW Gold et al., "Characteristics and Clinical Outcomes of Adult Patients Hospitalized with Covid-19—Georgia, March 2020," *Morbidity and Mortality Weekly Report* 69, no. 18 (2020): 545.

7. Zainab Shahid et al., "Covid-19 and Older Adults: What We Know," *Journal of the American Geriatrics Society* 68, no. 5 (2020): 926.

8. Eric E. Brown et al., "Anticipating and Mitigating the Impact of the Covid-19 Pandemic on Alzheimer's Disease and Related Dementias," *The American Journal of Geriatric Psychiatry* 28, no. 7 (2020): 712.

9. World Health Organization, "Weekly Epidemiological Update on Covid-19, 6 July 2021," https://www.who.int/publications/m/item/weekly-epidemiological-update-on-covid-19---6-july-2021.

10. LJGR Morawska et al., "Size Distribution and Sites of Origin of Droplets Expelled from the Human Respiratory Tract During Expiratory Activities," *Journal of Aerosol Science* 40, no. 3 (2009): 256.

11. Balasankar Ganesan et al., "Impact of Coronavirus Disease 2019 (Covid-19) Outbreak Quarantine, Isolation, and Lockdown Policies on Mental Health and Suicide," *Frontiers in Psychiatry* 12 (2021): 1.

12. Caroline Bradbury-Jones and Louise Isham, "The Pandemic Paradox: The Consequences of Covid-19 on Domestic Violence," *Journal of Clinical Nursing* (2020): 1.

13. Times of India, "Tamil Nadu Police Book 39,000 for Section 144 Violation," 2020.

14. Olivier Coibion, Yuriy Gorodnichenko, and Michael Weber, "Labor Markets During the Covid-19 Crisis: A Preliminary View," (National Bureau of Economic Research, 2020).

15. Guanghai Wang et al., "Mitigate the Effects of Home Confinement on Children During the Covid-19 Outbreak," *The Lancet* 395, no. 10228 (2020): 945.

16. Muhammad Arif Nadeem Saqib et al., "Effect of Covid-19 Lockdown on Patients with Chronic Diseases," *Diabetes & Metabolic Syndrome: Clinical Research & Reviews* 14, no. 6 (2020): 1621.

17. Samantha K. Brooks et al., "The Psychological Impact of Quarantine and How to Reduce It: Rapid Review of the Evidence," *The Lancet* 395, no. 10227 (2020): 912.

18. Christine M. Lee, Jennifer M Cadigan, and Isaac C Rhew, "Increases in Loneliness among Young Adults During the Covid-19 Pandemic and Association with Increases in Mental Health Problems," *Journal of Adolescent Health* 67, no. 5 (2020): 714.

19. MK Narayanan, "The Spectre of a Post-Covid-19 World," *The Hindu* 2020.

20. Ellen Yard et al, "Emergency Department Visits for Suspected Suicide Attempts among Persons Aged 12–25 Years before and During the Covid-19 Pandemic—United States, January 2019–May 2021," *Morbidity and Mortality Weekly Report* 70, no. 24 (2021): 888.

21. Samuel F. Acuff et al., "Temporal Precedence of Self-Regulation over Depression and Alcohol Problems: Support for a Model of Self-Regulatory Failure," *Psychology of Addictive Behaviors* 33, no. 7 (2019): 603.

22. Cindy H. Liu et al., "Factors Associated with Depression, Anxiety, and PTSD Symptomatology During the Covid-19 Pandemic: Clinical Implications for Us Young Adult Mental Health," *Psychiatry Research* 290 (2020): 113172.

23. Brigid Delaney, "Drinking in Coronavirus Isolation: Experts Warn Australians to Monitor Their Intake," *The Guardian* 2020.

24. BBC News, "Coronavirus: Shoppers Stock up on Alcohol Amid Lockdown," 2020.

25. Tara M. Dumas, Wendy Ellis, and Dana M. Litt, "What Does Adolescent Substance Use Look Like During the Covid-19 Pandemic? Examining Changes in Frequency, Social Contexts, and Pandemic-Related Predictors," *Journal of Adolescent Health* 67, no. 3 (2020): 354.

26. Scott Graupensperger et al., "Changes in College Student Alcohol Use During the Covid-19 Pandemic: Are Perceived Drinking Norms Still Relevant?," *Emerging Adulthood* (2021): 1.

27. Derek D. Satre et al., "Addressing Problems with Alcohol and Other Substances among Older Adults During the Covid-19 Pandemic," *The American Journal of Geriatric Psychiatry* 28, no. 7 (2020): 780.

28. Marisa R. Eastman, Jessica M. Finlay, and Lindsay C. Kobayashi, "Alcohol Use and Mental Health among Older American Adults During the Early Months of the Covid-19 Pandemic," *International Journal of Environmental Research and Public Health* 18, no. 8 (2021): 4222.

29. Bradbury-Jones and Isham, *Pandemic Paradox*, 1.

30. Emma Graham-Harrison, Angela Giuffrida, and Helena Smith, "Lockdowns around the World Bring Rise in Domestic Violence," *The Guardian* 2020.

31. June Kelley and Tomos Morgan, "Coronavirus: Domestic Abuse Calls up 25% since Lockdown, Charity Says," *BBC* 2020.

32. Bradbury-Jones and Isham, 1.

33. Qin Gao and Xiaofang Liu, "Stand against Anti-Asian Racial Discrimination during COVID-19: A Call for Action," *International Social Work* 64, no. 2 (2021): 261; Suyeon Lee and Sara F. Waters, "Asians and Asian Americans' Experiences of Racial Discrimination during the COVID-19 Pandemic: Impacts on Health Outcomes and the Buffering Role of Social Support," *Stigma and Health* 6, no. 1 (2021): 70; Drishti Pillai, Aggie J. Yellow Horse, and Russell Jeung, "The Rising Tide of Violence and Discrimination Against Asian American and Pacific Islander Women and Girls," Retrieved July 16, 2021 from https://stopaapihate.org/wp-content/uploads/2021/05/Stop-AAPI-Hate_NAPAWF_Whitepaper.pdf

34. Neil G. Ruiz, Juliana J. Horowitz, and Christine Tamir, "Many Black and Asian Americans Say They Have Experienced Discrimination Amid the COVID-19 Outbreak." Retrieved July 16, 2021 from https://www.pewresearch.org/social-trends/2020/07/01/many-black-and-asian-americans-say-they-have-experienced-discrimination-amid-the-covid-19-outbreak/

35. Minh Hao Nguyen et al., "Changes in Digital Communication during the COVID-19 Global Pandemic: Implications for Digital Inequality and Future Research," *Social Media+ Society* 6, no. 3 (July-September 2020): 1.

36. Ruiz et al., *Experienced Discrimination*, 2020.

37. Lindsay Y. Dhanani, and Berkeley Franz, "Unexpected Public Health Consequences of the COVID-19 Pandemic: A National Survey Examining Anti-Asian Attitudes in the USA," *International Journal of Public Health* 65, no. 6 (2020): 747.

38. Charissa S. L. Cheah et al., "COVID-19 Racism and Mental Health in Chinese American Families," *Pediatrics* 146, no. 5 (2020): e2020021816; Piotr Rzymski and Michał Nowicki, "COVID-19-Related Prejudice toward Asian Medical Students: A Consequence of SARS-CoV-2 Fears in Poland," *Journal of Infection and Public*

Health 13, no. 6 (2020): 873; Cary Wu, Yue Qian, and Rima Wilkes, "Anti-Asian Discrimination and the Asian-White Mental Health Gap during COVID-19," *Ethnic and Racial Studies* 44, no. 5 (2021): 819; Mengxi Zhang et al., "Discrimination and Stress Among Asian Refugee Populations During the COVID-19 Pandemic: Evidence from Bhutanese and Burmese Refugees in the USA," *Journal of Racial and Ethnic Health Disparities*, (2021): 1.

39. Russell Jeung, Aggie J. Yellow Horse, and Charlene Cayanan, "Stop AAPI Hate National Report, 3/19/20–3/31/21," San Francisco, CA: Stop AAPI Hate Report Center. Retrieved July 15, 2021 from https://stopaapihate.org/wp-content/uploads/2021/05/Stop-AAPI-Hate-Report-National-210506.pdf.

40. Wu et al., *Anti-Asian Discrimination*, 819.

41. Cheah et al., *Racism and Mental Health*, e2020021816.

42. Aggie J. Yellow Horse et al., "Stop AAPI Hate National Report, 3/19/20–6/30/21," San Francisco, CA: Stop AAPI Hate Report Center. Retrieved July 15, 2021 from https://stopaapihate.org/wp-content/uploads/2021/08/Stop-AAPI-Hate-Report-National-v2-210830.pdf.

43. Angela R. Gover, Shannon B. Harper, and Lynn Langton, "Anti-Asian Hate Crime During the COVID-19 Pandemic: Exploring the Reproduction of Inequality," *American Journal of Criminal Justice* 45, no. 4 (2020): 647.

44. Bob Filbin, "*Bob's Notes on COVID-19: Mental Health Data on the Pandemic*," Crisis Text Line. Retrieved July 20, 2021 from https://www.crisistextline.org/data/bobs-notes-on-covid-19-mental-health-data-on-the-pandemic

45. Sungchul Park et al., "The Effects of the Affordable Care Act on Health Care Access and Utilization among Asian American Subgroups," *Medical Care* 57, no. 11 (2019): 861; Francis G. Lu, "The Poor Mental Health Care of Asian Americans," *The Western Journal of Medicine* 176, no. 4 (2002): 224.

46. Alexia Fernandez Campbell and Alex Ellerbeck, "Federal Agencies are Doing Little about the Rise in anti-Asian hate," The Center for Public Integrity. Retrieved July 20, 2021 from https://publicintegrity.org/health/coronavirus-and-inequality/federal-agencies-are-doing-little-about-the-rise-in-anti-asian-hate/; Matt Loffman, "Asian Americans Describe 'Gut Punch' of Racist Attacks during Coronavirus Pandemic | PBS NewsHour," PBS 2020.

47. Bongki Woo and Jungmi Jun, "COVID-19 Racial Discrimination and Depressive Symptoms among Asians Americans: Does Communication about the Incident Matter?" *Journal of Immigrant and Minority Health*, (2021): 1.

48. Jeung et al., *AAPI Hate National Report*, 2021.

49. Jun He et al., "Discrimination and Social Exclusion in the Outbreak of COVID-19," *International Journal of Environmental Research and Public Health* 17, no. 8 (2020): 2933; Gao and Liu. *Anti-Asian Racial Discrimination*, 261–64.

50. William F. Owen, Richard Carmona, and Claire Pomeroy, "Failing Another National Stress Test on Health Disparities," *JAMA* 323, no. 19 (2020): 1905.

51. Thomas K. Le et al., "Anti-Asian Xenophobia and Asian American COVID-19 Disparities," *American Journal of Public Health* 110, no. 9 (2020): 1371.

52. Hyeouk Chris Hahm et al., "Racially Diverse US Young Adults' Experience of COVID-19-Related Anti-Asian Discrimination: Types and Emotional Reactions,"

Preprint. In Review; iun-Ruey Hu, Margaret Wang, and Francis Lu, "COVID-19 and Asian American Pacific Islanders," *Journal of General Internal Medicine* 35, no. 9 (2020): 2763.

53. Shinwoo Choi, "'People Look at Me like I AM the Virus': Fear, Stigma, and Discrimination during the COVID-19 Pandemic," *Qualitative Social Work* 20, no. 1–2 (2021): 233; Rzymski and Nowicki, *COVID-19-Related Prejudice*, 873.

54. Le, *Anti-Asian Xenophobia*, 1371.

55. Owen, *Health Disparities*, 1905.

56. Russell Jeung, "Incidents of Coronavirus Discrimination March 26–April 1, 2020," https://stopaapihate.org/wp-content/uploads/2021/04/Stop-AAPI-Hate-Report-2Weeks-200403.pdf.

57. Gover, *Anti-Asian Hate Crime*, 647.

58. Tyler T. Reny and Matt A. Barreto, "Xenophobia in the Time of Pandemic: Othering, Anti-Asian Attitudes, and COVID-19," *Politics, Groups, and Identities*, (2020): 1.

59. Leonard Schild, "'Go Eat a Bat, Chang!': On the Emergence of Sinophobic Behavior on Web Communities in the Face of COVID-19," In *Proceedings of the Web Conference* (2021): 1122.

60. Dhanani, *Anti-Asian Attitudes*, 747; Zhang, *Discrimination and Stress*, 1.

61. Rzymski, *COVID-19-Related Prejudice*, 873.

62. Gilbert C. Gee et al., "Racial Discrimination and Health Among Asian Americans: Evidence, Assessment, and Directions for Future Research," *Epidemiologic Reviews* 31, no.1 (2009): 130.

63. Lee, *Racial Discrimination*, 70; Dhanani, *Unexpected Public Health Consequences*, 747; Rzymski, 873.

64. Lillian Comas-Díaz, Gordon Nagayama Hall, and Helen A. Neville, "Racial Trauma: Theory, Research, and Healing: Introduction to the Special Issue," *American Psychologist* 74, no. 1 (2019): 1.

65. Le, 1371; Devon E. Hinton and Baland Jalal, "Dimensions of Culturally Sensitive CBT: Application to Southeast Asian Populations," *American Journal of Orthopsychiatry* 89, no. 4 (2019): 493.

66. Wei-Chin Hwang and Sharon Goto, "The Impact of Perceived Racial Discrimination on the Mental Health of Asian American and Latino College Students," *Cultural Diversity and Ethnic Minority Psychology* 14, no. 4 (2008): 326; Gilbert C., Gee et al., "A Nationwide Study of Discrimination and Chronic Health Conditions Among Asian Americans," *American Journal of Public Health* 97, no. 7 (2007): 1275.

67. Justin A. Chen, Emily Zhang, and Cindy H. Liu, "Potential Impact of COVID-19–Related Racial Discrimination on the Health of Asian Americans," *American Journal of Public Health* 110, no. 11 (2020): 1624; Yao Li and Harvey L Nicholson, "When 'Model Minorities' Become 'Yellow Peril'—Othering and the Racialization of Asian Americans in the COVID-19 Pandemic," *Sociology Compass* 15, no. 2 (2021).

68. Filbin, *Mental Health Data*, n/a; Francis G. Lu, "The Poor Mental Health Care of Asian Americans," *The Western Journal of Medicine* 176, no. 4 (2002): 224.

69. Sylvia L. Mikucki-Enyart and Katheryn C. Maguire, "Introduction to the Special Issue on Family Communication in the COVID-19 Pandemic," *Journal of Family Communication* 21, no. 3 (June 2021): 145.

70. Kimberly K. Walker et al., "Mothers' Sources and Strategies for Managing COVID-19 Uncertainties during the Early Pandemic Months," *Journal of Family Communication* 21, no. 3 (June 2021): 205.

71. Elizabeth Johnson Avery and Sejin Park, "Perceived Knowledge as [Protective] Power: Parents' Protective Efficacy, Information-Seeking, and Scrutiny during COVID-19," *Health Communication* 36, no.1 (2021): 81.

72. Marina Merkaš, Katarina Perić, and Ana Žulec, "Parent Distraction with Technology and Child Social Competence during the COVID-19 Pandemic: The Role of Parental Emotional Stability," *Journal of Family Communication* 21, no. 3 (June 2021), 186.

73. Carla Ickert et al., "Maintaining Resident Social Connections during COVID-19: Considerations for Long-Term Care," *Gerontology and Geriatric Medicine* 6, (October 2020): 1.

74. Anzhela Popyk and Paula Pustułka, "Transnational Communication between Children and Grandparents during the COVID-19 Lockdown: The Case of Migrant Children in Poland," *Journal of Family Communication* 21, no. 3 (June 2021): 223.

75. Hannah E. Jones et al., "Assessing the Effects of COVID-19 on Romantic Relationships and the Coping Strategies Partners Use to Manage the Stress of a Pandemic," *Journal of Family Communication* 21, no. 3 (June 2021): 152.

76. Brian J. Houston, "COVID-19 Communication Ecologies: Using Interpersonal, Organizational, and Mediated Communication Resources to Cope with a Pandemic," *American Behavioral Scientist* 65, no. 7 (February 2021): 887.

77. Mina Choi and Hyesun Choung, "Mediated Communication Matters during the COVID-19 Pandemic: The Use of Interpersonal and Masspersonal Media and Psychological Well-Being," *Journal of Social and Personal Relationships* 1, (July 2021): 1.

78. Jennifer Ihm and Chul-Joo Lee, "Toward More Effective Public Health Interventions during the COVID-19 Pandemic: Suggesting Audience Segmentation Based on Social and Media resources," *Health Communication* 36, no. 1 (2021): 98.

79. Ian Grey et al., "The Role of Perceived Social Support on Depression and Sleep during the COVID-19 Pandemic," *Psychiatry Research* 293, (November 2020): 113452.

80. Emily Charvat et al., "Navigating Pregnancy during the COVID-19 Pandemic: The Role of Social Support in Communicated Narrative Sense-Making," *Journal of Family Communication* 21, no. 3 (June 2021): 167.

81. Galit Nimrod, "Changes in Internet Use when Coping with Stress: Older Adults during the COVID-19 Pandemic," *The American Journal of Geriatric Psychiatry* 28, no. 10 (July 2020): 1020.

82. Samantha Nazione, Evan Perrault, and Kristin Pace, "Impact of Information Exposure on Perceived Risk, Efficacy, and Preventative Behaviors at the Beginning of the COVID-19 Pandemic in the United States," *Health Communication* 36, no. 1 (2021): 23.

83. Gregory Ezeah et al., "Measuring the Effect of Interpersonal Communication on Awareness and Knowledge of COVID-19 among Rural Communities in Eastern Nigeria," *Health Education Research* 35, no. 5 (October 2020): 481.

84. Jennifer M. First et al., "COVID-19 Stress and Depression: Examining Social Media, Traditional Media, and Interpersonal Communication," *Journal of Loss and Trauma* 26, no. 2 (2021): 101.

85. Fangsu Hou et al., "Gender Differences of Depression and Anxiety among Social Media Users during the COVID-19 Outbreak in China: A Cross-Sectional Study," *BMC Public Health* 20, no. 1 (2020): 1648.

86. Lu Tang and Wenxue Zou, "Health Information Consumption under COVID-19 Lockdown: An Interview Study of Residents of Hubei Province, China," *Health Communication* 36, no.1 (2021): 74.

87. Pranav Malhotra, "A Relationship-Centered and Culturally Informed Approach to Studying Misinformation on COVID-19," *Social Media+ Society* 6, no. 3 (July-September 2020): 1.

88. Nguyen, *Changes in Digital Communication*, 1.

89. Center for Disease Control, "Coping with Stress," Retrieved July 16, 2021 from https://www.cdc.gov/coronavirus/2019-ncov/daily-life-coping/managing-stress-anxiety.html

90. Petru Lucian Curşeu et al., "Death Anxiety, Death Reflection and Interpersonal Communication as Predictors of Social Distance towards People Infected with COVID 19," *Current Psychology*, (March 2021): 1.

91. Woo and JunJun, *Racial Discrimination*, 1.

92. Lee, 70.

93. John P. Crowley et al., "Uncertainty Management and Curve Flattening Behaviors in the Wake of COVID-19's First Wave," *Health Communication* 36, no. 1 (2021): 32.

94. Sara Rubinelli et al., "Implications of the Current COVID-19 Pandemic for Communication in Healthcare," *Patient Education and Counseling* 103, no. 6 (June 2020): 1067.

95. Elaine Wittenberg et al., "Opportunities to Improve COVID-19 Provider Communication Resources: A Systematic Review," *Patient Education and Counseling* 104, no. 3 (March 2021): 438.

96. Lucy E. Selman et al., "Bereavement Support on the Frontline of COVID-19: Recommendations for Hospital Clinicians," *Journal of Pain and Symptom Management* 60, no. 2 (August 2020): e81.

97. Nour Mheidly et al., "Effect of Face Masks on Interpersonal Communication during the COVID-19 Pandemic," *Frontiers in Public Health* 8, (December 2020): 898.

98. Nurit Guttman and Eimi Lev, "Ethical Issues in COVID-19 Communication to Mitigate the Pandemic: Dilemmas and Practical Implications," *Health Communication* 36, no. 1 (2021): 116.

99. Robin M. Kowalski and Kelly J. Black, "Protection Motivation and the COVID-19 Virus," *Health Communication* 36, no. 1 (2021): 15.

100. Robert Hornik et al., "Association of COVID-19 Misinformation with Face Mask Wearing and Social Distancing in a Nationally Representative US Sample," *Health Communication* 36, no. 1 (2021): 6.

101. Malhotra, "A Relationship-Centered and Culturally Informed Approach," 1.

102. Nguyen, 1.

103. Amy Henderson Riley et al., "Entertainment-Education Campaigns and COVID-19: How Three Global Organizations Adapted the Health Communication Strategy for Pandemic Response and Takeaways for the Future," *Health Communication* 36, no. 1 (2021): 42.

104. Christine Elers et al., "Negotiating Health amidst COVID-19 Lockdown in Low-Income Communities in Aotearoa New Zealand," *Health Communication* 36, no. 1 (2021): 109.

105. Grey, *Perceived Social Support*, 113452.

Chapter 8

Religious Communication in the Age of COVID-19

Dennis D. Cali

As have many interdisciplinary fields emerging during the digital age,[1] religious communication has risen through the interfaces between established areas of scholarship in advancing new lines of inquiry and teaching. Similar to other transdisciplinary or multidisciplinary areas, religious communication may be regarded as rhizomatic in its investigation of multiple facets of human experience. Writing of media ecology, for instance, Robert MacDougall, Peter Zhang, and Robert K. Logan describe what applies as well to religious communication: attempting to identify a comprehensive framework for such a field is "like urban planning for gypsies."[2] Still, religious communication scholars do attempt such planning, or in the case of this chapter, theorizing, with those who examine such discourse finding useful the definition of the term "religion" proffered by cultural anthropologist and rhetorician Clifford Geertz. In his definition, one notices the prominent placement of "a system of symbols," conferring particular relevance to the field of communication: "A religion is a *system of symbols which acts to establish powerful, pervasive, and long-lasting moods in men* by formulating conceptions of a general order of existence and clothing those conceptions with such an aura of factuality that the moods and motivations seem uniquely realistic."[3] Importantly, implied within that same phrase, "system of symbols," is the notion of *shared* conceptions and *shared* systems, which grounds the notion of religion squarely in the realm of the cultural, where sharing of conceptions occurs. Professors of religious communication thus often frame "religion" in terms of cultural systems. "Religious communication," therefore, is that area of communication that studies those *cultural* systems of symbols that act in function of the actions Geertz has delineated.

As can be seen, religious communication as a subfield within the larger communication discipline is a complex construction; nevertheless, with the above as our starting point, I proceed with this chapter in five key sections. First, I point to significant contributors to the development of the field; second, I outline the key axes of discussion within the field; third, I identify key themes or principles in the field; fourth, I argue that the field of religious communication is particularly relevant to our contemporary pandemic-induced social condition (indeed, as the world has endured the COVID-19 pandemic, the field seems more pertinent than ever as the interplay of religion and popular culture intensified). Finally, I conclude with suggestions for future research and teaching in this area.

PIONEERS IN THE FIELD

The subdiscipline of religious communication can be distinguished by forerunners in the field and through key contributions that anticipate a line of inquiry that we call today "religion and popular culture." According to *The Routledge Companion to Religion and Popular Culture,* one publication that can be considered the early stages of the field because it instantiates the kind of work that today can be placed under the aegis of "religion and popular culture" is Robert L. Short's 1965 publication of *The Gospel According to Peanuts*. That publication uses cartoonist Charles M. Schulz's characters to explain the Christian faith.[4] Sales of more than 10 million copies attest to a popular acceptance of the religion-popular culture marriage. The decade of the 1960s in which Short's book was released is known as a transformative period during which the culture saw dramatic shifts in the conferral of authority. In the Catholic world, for example, the Second Vatican Council gave new prominence to the role of the laity in the affairs of the church. In that same vein, espying "the gospel" in a popular culture form, the cartoon, may mark the genesis of the rise of religion and popular culture as a distinct area of inquiry. Short's book was an early instance of mining "religious" undertones in an artifact of popular culture. In his 2007 essay, "Reflections on the Past and Future of the Study of Religion and Popular Culture," Jeffrey H. Mahan worked both to codify the field extant at that time and to inscribe the *Peanuts* book as a harbinger of the field.[5] And in 2015, editors John C. Lyden and Eric Michael Mazur in the above mentioned *Routledge Companion* brought together scholars to define the field; to identify its methodology; to point to religious encounters with popular culture, material culture, and space; and to illustrate representations of religion in the media, including in that media of non-Western cultures.[6] Attempts such as that of Mahan and Lyden and Mazur at marking the contours of the field also demonstrate its multidisciplinary, multimethodological, and multimedia nature. As in the field of media ecology, born in the last half of the 20th Century, religious communication as a field yields distinct insight while erasing prior disciplinary boundaries. In fact, it may be said that the most novel insights of the field lie at the margins of traditional disciplines and social spheres.

Perhaps greatest insight as to the nature of the field lies in persons whose work is most consulted in the field. One such leader of the field is Jeffrey H. Mahan, co-author along with Bruce David Forbes, of *Religion and Popular Culture in America*.[7] His contributions to the nascent field began during his seminary and graduate school years in the late 1970s and early 1980s, during which time he combined work in religion and society with work being done in his school's film department. His dissertation combined interest in religious studies with interest in detective novels. Working with Forbes, Mahan cofounded the Religion and Popular Culture Group at the American Academy of Religion and co-edited the popular *Religion and Popular Culture* volume. Another key figure in the emerging field is Stewart Hoover. In Hoover's work, one finds a central concern with the confluence of media and religion. In particular, his co-edited volume *Rethinking Media, Religion and Culture* focuses on the intersections of media, culture, and religion.[8] One chapter, for example, explores media and religion in the construction of culture. Another chapter examines the role of media as a site of resacralization of contemporary cultures.[9]

The religion-culture nexus plays out as well in several journals dedicated to the study of religious communication, whether exploring connections between religion and culture in film and in other popular media and in other interpretive communities. *The Journal of Religion and Popular Culture; The Journal of Religion and Film; The Journal of Religious Communication,* and the *Journal of Media and Religion* all locate their investigations at the intersection of religion and culture. One can find this same dialectic in various professional societies (e.g., The International Society for Media, Religion, and Culture; the Religious Communication Association) or divisions and interest groups (e.g, the Religious and Media Interest Group in the Association for Education in Journalism and Mass Communication).

Consistent with the nature of the field as intrinsically multifaceted, my interest in capturing the broad contours of the field is not primarily in religion or in popular culture but precisely in their interplay, the nexus, which is to say in the symbolic expression of religion in culture and of culture in religion. In that vein, I have adopted the framework proposed by Forbes and Mahan of "four relationships between religion and popular culture" in classifying the nature of scholarship conducted in the field.[10] Below I define each of those relationships and highlight studies within each category that illustrate both the category, or "relationship," and, therein, the kind of work carried out in the field.

DIALECTICS IN RELIGIOUS COMMUNICATION

In attempting to frame the multidirectional pursuits in the field of Religion and Popular Culture, I adopt the categories of Forbes and Mahan. Besides structuring their book *Religion and Popular Culture in America*, 3rd edition,[11] these dialectal relations function to capture the entire conspectus of the field at large. Most importantly, they reveal a dynamic tension between the two social spheres of religion and popular culture that is intrinsic to its study.

Religion in Popular Culture

Religious themes, language, imagery, and subject matter are ubiquitous in popular culture. For the past several decades, one could find examples among the super heroes in comic books; in angels such as in the CBS Television's series *Touched by an Angel* and NBC's *Highway to Heaven*; in prayer in sports locker rooms; and in the portrayals of Catholics, Muslims, and Jews in theater, film, novels, and television detective and comedy series, such as Angel Studio's *The Chosen*, Amazon's *The Baker and the Beauty*, and WestWind Picture's *Little Mosque on the Prairie*.

The theme of Religion in Popular Culture is widely exhibited also in family communication studies. There one finds a myriad of studies on how parents listen to their children; on building encouragement; on resolving conflicts; on building and sustaining relationships; on fostering trust, and the like. For example, Colleen Warner Colaner sought to understand the correlation between parents' religious views, in terms of progressive or conservative, and the communication patterns within their respective families.[12] She found that those holding more progressive evangelical views demonstrated more conversation-oriented communication patterns whereas those holding more conservative religious views demonstrated more conformity-oriented communication patterns within their families.

Moreover, one finds abundant publications exploring religion in news media ranging from portrayals of Catholics, evangelicals, protestants, the Amish, and The Church of Latter-day Saints, to the portrayal of religion in general by major news media outlets. Publications such as these are particularly relevant to this category as mass media is a driving force behind the dissemination of popular culture throughout the world. Publications such as these, that examine the representation of religion in the news, offer valuable insights into attitudes and interpretations of religion in popular culture. For instance, in one study Joni Y. Sasaki and Heejung S. Kim explore the nexus of religion and popular culture while investigating how acceptance of and adjustment to difficult situations, or "secondary control," strengthens social relationships in religious communities.[13] Their study compared how European American communities adopt religious perspectives in strengthening personal agency whereas Korean Americans tended to adopt religious perspectives in strengthening social affiliation.

During the period of the Pandemic, the interface of religion in culture concerned the tension between some church officials who countenanced open services and uninterrupted worship and civic authorities imposing strictures to protect public health. Within legal battles between the First Amendment and recommended and mandated safety and health standards of the Centers for Disease Control and the Occupational Safety and Health Administration came the reminder that religion occupies a vital role in popular culture.

Popular Culture in Religion

In this category, I find such scholarly explorations as those concerning the McDonaldization of Church[14] and Meeting Jesus at Starbucks.[15] Studies such as these review how entertainment values of the popular culture might be deployed in "selling Jesus." I also find articles and books that borrow from popular marketing strategies for branding church outreach and for evangelizing. Also found in this category are publications (books and journal articles) on religious themes (e.g., sin and virtue) and slogans in advertising; imagery in advertising; the various modalities of communication (signs, internet, telemarketing, direct mail); the commodification of religion; branding of religion; attitudes and perceptions of religious advertising; and focused studies on Korean, Catholic, and Southern Baptist use of media. One such study is Donald Gene Beehler's "Christian Public Relations Strategies and 'The Last Temptation of Christ.'"[16] In his thesis, Beehler seeks to develop a novel public relations strategy for religious groups to relate with "secular news media." Mara Einstein's *Brands of Faith: Marketing Religion in a Commercial Age*, is another such publication, one in which she describes religion as a "product to be sold."[17] She goes on to give an account of a blend of popular culture and religion as a result of an expansion in religious marketing, citing examples such as Rick Warren, Joel Osteen, and Oprah Winfrey.

When considering popular culture in religion I also find concern for imagery, iconography, graphic design, beauty, and aesthetics of the sacred; signs and symbols, narrative painting; spiritual seeing; paintings and windows; and particular artistic sites (e.g., Notre Dame in Paris) and their windows and painting. Much of the scholarly literature in this area focuses on periods (e.g., 16th Century, Renaissance); on the art of a particular religion (e.g.,

Orthodox, Catholic, Russian Byzantine); or on particular geographic location (e.g., Santa Fe, Ethiopia, the Pacific, Cappadocia). I also see in this category studies of faith expression and faith formation. Some studies in this category focus on particular Biblical scenes or scenes in the life of saints.

The category of Popular Culture in Religion also consists of biographical studies. Here one finds history and ethnographies, lives and especially legacies of saints, profiles of missionaries (including women, African), evangelists, and even TV anchors.

Many of the studies in this category present as handbooks or guidance and, as such, tend to be skills-oriented. One finds various forms of church documents, including handbooks, reviews, literary sources, pastoral instruction and plans, magisterial guidance (e.g., the Vatican's Church and the Internet); and statements (National Council of the Churches of Christ U.S.A). The vast majority of such documents tend to be Vatican documents.

This category includes, also, studies on the incorporation of art, theater, and dance within religious services and liturgies. Such studies examine the performance of religion: how the arts of acting, dancing, and dramatizing might be incorporated into religion to enhance theological understanding and liturgical experience. For example, Katherine J. Frederic[18] makes the case, as does Gordon Graham,[19] for liturgy AS drama while Kurivilla George[20] seeks to recover drama in liturgy. In his dissertation, Matthew S. Farlow examines the theologies of Hans Urs von Balthasar and Karl Barth as a participation in God's drama.[21] Also included in this category are studies of the adoption of cartoons, clip art, graphic novels, and other pictorial forms as genres for expression of faith. Those studies that operate on the more theoretical level explore how the discoveries of communication theory might be utilized in preaching and in evangelizing. Similarly, they undertake to apply mass media theory in promotion of religious values.

Publications describing instances in which the church has adopted various forms of print media also exhibit the theme of Popular Culture in religion. Such publications discuss the way Christian print media outlets "shape an evangelical identity"; take inventory of the goals and values of Christian print media; and the choices associated with editing a Christian magazine. For example, in 2010 Phillis E. Alsdurf examined *Christianity Today Magazine* "as both an ideological tool, and a journalistic enterprise" to understand the magazine's role in the rise of evangelicalism.[22]

During the Pandemic, nowhere was the presence of popular culture in religion more evident than in the adoption of safety recommendations in houses of worship. Added to Muslim hijabs and Catholic mantillas were face masks and shields of a variety of fabrics. And social distancing practices typical at department stores and restaurants during the period of time in which they remained open were seen as well in houses of worship as congregants staggered their placement in pews. Moral debates were waged in social commentary and on social media as people invoked the language of good and evil to assert the righteousness or freedom of being vaccinated or not being vaccinated and to characterize those who took opposing positions often in terms of poorly formed consciences. In these instances, people assumed a deific posture, conferring judgment and assigning penance. The thin veil separating religion and popular culture was thus parted.

Popular Culture as Religion

Many people have described sports as performing a religious function with their rituals, their canonical figures whose statues appear in the stadiums; tailgating as performing a ritualistic and communitarian functions, etc. Disney as American Civil Religion; Elvis as Christ figure, science books as religious texts, and shopping malls as temples for American capitalistic "religion." In the category of Popular Culture AS Religion, we find elements of the Popular Culture, while outwardly secular, to perform a religious function— or to function religiously. Here we find studies of sacred stories and myths; rituals; and other cultural elements that invoke the sacred or that function to promote transcendence, communion, or rites of passage. This category, for example, argues how a playwright can function as a priest and how dance can be experienced as a spiritual practice. Studies along these lines explore a relationship between the body and the sacred ("moving the body to stir the soul," encountering God through dance and movement as sacred practice). Sports studies figure prominently in this category. Many such studies explore the kind of sacredness that sports enthusiasts accord to sports stadiums such as Yankee Stadium or Wrigley Field in Chicago. Such arenas often feature large statues of heroic figures in the respective sports, "canonizing" them as saintly models in the sport.

Such studies also make the case for how certain public spaces achieve religious ends inasmuch as they function as centers of renewal. The shopping mall, for example, is the subject of considerable study on how the arches or solarium or high ceilings mirror sacred temples and gather people around common enterprise. It comes as no surprise, then, that publications discussing new media and social media heavily display the theme of popular culture as religion. One such publication discusses the religious features and function of new media, characterizing it as "a god of sorts." Eleonora Duvivier-Dodds claims that this religion "creates its own paradise and predestination" its own "cosmology that shapes our circumstances" and offers a "destiny in which reality and fiction become one through artifice."[23] Though extremely radical, her claims ultimately point to the many ways new media can act as religion. Publications are concerned with the religious function of social media. For example, one publication discusses the way social media acts as a set apart, or sacred, space. One publication describes blogging as a ritualistic act. Another characterizes digitally connected communities such as Facebook as religious.

Religion and Popular Culture in Dialogue

The dialog, or even dialectic, of religion and popular culture holds the two spheres as separate but puts them in a kind of conversation (e.g., applying religious ethics to some moral dilemma in popular culture or exploring how popular culture might inform a religious perspective). A significant body of literature concerning ethical practice in media and in society at large can be found to illustrate the tension and sometimes the collaboration between the spheres of religion and popular culture. Especially present are studies of ethics within public relations, marketing, and branding. I see this, for instance, in Thomas A. Klein and Gene R. Laczniak's "Applying Catholic Social Teachings to Ethical Issues in Marketing."[24] A major current of such studies considers the ethical implications wrought through technological advancements; for example, Brian Brock explores Christian Ethics in a Technological Age.[25]

Related to ethics considerations in mass media and public life are a swath of studies that undertake a critique of media. They study values that underlie and are sometimes explicitly conveyed in media programming. Such studies include considerations of the value that "efficiency" is accorded in the media. It also includes studies of religious expression within political discourse as well as within portrayals in television programs (e.g., *Dr. Phil*, *South Park*) and through characters cast as "religious." This area of study also examines the secularization of the media and how the sacred is conveyed in postmodernity.

"New Media" also captures the attention of religious communication scholars. They pursue such matters as attitudes toward technology throughout church history, exploring the advantages and disadvantages and the ethical implications of culture conditioned by technology. Religious Communication scholars also take up other such forms of popular culture as tattoos.[26]

Another area of religion and popular culture studies consists of publications discussing questions surrounding biblical translations, religious images, and "ministry" related communication via digital media through the lens of orality v literacy.[27]

The study of "dialogue" between religion and culture extends to radio studies as well, such as in Yoon Kyoung Han's 2002 Mass Communication thesis, entitled *American Public Radio and Christian Radio: Historical Research and Suggestions for CBS in Korea*. In this study, cultural distinction illuminates religious communications.[28]

I have seen it also in rhetorical studies that place religion and popular culture in conversation. Often these explore congruence or conflict. For example, this bibliography entry offered some really interesting publications involving dialogue between Christianity and feminism, homosexuality, and hip-hop. "Identities" seems a central concern of studies in this category. One can see the interdisciplinarity of rhetorical studies here that is reflective of the broader field of religion and popular culture. Such studies investigate discourse, music, and theater as just three areas in which the religion-popular culture nexus is explored.[29] The characteristic that cuts across these somewhat disparate studies is that "religion" and "popular culture" stand not in confluence but as spheres that stand apart from each other and work to bring perspective to each other. Instead of a merger or incorporation of one into the other, one might be the "topic" of the other. "Religion" and "popular culture" are, as such, kept at bay from each other in a dialectic of difference that brings perspective from one to the other.

Where such "dialogue" manifested during the Pandemic was through public stands that religious officials took. Pope Francis, for example, puzzled by the hesitancy of some people in the Church, urged them to get vaccinated. Said the pontiff, "Vaccination is a simple but profound way of promoting the common good and caring for each other, especially the most vulnerable." He called being vaccinated "an act of love."[30] On the other hand, some religious communities resisted getting the vaccine. According to the Pew Research Center, a survey conducted February 16–21, 2021, showed that 45% of white Evangelicals said they would not be vaccinated and that 33% of Black Protestants would not take the jab, either. Complicating our understanding of the matter, Reverend Russell Moore stated that the resistance was due not to religious belief, but rather to distrust among religious people in public services and to the wave of disinformation and misinformation that strains the social fabric.[31]

KEY PRINCIPLES OF THE FIELD

In reviewing the above four categories of scholarship concerning the interface of religion and popular culture—Religion in Popular Culture; Popular Culture in Religion; Popular Culture as Religion; and Religion and Popular Culture in Dialogue—as advanced by Forbes and Mahan, I find four principles to underlie the literature. Although typically not explicitly stated, they form the underpinnings of the emerging discipline. The four principles presented in turn are Communitas, Liminality Hierophany, and Myth. I present them first by way of an overview and then show in the ensuing section how they obtained during the Pandemic.

Communitas

In 1969 Victor Turner explained the close relationship between Communitas and Liminality (which will be covered below).[32] His work is extended in Edith Turner's 2012 work that further explores the relationship.[33] Victor Turner especially refers to a certain esprit de corps that forms among unstructured communities. Where communitas is present, members of the community feel among themselves to be relatively equal. Communitas is manifested in rituals and festivals and similar occasions which reify a community by marking it in space and time. The ritualistic nature of such events, intrinsic to communitas, commemorate what is distinct about the community and shore up the "we-ness" of the community. Where there is communitas, members of the community feel "in the zone," "at-home," and are renewed in their identification with the community. For Edith Turner, "Communitas is togetherness itself."[34] A small community of Italian descent in Southern Louisiana, for example, holds a "Little Italy" festival, where everyone by virtue of their Italian heritage enjoys an equal seat at the table. People can report a feeling of communitas at sports events, at music concerts, and, of course, at religious services. Amidst the stresses of daily life, communitas confers an awareness of being distinctly linked with others. Especially occurring in unstructured conditions, communitas is particularly apparent following tragedies or disasters. In the wake of 9/11, for example, the nation enjoyed a period of unity as people gathered in common grief and support. People can feel communitas as well when a family member or co-worker loses a job or suffers some other defeat. Such a phenomenon endures in communities where acceptance and belonging and a sense of being set apart from the larger community are nurtured.

Communitas as a quality of religious experience suffered the most among religious observers during the Pandemic as people were effectively shut out of their places of worship. Online worship formats lacked the sacred surroundings and the presence of fellow congregants that normally conduce to a spirit of togetherness. Worship was stripped of community, leaving congregants generally in a congregation of themselves.

Liminality

Deriving from the Latin root "limen," or "threshold," such as the space one crosses in passing through a doorway, the term connotes a period of time in which individuals are set apart from a larger community while undergoing a period of discernment and engaging in a process of formation. The person is "not yet" in the community but has also stepped out of the larger community; the period is thus a dark time, a kind of incubation or purgation. An example of this are rites of passage, which have the effect of both humbling the uninitiated and fostering bonds among themselves and with the community in which they seek entrance. Such a period tends to be highly stylized, often invested with religious or spiritual symbolism. "Pledges" to fraternities and sororities on college campuses traverse through this period throughout their pledgeship as they carry out tasks, indicating that they are not yet initiated members. In the religious realm, such rites of passage actually bear the name of "rites." For example, people seeking entrance in the Catholic Church typically engage in a program called the "Rite of Christian Initiation."

Perhaps the strongest of religious dimensions during the Pandemic occurred in the liminal when religious observers were shut out of their religious traditions. Such ritualistic services were interrupted by COVID and observers had not yet returned to the "normalcy" of their religious practice. The more scripted language of religious service eroded into makeshift prayer. One can conjecture that the deprival of ritual may have spurred greater interest in books on transcendence, sacramentality, communion, salvation, and the search for meaning while others likely turned to diversions such as TV binge-watching and video-game playing.

Hierophany

A third principle that often characterizes a certain quality described in the literature of religion and popular culture is hierophany. Of Greek origin, consisting of "hiero," meaning "sacred" and "phainein," meaning "to show," the concept refers to the manifestation of the sacred. Like the quality of communitas that is felt, hierophany indicates a space set apart from the ordinary world in which one's gaze is directed toward a focal point. One experiences hierophany upon entering a grand cathedral or temple as light beams through stain glass windows darkened by years of incense. One might experience it as well in touring the remains of some historic or tragic site. Hierophany is a sensorial phenomenon that engenders a mode of consciousness. As a religious experience, one's attention is directed toward the transcendent, and one feels oneself to be a part of a grand design and to be firmly inserted into a larger community. In the secular realm, one might experience it in baseball bleachers while smelling fresh cut grass and hearing the crack of a bat or looking up at statues of sports legends in an historic stadium. Shopping malls, too, contain elements that would engender a sort of hierophany: water fountains, vegetation, arches and expansive doors, music. All would center patrons and insert them in local but cosmic experience.

In place of arched doorways and stained glass windows, religious observers were left to invent their own sacred spaces. Although some may have on occasion lit a candle or gathered in a family circle, when houses of worship were closed, most religious observers were left either without formal religious observance or became tethered to their electronic devices in search of a televised service or inspirational message. Space acquired a new salience through the absence of physical markers of holiness.

Myth

Binding all such qualities in religious experiences, or in experiences that function religiously but are otherwise secular, are implicit or explicit narratives about the sacred and humanity's relationship to the sacred. Such narratives often present as myths. In the literature of religion and popular culture, "myth" does not mean untrue. In fact, it may be more accurate to say that myths express deeper truths or more transcendent truths that strain beyond human grasp through merely empirical means. Some myths are psychological in nature. Joseph Campbell's monomyth, for example, expresses persons' inner struggle to be fully integrated. Other myths orient cultures' perception of time—historically or cyclically, for example. But a common function of myth is to forge a relationship between the lived immanent reality and a religious worldview that contains elements of creation, transformation, redemption, and the after-life and guide people in the basic human experiences of love, sex, pain, death, and the like. Judeo-Christian religion, for example, re-enacts the myth of Exodus at the Passover or the death and resurrection of Jesus during Easter.

Throughout the Pandemic, the narratives of religious stories that supported rituals, theology, and ethics were overshadowed by myths of another sort: those launched to discredit public officials, to assign fault for the spread of COVID, to discount or to tout medical cures, and the like. In place of stories of supernatural beings and events to which religious observers typically looked to reinforce their beliefs, other myths asserting false ideas, beliefs, and conspiracies acquired greater salience. I noticed this, especially, in the demonizing of Anthony Fauci, director of the National Institute of Allergy and Infectious Diseases and the Chief Medical Advisor to the President. In a transformation of the American culture's Judeo-Christian mythos, Fauci morphed from the nation's exalted chief medical counselor to alleged Congressional perjurer. Even the Centers for Disease Control acquired the role of agent of deception as critics cried foul on the shifting definition of "vaccine." The nation's narrative of salvation from sin gave way to the morality play of protection from COVID.

POPULAR PANDEMIC CULTURE IN RELIGION AND RELIGION IN POPULAR PANDEMIC CULTURE

Drawing upon the four themes of religious communication proposed above, I turn now to reflections on what this area of the field might offer the larger community racked with the disruptions of the COVID pandemic. These principles help to identify societal response to the Pandemic and suggest ways for healthy coping.

Communitas

At the core of the notion of communitas is a sense of connection. As schools, churches, restaurants, and other businesses were forced to shut down, everyone turned increasingly to online connection. Whether through Learning Management Systems such as Blackboard or Canvas; through live streams of church services; or online food ordering, people took to the Internet in a quick shift to digital connection.

And yet, what was the nature of that connection? Did we grow to understand one another better? Did our relationships become stronger? Did our organizations enjoy a healthier esprit de corps? If we are honest with ourselves, I think we would, in most cases, have to answer "No." Speaking from my own experience, I felt like a drone hovering over the various church sites that presented the Catholic mass through live stream. I was in some weeks at the Casa Santa Maria, where Pope Francis celebrated mass with English translation by an American nun; at other weeks at the Basilica of the National Shrine of Elizabeth Ann Seton; and at other times at random places across the country. And while the "pilgrimage" across these various church sites held a certain exotic appeal, one factor stood out in my religious experience: I participated in the mass alone.

In this regard, the very collective nature of the worship experience was undercut. Gone was the orchestral sitting, standing, kneeling, and standing again postures that united congregants like dancers in a Broadway musical. Gone was the proximity of the usher with the limp or the widow with too-strong perfume who placed me in the company of familiars, of family. Gone was the procession to the altar that lined up worshipers in unison.

Religious communication helps us to understand that communitas suffered as a result of virtual church. And what was lost in the explicitly religious realm was lost as well in the quasi-religious (i.e., in other social spheres were a sense of *we*-ness grounds the experience). If we view the college experience as the quasi-religious, we can look at the transition to online education as an example. So, prepandemic, in a classroom, I could spot someone who was down or notice that someone was absent in online course delivery. During the Pandemic, with online the medium of instruction, I could detect a student's state of being only through inference and indirectly. I learned, for example, that some students act out their anxiety by withdrawing—something I discovered only after a series of missed assignments—while others went into overdrive and harangued me with an avalanche of emails. But this was not a communal experience. It was, in fact, the undoing of community. And one does not need results of a Pew study that examined the effects of the lockdown to recognize the mental and emotional toll it took on people. Each of us probably knows more than one person, particularly students,[35] who demonstrated increased anxiety, fatigue, and loneliness—qualities not felt when communitas reigns.

But beyond helping us to recognize what suffered during the lockdown, religious communication and the studies of religion and popular culture can also point us to areas where communitas might be restored or at least sustained during periods of social disintegration. What we learn from the literature of religious communication are the essentials of what unites people. So , for example, we reframe our online communication from the conceptualization of it as messages tapped out on a keyboard to an act of connection. We foreground the person(s) at the other end of the communication line (as well as those with whom we live). We attend to the affordances of the Learning Management System and plan, for example, to see each other, synchronously when possible, to establish a more holistic connection. And we look to create something of an environment conducive to interaction and community.

Liminality

The period of suspense began as we waited to see how the schools and houses of worship and public spaces might operate and has run until the period continuing today, as we wonder how closely we should sit next to someone or worry about the person who just coughed next to me, is nothing if not a period of liminality. This anxious period of waiting, of uncertainty, held us between the routine of the pre-pandemic and the not-yet-known condition of post-pandemic. It was a period in which most of us lost our moorings or at least found our moorings shaken.

Among many discomfiting situations that we encountered during this liminal period of the Pandemic was the dissolution between "home" and "work" life. In my case, my home study is virtually adjacent to the kitchen, separated by only a short hallway. Within the same period of day, I could be recording a lecture and returning to the fridge. Similarly, I could don a dress shirt and tie for camera viewing while wearing my moisture-wicking gym shorts. While many might laud the comfort and conveniences of our more relaxed working conditions, they thrust us into a Dionysian mode of existence, disrupting the more rational and structured regimen that had accorded our life some Apollonian scaffolding. Pushing this further, one could make the case that the absence of the more ordered routines of our work life plunged us into a kind of hell—a hell of not yet being within the workplace, religious, or other civic community of which we were a member. I remember a wise spiritual director saying of such transitional periods that they were the loneliest period in all of human experience because we are neither where we were before or where we will be later but are, instead, in a very real sense, "in the middle of nowhere."

What the literature of religious communication, and that of religion and popular culture, teaches us about communitas can offer guideposts in traversing this threshold period. We learn from the absence of what fosters communitas what liminality lacks. And this can suggest to us steps we might take to engender some of these qualities in this period between one thing and another. We could point, for example, to productive and restorative activities that many took up (or returned to) while waiting for life to return to "normal." Many, for instance, reported spending more time in their gardens, taking more walks, cooking up meals from scratch, playing more with their children or pets.

Such provided instances of connectivity—with the earth, with nature, with their bodies, with their environment. And many were, in fact, able to reconnect with friends set "out of sight" by the demands of location-based jobs. In other words, religious communication gives us the language for describing means of productive and creative adjustment to the pangs of being shut out of environments where communitas might more easily be fostered.

Hierophany

The physical manifestation of the sacred occurred on two fronts during the Pandemic. We experienced it in its withdrawal from our access. Unable to gaze upon stained glass windows, arched walkways, assembly of people, and other signs and symbols of the sacred had the effect of increasing our consciousness of them. They loomed larger in our inability to draw close to them; and we missed them. Katia Rubio lamented the loss of the ritualistic dimension of the 2020 Tokyo edition of the Olympic Games, the rich symbolism in the fields of competition that confers on them a certain sacredness, when those games were suspended because of the COVID-19 pandemic.[36] The lines of procession as the games began, the arenas that enclosed the events, and the platforms where flags were raised all functioned as ritualistic sites that imparted a certain sacred quality to the Olympics but were missing from public consciousness when the Tokyo games were canceled.

At the same time, kept out of places we had frequented, during the Pandemic, we were afforded more time to "smell the roses": to encounter hierophany on another front. We could notice the light glistening on the lake, the tree leaves changing colors, the playfulness of our pets. In other words, we became more aware of how the line of trees formed cathedralic steeples. We saw something sacred even in the slowing down of time, the lingering, entailed in talking with our significant others. We also became more aware of the suffering of loved ones, those suffering loss of income from layoffs and shutdowns. We saw it, also, in friends and relatives unable to receive guests and left alone to their cells. During the Pandemic, many adapted ritualized customs to their natural and domestic environment. The ritualized homily or sermon was often live streamed, turning one's computer screen into sacred site. For others, tailgates served as sacred site as people who had ritualistically watched films at movie theaters began to view them, instead, from their vehicles. Still others created new family rituals such as playing board games, engendering a hierophany out of a table top.[37] Many of us have witnessed the drive-by birthday party or graduation ceremony in which cars drove past the home of the person being celebrated and either honked their horns or bellowed "Happy birthday" or "Congratulations." Each of these was an effect to recover a sacred space that had been shut down by COVID closures.

Such awareness awakened in us the presence of the divine outside the hollowed structures of religion. While religious observers longed to return to their houses of worship, a different manifestation of the sacred caught us by surprise. The walls of worship were thus extended.

Religious communication equips us to discover how the sacred presents itself ubiquitously. We learn to find hierophany in a garden, in a conversation, in a song, in a gathering of friends. Such awareness does not require enrollment in a Religious Communication class, of course, but to the extent that all education in the humanities and liberal arts aims to liberate the human spirit, to equip students to make meaning of their experience, a course in Religious Communication can go a long way in that very liberation, particularly needed during the period of heightened anxiety or malaise occasioned by the Pandemic. It can point students to areas of life where their spirits might be elevated, where they achieve communion with their environment and with their creator and one another.

Myth

A common lamentation of social commentators is the loss of a "grand narrative." The notion of "shared" system, (in Western society most prominently lived out in Abrahamic religions and, in general, in "the American way"), has splintered in modern society. The Pandemic exacerbated the erosion of the shared narrative as attention was directed toward concern about religious freedom and the right to assemble. When religious figures spoke on the issue of lockdowns, they often pitted their position against civil authorities, sometimes assigning malicious motive to public leaders. As the Pandemic wore on and continues still, polarization on other issues wielded further damage to a shared narrative and gave way to conspiracy theories and to variations on apocalyptic myths.

The absence of a shared grand narrative during the Pandemic left the culture without a centralized moral act around which to coalesce. There were no state funerals as the nation had when television covered the burial ritual of President John F. Kennedy; no Aeschylus-like figure to transform the pain of tragedy into a rallying cry, as President Ronald Reagan did in his famous eulogy of Challenger space shuttle astronauts in speaking of them as "'slip[ping] the surly bonds of earth' to touch the face of God"; no national leader to register the nation's pain as President George W. Bush did at Ground Zero a few days following the September 11, 2001, terrorist attacks in shouting through a bullhorn, "I can hear you." Beyond the absence of such ritualized mythos, our national institutions promoted a veritable retreat into our individual silos as we were told to practice social distance and to quarantine. And with this isolation came heightened anxiety, distress, sadness, and loneliness.[38]

Commentators have begun to consider how the social fabric might be rewoven. Sociologist Eric Klinenberg has sought to combat the isolation that resulted from lockdowns and social distancing by calling people to "knock on our neighbor's door," in promoting "civic bonds and collective sacrifice."[39] Such pursuits seek to restore a grand narrative, a national mythos, to rescue the culture from the social isolation wrought by COVID-19.

Religious Communication can help to establish the role of grand narratives in the preservation of culture as well as how those narratives evolve and even erode. And as students contemplate the story underlying cultural experience, they come to understand the inextricable connection between culture and religion. Many consulted Greek mythology for guidance on coping with the strains imposed by COVID-19. A theater company, for example, sought to bring catharsis to the traumatized culture through its performance of Greek tragedy.[40]

SUGGESTIONS FOR FUTURE RESEARCH AND TEACHING

While causing tremendous disruption across multiple spheres of our society, the Pandemic also unveiled the centrality of religion in American culture.

Facets of cultural experience that are religious in nature became more prominent partly through their absence as houses of worship and religious practices were curtailed. "Religion," then, came to be seen as fundamental to human experience. I believe what we have seen offers even greater reason for a course in Religious Communication to be incorporated into Communication Studies curricula, and there are multiple reasons: It could help us to understand better the importance of the synodal sense of togetherness. It could help us grasp the interconnectedness of religion and popular culture. It could help us expand our sense of the sacred both in designated religious places and in more surprising sacred spaces. Such a course would include in its scope sacred "media" of all sorts: cathedrals, shopping malls, film, novels, sports, and other pop-cultural sites where the sacred is manifest.

A course in religious communication during a lockdown might thus direct students in discovering elements of religious experience in new locations. In my own family, for example, we adopted a "reading hour" each evening as a time for pausing and coming together. Others took advantage of the extra at-home time to take walks around the neighborhood. A course in religious communication could lead students in discovering systems of shared moments of community, sacredness, and belief within spheres of existence that lie outside of the traditional houses of worship. Students could also explore how communitas might be experienced when the community is non-institutional as they examine the formation of new rituals or return to previously abandoned ones. Likewise, liminality acquires new tonality when all members of a group are thrust into a period of "time out of time" as people simultaneously wait to return to "normalcy" while also establishing new ways of being and working (e.g., conducting more work from home; taking more classes online; communicating more via video platforms such as Skype, Zoom, and Google Meet). In other words, professors can take advantage of lockdowns imposed by the Pandemic to help students discover sacrality in the secular.

On the scholarly front, the Pandemic has invited researchers to investigate how the activities overlapping religion and culture might better withstand the perils of such wide-scale disturbance. Future research could scrutinize sectors of society that were able to preserve communitas for insight into engendering it. Likewise, they could investigate the conditions that imperil it when a biological phenomenon grips society. Another area to investigate could be to explore what happens to people when their religious and other traditions and practices are disturbed with a view toward optimizing the liminal period. And further analysis could be turned in pursuit of understanding better what inclines people toward the sacred, and how they recognize in otherwise prosaic events qualities that incline toward the sacrosanct.

More focused study could center around the four principles of the field discussed above. The notion of communitas seems particularly crucial to study in the face of intensifying divisiveness in our culture. If religious communities, where communitas might be expected to thrive, have their public services curtailed, or if formal religious practice begins to wane, scholars would make a valuable contribution to the literature if they could point us to new areas in which communitas might be experienced. In the educational sphere, for example, scholars could examine how the sense of community normally established in face-to-face formats might be engendered in online course delivery. Scholars might also study how the sense of isolation occasioned by the lockdowns might be overcome, at least partially, through participation in online video presentations, such as cooking videos, in which the person(s) conducting the cooking demonstration interacts with viewers. Scholars might also study what happens to the sense of communitas when individuals who had been kept away from their places of worship return to those places: does communitas pick up where it left off? Is it unrecoverable? Does it return stronger from having been temporarily withheld?

Also in the area of liminality, scholars see in the lockdowns a new kind of transition period. Unlike a typical rite of passage in which one generally volunteers to take part, what happens when the state of transition is imposed from government mandates? Are the qualities that people undergo different in this kind of liminality? Likewise, in the in-between period of lockdowns, does the religious impulse percolate from within as people invent their own rituals to supplement those in which they had engaged or do they sink into a kind of despair in the absence of formalized rites of passage? Another potential fruitful area of study of liminality could be the exploration of how the liminal space of lockdown served to stimulate activity as it provided a pause from routine. In what way can liminality bring light to the banal, to the everyday spaces and activities that had been part of the convention? Our understanding of the value of pausing, of lingering, of hovering could be enriched as scholars come to understand better the "religious" function they perform as a kind of "sabbath" from the technologized rat race.

Another possible area of inquiry could be the pursuit of the experience of hierophany. Communication scholars might examine how cultures change as they move from religiously oriented to primarily secular. The demise of traditional religion has coincided with the rise of cult-like commitment to "wokeness," which functions as a kind of substitute for hierophany. People adopt new value systems of intersectionality, gender fluidity, and critical race theory as sites of morality. What these progressive values point to, however, are abstractions; they are "social" causes that manifest locally only in protests, which are often raucous and destructive. In the face of these emergent values, communication scholars urgently need to search out new sacred sites that offer people the opportunity to transcend the ephemeral concerns of a wounded culture. Alongside churches, synagogues, and mosques, communication scholars could point to other natural landmarks of sacrality. Besides natural sites such as hills and trees and rocks that are part of creation, communication scholars could explore how cultural sites function religiously. Such sites could include sports stadiums such as Lambeau Field in Green Bay, Wisconsin, or entertainment sites such as the Grand Ole Opry in Nashville, Tennessee, or "intentional" communities such as "Love Valley" in North Carolina as well as film, music, and print cultural discursive forms. Communication scholars can find in such spaces a religious impulse that tends toward community, that turns on ritual, that exhibits traditions embodying values, and communication scholars can mine such sites to illuminate how religious experience is conferred symbolically. At the same time, the highly symbolic nature of traditional religious sites could also be recovered through new information on the history and geographical contexts of these sacred sites. In other words, bringing context to traditional religious sites could enrich understanding of how sacred sites are situated.[41]

Finally, myths might also be profitably studied to enhance our understanding of how cultures adapt to ruptures in society wrought not only through lockdowns but also through the large-scale changes that media carry with them. Restoring grand narratives could contribute substantially to a sense of community, continuity, and hopefulness. In this regard, rituals can play an important role. As Byung-Chul Han observes, "Rituals give form to the essential transitions in life."[42] As rituals such as funerals and weddings and attendance at religious services were disrupted during the Pandemic, people were for a time without the mediating function that myths and rituals perform between the vicissitudes of lived experience and enduring values. Scholars would contribute substantially to a world torn asunder by the Pandemic and by other decentralizing forces of media by exploring ways in which people can achieve a "sacred silence" in the midst of a fast-changing world. We know that people seek to fill the void that shared ritualistic activities perform as manifest in "binge-watching" television series and in addictive tendencies in playing video games. In this regard, scholars could investigate residual forms of grand narratives and new myths that emerge when people are deprived of rituals to which they had become accustomed. More importantly, scholars would be advised to study the narcissistic tendencies that behaviors such as binge-watching promote inasmuch as they center a person on individual media consumption and to investigate activities that promote shared experience, transcendent narratives, and those in which joint ritualized gestures foster a common good instead of the more inward activities in which individual identity is foregrounded. The study of myths is necessary to combat the compulsion to manage highly individualized identities and to restore a sense of community that is compromised through individualistic identity management.

Religion in American has faced strong headwinds in recent history. The proliferation of technology has militated against communal experiences such as religious rituals as it has promoted more customized and individualized behavior in using our electronic devices. And yet, it is precisely this dismemberment of community that calls for study of how shared symbols and values might be recovered. The massive disruptions wrought by COVID-19 dealt another strong blow to religious experience, and yet aroused at the same time an appetite for that which confers meaning in human experience, found both within religious institutions that endure as well as those that might be experienced within ordinary spaces not otherwise thought of as "religious."

Through this chapter I have sought to mine explorations of religious communication. In doing so, I have made reference to the plethora of studies within the field of communication. Certainly one can see how "religion" is salient within various spheres of the field, ranging from rhetoric to mass communication; as such, it merits prominent placement in communication curricula. We can see the complexity of such educational explorations of religious communication especially in the dialectics or axes of investigation between "religion" and "popular culture." Thus, as communication scholars undertake to design courses in religious communication or to chart new areas of scholarly inquiry, they are advised to remain mindful of the tensions between those two axes and to navigate those tensions with a view toward deepening our understanding of the religious impulse that lies within us all. The field of communication is uniquely equipped to illuminate those impulses and thus to contribute to our understanding of the human experience.

NOTES

1. For example, genomics, media ecology, biomedical informatics, and human resource development.

2. In Robert C. MacDougall, Peter Zhang, and Robert K. Logan. "Preface: Probing the Boundaries of Media Ecology," *Explorations in Media Ecology* 12, Nos. 3 & 4, (December, 2013):155.

3. Clifford Geertz, *Religion as a Cultural System* (London: Tavistock, 1966), 4. Emphasis mine.

4. Robert L. Short, *The Gospel According to Peanuts* (Louisville, KY: Westminster John Knox Press, 1965).

5. Jeffrey H. Mahan, "Reflections on the Past and Future of the Study of Religion and Popular Culture," in *Between Sacred and Profane: Researching Religion and Popular Culture*, ed. Gordon Lynch (London: I.B.Tauris & Co Ltd., 2007), 47–62.

6. John Lyden, and Eric Michael Mazur, eds., *The Routledge Companion to Religion and Popular Culture* (New York City, NY: Routledge, 2015).

7. Bruce David Forbes and Jeffrey H. Mahon, *Religion and Popular Culture in America*, 3rd ed, (Oakland, CA: University of California Press, 2017).

8. Stewart Hoover and Knut Lundby, eds, *Rethinking Media, Religion, and Culture* (Thousand Oaks, CA: SAGE Publications, Inc., 1997).

9. Stewart also heads the Center for Media, Religion and Culture (https://www.colorado.edu/cmrc/research). The Center's website offers a bibliography of key sources within a period of 2004–2014 related to the field, many of which are authored by Stewart himself. Steward Hoover maintains a website of "related links" on the navigation bar of "Stewart's Archives." The URL to Stewart's archives is https://www.colorado.edu/cmrc/resources/related-links.

10. Forbes and Mahon, *Religion and Popular Culture*.

11. Ibid.

12. Colleen Warner Colaner, "Exploring the Communication of Evangelical Families: The Association Between Evangelical Gender Role Ideology and Family Communication Patterns," *Communication Studies* 60, no.2 (April 2009):97–113,

13. Joni Y. Sasaki and Heejung S. Kim, "At the intersection of culture and religion: a cultural analysis of religion's implications for secondary control and social affiliation" *Journal of Personal and Social Psychology* 101, no. 2 (December 2010):401–414.

14. John Drane, *The McDonaldization of the Church: Consumer Culture and the Church's Future* (Smyth & Helwys: Macon, GA, 2001).

15. J. Patrick Vaughn, *Meeting Jesus at Starbucks: Good news from those done with church.* (Pinnacle Leadership Press: Chapin, SC, 2018).

16. Donald Gene Beehler, "Christian public relations strategies and 'The Last Temptation of Christ': A case study," M.A. thesis, California State University, San Bernardino, 1990.

17. Einstein, Mara. *Brands of faith: Marketing religion in a commercial age.* (New York: Routledge), 2007.

18. Katherine J. Frederic, *Acting on faith: the dramatization of Christian liturgy.* [s.n.], 2002.

19. Gordon Graham, (2007). "Liturgy as Drama." *Theology Today*, 64, no. 1 (April 1, 2007): 71–79.

20. Kurivilla George. *From people's theater to people's eucharist: recovering the drama of Christian worship.* (Delhi, India: ISPCK), 2002.

21. Farlow, M. S., & St. Mary's College (Scotland). Institute for Theology, I. and the A. (2011). *The dramatising of theology: humanity's participation in God's drama with particular reference to the theologies of Hans Urs von Balthasar and Karl Barth.* http://hdl.handle.net/10023/2102 (Ph.D. Diss., University of St. Andrews, November 30, 2011).

22. Phyllis E. Alsdurf, "The Founding of Christianity Today Magazine and the Construction of An American Evangelical Identity," *Journal of Religious & Theological Information* 9, nos. 1–2 (2010):20–43

23. Eleonora Duvivier-Dodds, *The spectacled angel: the religion of technology (*New York City: NY: Vantage Press 1996): 10.

24. Thomas A. Klein and Gene R. Laczniak. "Applying Catholic social teachings to ethical issues in marketing." E-poublications@Marquette, 2009, https://epublications.marquette.edu/cgi/viewcontent.cgi?referer=&httpsredir=1&article=1027&context=market_fac

25. Brian Brock. *Christian ethics in a technological age.* (William B. Eerdmans Publishing Company: Grand Rapids, Michigan) 2010.

26. See, for example, M. Firmin, ML. M. Tse, J. Foster, & T/ Angelini, Christian student perceptions of body tattoos: a qualitative analysis. *Journal of Psychology and Christianity,* 27, no.3 (2008):195–204; D. Jasper, *The sacred body: asceticism in religion, literature, art and culture* (Waco, TX: Baylor University Press, 2009); and J. A. Rush, *Spiritual tattoo: a cultural history of tattooing, piercing, scarification, branding, and implants* (Berkeley, CA: Frog Books, 2005).

27. Chávez, K. R. "Beyond Complicity: Coherence, Queer Theory, and the Rhetoric of the 'Gay Christian Movement.'" *Text & Performance Quarterly,* 24, nos. 3 and 4 (2004): 255–275. https://doi.org/10.1080/1046293042000312760

28. Yoon Kyoung Han, "American public radio and Christian radio: historical research and suggestions for CBS in Korea" (Ph.D. diss., University of Wisconsin-Milwaukee, Fall 2002).

29. Browne, G. H. (1993). Feminist Rhetoric and Christological Discourse: Conflict or Conversion. https://www.euro-book.net/book/tw9hNwAACAAJ/feminist-rhetoric-and-christological-discourse

30. Associated Press, "In A Message To Americans, Pope Francis Says Getting Vaccinated Is 'An Act Of Love,'" *NPR,* August, 18, 2021, https://www.npr.org/sections/coronavirus-live-updates/2021/08/18/1028740057/in-a-message-to-americans-pope-francis-says-getting-vaccinated-is-an-act-of-love

31. Adelle M. Banks, "Russell Moore: Sickness, death from COVID-19 likely reducing some vaccine hesitancy," *Religious News Service,* August 10, 2021, https://religionnews.com/2021/08/10/russell-moore-sickness-death-from-covid-19-likely-reducing-some-vaccine-hesitancy/

32. Victor Turner, *The Ritual Process: Structure and Anti-Structure.* (New York: Routledge, 1969).

33. Edith Turner, *Communitas: The Anthropology of Collective Joy.* (New York: Palgrave Macmillan, 2012).

34. Edith Turner, 4.

35. See, for instance, Edward Lempinen, "Student depression, anxiety soaring during pandemic, new survey finds," *Berkeley News,* August 18, 2020, https://news.berkeley.edu/story_jump/student-depression-anxiety-soaring-during-pandemic-new-survey-finds/

36. Katia Rubio. "The Olympic games as hierophany: Rite and ritual, a tradition, more than a championship." *Olympianos, Journal of Olympic Studies,* 24, no. 40, http://olimpianos.com.br/journal/index.php/Olimpianos/article/view/99/65

37. NPR. The Coronavirus crisis, PHOTOS: How the world is reinventing rituals. September 19, 2020, https://www.npr.org/sections/goatsandsoda/2020/09/19/909275936/photos-how-the-world-is-reinventing-rituals

38. Sloane Shearman. The Mythos of Pandemic. March 30, 2020. Erraticus.com., https://erraticus.co/2020/03/30/mythos-pandemic-coronavirus-kennedy-onassis/

39. Ezra Klein, "What social solidarity demands of us in a pandemic," *Vox*(April 3, 2020). https://www.vox.com/podcasts/2020/4/3/21204412/coronavirus-covid-19-pandemic-social-distancing-social-solidarity-the-ezra-klein-show

40. Elif Batuman. "Can Greek tragedy get us through the pandemic?" *The New Yorker,* September 1, 2020, https://www.newyorker.com/culture/culture-desk/can-greek-tragedy-get-us-through-the-pandemic

41. See, for example, the study of pilgrimages to the Monastery of Aostolos Andreas (Cyprus) in Evgenia Mesaritou. Non-"Religious" Knowing in Pilgrimages to Sacred Sites. *The New Yorker* 1, no. 1 (nd):105–133, https://www.berghahnjournals.com/view/journals/journeys/21/1/jy210106.xml

42. Buyng-Chul Han, *The disappearance of rituals.* (Polity Press: Medford, MA) 2020.

Chapter 9

"Saturday Nite Is Dead" at Least for a While

Changes in Popular Culture Theory during a Time of Crisis

David Nelson and Kimberly Kulovitz

When members of the public think about popular culture, they usually reference music, memes, videos, fashion, food, etc. Popular culture studies is a broad field in scope, and it can be challenging to define as it is applied across several disciplines. For example, John Storey[1] reflects on several scholars' thoughts regarding defining popular cultures and suggests embracing popularity, high culture, cultural products, authenticity, and postmodernism. All of this contributes to trying to define popular culture as a formidable task. As Tony Bennett stated, "the concept of popular culture is virtually useless, a melting pot of confused and contradictory meanings capable of misdirecting inquiry up any number of theoretical blind alleys."[2] Others have also made similar observations. For example, Marcel Danesi also addresses the difficulties of creating a definition or explaining popular culture since it has so many divisions and categories.[3] Ray Browne stated that any attempt to define popular culture is a futile task for scholars to agree upon, but instead, popular culture is a broad assumed experience.[4] John Fiske views "popular culture is not consumption, it is the active process of generating and circulating meanings and pleasures within a social system."[5] Multiple factors influence trying to define what popular culture is.

Popular culture is difficult to define because it crosses various academic disciplines, cultures, quantitative and qualitative values, influences, and experiences scholars have. Additionally, those who look to attach a meaning to popular culture are informed through critical perspectives of their fields of study. Storey makes the point that popular culture can be viewed as "an empty conceptual category, one that can be filled in a wide variety of often conflicting ways, depending on the context of use."[6] When establishing what popular culture is, what metrics must be considered? Is it time, technology, or gatekeepers/those who are in power? We will not attempt to define popular culture because that would be an arduous charge, but instead, we look at what informs how popular culture is defined as the lens through which popular culture is viewed.

As a field of study, popular culture is by its nature transdisciplinary and has found a home in several academic areas such as math, geology, communication, sociology, anthropology, and economics. We argue that the popular culture theories are still relevant, no matter their field, but that society has dramatically changed. The change affects how popular culture studies are taught, how research is conducted, and how it is consumed, used, and created. These alterations will have short and long-term effects to the lenses used in examining popular culture. With this in mind, we proceed by covering five main sections: Theoretical Views of Popular Culture; Defining the COVID Bubble; Pop Culture, COVID, and Research; Pop Culture, COVID, and the Classroom; and Predictions for the Future of Popular Culture Research and Teaching.

THEORETICAL VIEWS OF POPULAR CULTURE

To examine how COVID-19 impacts popular culture theory, we explore how it has altered some theoretical lenses used when viewing, creating, and researching popular culture. The lens creates a researcher's foundation for any arguments or new knowledge. Perspectives used to address those lenses could include time, gender, technology, geography, economics, and field of study. Lenses can be specific and narrow, but COVID-19 has created an omnipresent influence that affects everyone, particularly popular culture. To explore this, we discuss in broad strokes how the popular lens culture is impacted by the COVID-19 pandemic while concomitantly arguing popular culture is not shaped by definition but through individual lenses.

Our particular research areas, thus the lenses through which we view popular culture and pandemic interaction, include humor, video games, and social media; changes in theories within those areas of popular culture do not represent all changes within popular culture theory. The lens through which theory is viewed and based on ontological and epistemological practices guides a researcher's field and how problems are explored and collected. Therefore, it is crucial that we define what we mean when the term lens is used. Doing so will help understand the impact that a lens brings to popular culture theory on what needs to be considered. At the time of writing this, and due to world events, we are entering a new cycle that will change explanations, frontiers, and opportunities for generating new knowledge and how it is identified.

A lens can be defined as how a topic is viewed. It provides a carefully chosen standpoint to outline and profile a moment or effect of examining. Fred Niderman and Salvatore March argue that a lens is a tool for mapping to help create and structure theory to help transform, target a province, and add purpose to a theory.[7] In short, a lens provides the foundation that guides the framework for theory to support authors' application of their thinking. The lens helps guide not theory but the questions researchers wish to ask about popular culture and theory. COVID has changed how we use and create popular culture, explicitly impacting how scholars approach pop culture and how instructors integrate pop culture in the classroom. Simultaneously, there has been an abrupt shift in how we respond to pop culture. Internet and mobile technologies have altered where people find information during times of crisis, such as how people consume music, where audiences discuss politics, or where they obtain the latest fashion trends. Any shift in technology where new mediums alter modes of communication creates disruption. For example, in contrast to previously waiting for a specific time and day to watch or record a show, streaming services such as Netflix and Amazon Prime transformed how audiences consumed movies and television with the ability to watch a show on-demand or to even binge-watch a whole season without waiting. Although prepandemic, it is essential to consider whether such shifts will be permanent or revert to old habits.

Certainly, the pandemic has broadened our perspective of what should be considered pop culture and how pop culture communities will interact in the future. Regardless of whether the COVID Bubble (defined more fully in a separate section below) will break, as the field of popular culture advances, several considerations need to be acknowledged when examining how the COVID Bubble could affect it. In simple terms, we can define the COVID Bubble as the window of time that has created a disruption and restrictions for the workplace, economic activities, communication between people, and entertainment for society and individuals during the COVID-19 pandemic. Scholars should reflect on how times of crisis such as 9/11, the great depression, wars, and so on have created disruptions in popular culture. Times of crisis help fashion lenses to address these shifts within a theory. Researchers need to consider the theory that defines the situation and the time and place being examined.

According to Ward Goodenough, culture has organized experiences that in turn become societal lenses and set the standards that become the society lens.[8] Those standards established by a culture help shape popular culture that becomes the lens through which researchers work. This can be viewed in how technology is used with music production changing the standards and expectations of producers and listeners of several music genres. For example, most music consumed is currently streamed or downloaded and eliminates the need for physical distribution of music to stores. The societal change in music consumption significantly minimizes the need for independent artists to be signed to a record company to get their music to a potential audience.

In contrast, Paul DiMaggio reasons that most popular culture is not molded by society's lens but are products of industries.[9] There are creators of cultural content, but cultural content is then co-opted and mass-produced by large companies and organizations. From this perspective, popular culture is viewed as a commodity that is sold to an audience. When an independent artist or style of music gains popularity, it is then copied, produced, and distributed by record companies to the public in order to capitalize on a trend. The increased reliance on technology to communicate and entertain the public has decreased the influence of regional and local cultural trends/culture. Another factor that impacts popular culture is the speed at which it is presented to an audience. The internet has become a way for companies/organizations to share their mass-produced content to the public quickly.

Popular culture is constantly in flux because it is always changing as Fiske argues that popular culture is driven "if the cultural commodities or texts do not contain resources out of which the people can make their own meanings of their social relations and identities, they will be rejected and will fail in the marketplace. They will not be made popular."[10] For something to become culturally vogue requires it serves both the producers and consumers of cultural commodities. Importantly, if popular culture is viewed as a produced and consumed product, it can be seen as a shift from the cultural to the materialistic and economic. Then, it could be argued that there is a constant struggle between mass-produced and bespoke popular culture.

From the above, we can see how popular culture is interpreted is up to one's area of discipline and areas of interest. Just thinking about it as a field of study, it could be argued that it crosses every discipline. With every discipline, some different lenses and perspectives impact how it interprets and applies theories. With such a variety of fields exploring popular culture and its theories, popular culture is not monolithic because a scholar's discipline can also shape meanings and interpretations. Even between the two authors of this chapter, though we work within the same communication discipline, we are examining different aspects and experiences of popular culture. The field has developed in niches and subsets of popular culture, so knowing how COVID will specifically impact every field and discipline is most certainly beyond the scope of this chapter.

Understanding the COVID pandemic's impact on popular culture theory should be looked at in a twofold approach that encompasses short and long-term effects on how it is viewed and researched. We maintain that both approaches to examine popular culture theory are impacted ontologically. We also argue that COVID has created changes in behaviors similar to those seen during the 1918 pandemic. Due to the COVID pandemic, changes include how groups and people gather and how we work, travel, and educate. Some of the changes that have occurred will be ephemeral; some will be perennial and need to be examined and understood in relation to their impact on popular culture and popular culture theory. Short- and long-term effects on the popular culture lens can be seen in teaching, research, creating, and consuming/using popular culture. An example can be seen in the use of memes, their meanings, and how they are used and viewed has changed as a communication means over the years. Memes have shifted from benign repeated catchphrases or images to sayings and images that carry political or social messages.

The way popular culture is shared has changed swiftly over the past three decades due to technological advancements such as computers and cell phones. Technology has always impacted how pop culture is generated, communicated, consumed, and shared. It can be argued that water cooler talk about events, ideas, and current trends have been replaced by checking one's social media on one's phone. Technology has helped create a marketplace for a cultural economy for anything relevant to a person and is not bound by time or geography. This shift has created an environment that allows people to share, design, and consume popular culture at an unprecedented pace. Technology historically has always been an accelerant to popular culture, whether it was the telephone, telegraph, movies, television, or the internet. It has advanced how fast a group or individual communicates, and with access, it has hastened how people learn about other cultures, fashion, or music.

The most significant impact that the COVID Bubble has had on popular culture theory is not about rewriting theories or definitions but how it shifted how technology was used and its effects on people's actions. For instance, shelter in place orders forced individuals to communicate in new and different ways. That resulted in changes to how people consumed, created, and shared information. The COVID Bubble has created an event that creates the lens to filter the theory when researchers do their work. As a result, scholars cannot look at popular culture theory as static statements of truth but living concepts or ideas that help understand a moment.

The lens that changes how scholars view, relate, and research includes one's academic background or area and the classroom and previously stated how people create, consume, and use popular culture. Consider how many educators had to make changes in teaching, and this shift impacted teachers, students, and parents. The pandemic has created a shift from teaching face-to-face to online or hyflex classrooms. The dramatic change from how classrooms operated created several short-term issues because there was an extensive reliance on technology. To help bring this into context, the traditional classroom fundamentally impacts how students and teachers communicate, how lectures are conducted, how classes meet, the taking and grading examinations, the turning in of assignments, and so on. To make a shift to the classroom occur, classroom technology was quickly adopted in response to the pandemic. The dramatic change that happened was a short-term solution to continue with the job of educating. We cannot predict what classrooms will look like in the future, but it would be safe to say that the pandemic will help shape them in some form or fashion. The classroom teaching paradigm shift also created changes for researchers, those who create content, and how individuals consume and use popular culture.

Culture shifts that happen during crisis times are not new and create short and long-term changes. When it comes to research, short-term impacts can be observed. It can be assumed that COVID halted some research because of safety and health reasons or the inability to access research because of the shelter in place restrictions. These and plenty of other similar issues are really about conducting research, and it is safe to assume that these problems will eventually be resolved. The long-term effects are issues that scholars should always consider when conducting research and applying or creating theories regarding popular culture in time and the times the research is conducted. Each discipline background, as well as personal experiences, brings a unique lens that can be applied. Time is what brings the change to popular culture theory and the research.

Technology has played a crucial role in communicating, working, creating, consuming, and sharing information. In the last twenty years, key impacts technology on breaking downtime and geographical boundaries, commerce, and means of production entertainment, news, and information. Since the outbreak of the pandemic, the Americans' amount of time spent online has increased, and over half of Americans say the internet has become indispensable.[11] The increase has happened on social media, chat apps, and streaming platforms.[12] Technology and internet use are not something new, but COVID is a catalyst for the increase. As a result, a transient situation has been created, thus allowing the researcher to examine and explain popular culture's impacts. Examples of other modern times of crisis that created temporary cultural shifts include hurricane Katrina, September 11, or the housing crisis of 2008. All of the events started to change with short and long-term impacts that can be seen and felt today. We would argue that the same can be said about COVID-19 and its implications to popular culture.

DEFINING THE COVID BUBBLE

The impact to popular culture theory and research will be seen in a concept to which we alluded above, the COVID Bubble, that window of time that has created a disruption and restrictions for such things as the workplace, economic actives, communication between people, and entertainment for society and individuals during the COVID-19 pandemic. This bubble is the cursory ontological effect and response COVID-19 has on researchers and research. It has disrupted the prepandemic rhythms of research, workflow, and possible data results collections. The COVID Bubble's interference has not created a change in popular culture theory but produced a window into a time that altered behaviors and habits. Those are viewed, interpreted, and researched within popular culture to consider how that changed during the COVID Bubble.

The COVID Bubble utmost is a change to a researcher's lens of popular culture, and those impacts are transitory. Will the COVID Bubble create lasting implications for academics and how they view popular culture theory? Maybe, but we will have to wait and see what those are. Perhaps we can look at the changes 9/11 or Hurricane Katrina brought to help speculate about the long-term effects, but we can see the short-lived influence it has. It is critical to identify the fundamental variables of the COVID Bubble, the first being COVID-19 and the use of technology, COVID-19 being the catalyst for the pandemic, and technology being the tool that allows society to communicate, work, teach, and entertain itself.

The implications of the COVID Bubble create thought-provoking changes and questions to popular culture research lenses. Has the reliance on technology accelerated a shift? Has it worked to create a monoculture because time and geographical boundaries are broken down? How should popular culture be evaluated, judged, and viewed due to the cultural behavior shift that has been created? Technology and its use within popular culture are not new, but what about the conditions that were created and why? How is the environment within popular culture different now than before the pandemic? Examining that element is key to framing technology's role within it while in a time of crisis. Within the context of technology being a lens to view popular culture, we should consider its role within the popular culture universe and the tribalism that it can create. The question that could be posed regarding this lens is whether or not, or to what degree, it made cultural tribalism more explicate or perhaps accelerated it. It is questioning how the lens should approach applying theory due to the pandemic situation.

The COVID Bubble has created a change in societal behavior and its reaction to work and maintaining a new normal under the circumstances. Keeping that in mind, the theory related to popular culture has not changed, but social norms, habits, and expectations have. Therefore, theories need to be framed in the context of the times they are used to study. It becomes the researcher's responsibility to frame the theory with lenses to help the field move forward. It should be the nature of the field to be able to ontologically examine anything within the popular culture to help understand its ever-changing nature.

POP CULTURE, COVID, AND RESEARCH

The public and private upheaval caused by the COVID-19 pandemic has produced a crisis response that will most likely continue to change the communication lenses we use to frame pop culture. Crisis communication, at least from a public relations perspective, may be understood by breaking it into three phases: precrisis, crisis response, and postcrisis.[13] At one end of the crisis communication continuum, precrisis includes planning for potential disasters and preventing any communication crises that may arise. Postcrisis encompasses behaviors such as crisis analysis, victim follow-up, learning, and healing on the opposite end of the continuum.[14] Thus, considering how pop culture has been affected by the pandemic, we must consider that we are currently in the crisis response stage, including the ongoing communication and mitigation efforts of public and private associations. At the time of this writing, we do not have the luxury of analyzing the postcrisis response or clarifying how we handle the current crisis response. However, we can examine the current ways in which the pandemic has shifted our use of pop culture within the various communities of interest. Researchers can conclude that the increase in media usage such as social media, films, music, and gaming has impacted pop culture with some certainty.[15]

During crises, particularly health crises, social trust and community resilience are essential qualities because of the crisis's high emotional responses.[16] Community resilience is part of the crisis response and relates to our ability to respond to a coherent group crisis. Responding as a group includes anticipating threats, reducing vulnerability, and the initial recovery from a crisis.[17] Essentially, if we have a community of people we trust behind us during a crisis, we can bounce back better and quicker and more readily withstand stress. Pop culture is in a unique position to gather communities of people with similar interests and outlooks.

It comes as no surprise that conferences across disciplines were canceled, postponed, or moved online during the pandemic, and although such face-to-face networking opportunities with colleagues have potentially diminished, the opportunity for pop culture research has arguably increased. Technology and pop culture are exponentially linked, and some may argue that modern pop culture does not exist without technology.[18] Additionally, the shift to virtual networking and conferences has been opened to those who may otherwise not have had access to the pop culture research conversation, such as junior scholars or those from schools with minimal professional development funds. For example, on average, the costs associated with a traditional face-to-face, in-country conference with plane travel and hotel range between $1,500 and $2,500. However, as a response to budget cuts in travel, travel restrictions globally, and other factors affecting conferences, several conferences that specifically address research on pop culture were (and still are) offering virtual conference registration for free, and expensive travel is unnecessary.

Prior to the pandemic, scholarly research was already shifting to collecting most data through online technology such as online survey platforms, participation solicitation through social media, and online IRB and ethics board approval processes. COVID-19 has accelerated this process for some, streamlined the process for others, and in some cases, prolonged the process. In addition, as more people seek out pop culture as a leisure activity or to survive the pandemic,[19] this opens up new opportunities for pop culture researchers to tap into.

POP CULTURE, COVID, AND THE CLASSROOM

Instructors of all kinds had to shift their classrooms rapidly to online instruction at the start of the pandemic, some of them making drastic changes that were well out of our comfort zones. These shifts created time management issues, routine interruption, burnout, and zoom fatigue, among many other effects. Unfortunately, the increased use of pop culture in the classroom has often been overlooked to stave off these effects and keep things interesting and engaging. Traditional activities in a traditional classroom, such as worksheets and small group games, were not feasible in an online or hyflex teaching environment, and previously unused technology helped facilitate pop culture integration. Although integrating pop culture in the classroom is nothing new (consider "edutainment" and "gamification," for example), pop culture integration increased significantly during the pandemic.[20] In the short term, instructors began using more integrative media such as TikTok and other cultural phenomena to illustrate concepts and ideas that were hard to demonstrate virtually.

While engagement in the classroom during the pandemic decreased overall,[21] exploratory studies suggest that students became more engaged, instructors felt less clumsy in the online format because of pop culture integration.[22] Of course, we can only speculate on the long-term effects of the increased use of pop culture in the classroom. Still, anecdotally, instructors seem more comfortable not only integrating pop culture into the classroom but are also significantly more adept at using technology to do so. Indeed, we all turned to pop culture during the pandemic to help with "distraction, inspiration, consolation, escapism, hope," and that seems to be continuing as we move through to the new normal.

Popular culture use in the classroom is just one of the individual lenses of popular culture due to COVID-19. The pandemic has unequivocally shifted the lenses that guide our individual frameworks for applying pop culture in our classrooms and how students perceive the integration and efficacy of pop culture in the classroom space. Simultaneously, our perspectives and interpretations of what pop culture is and how it relates to technology have shifted as well; the "new normal," so to speak.

PREDICTIONS FOR THE FUTURE OF POPULAR CULTURE RESEARCH AND TEACHING

There is no doubt that the pandemic has significantly altered the way scholars and instructors approach popular culture research and teaching. The critical questions regarding this shift is *how* it has changed research and teaching and *if* that shift will be permanent. Our prediction for the future is that this period of change in popular culture will not be permanent but will have some lasting effects that may shift later perspectives. Although we still do not benefit from viewing the pandemic from a historical standpoint, we are beginning to shift into a post-pandemic/postcrisis response stage. Public mask mandates have recently been lifted or loosened. We are starting to see people return to comfortable everyday routines such as dining out and attending large outdoor events, among other "normal" or pre-pandemic activities. As people shift to more comfortable habits, we will see less focus on alleviating stress and boredom and more transition to face-to-face communities and activities.

As we see these changes taking place socially, popular culture research and teaching will be directly affected. As we move back into the classrooms face-to-face, instructors will most likely be converting back to more traditional methods of classroom engagement while retaining some elements of online and hyflex instruction. For example, instructors now comfortable with the online and hyflex teaching methods required by the pandemic can deliver and integrate pop culture elements into their classrooms using technology they did not have access to prior to the pandemic. As we move into the post-pandemic period of research, we will see similar changes. Scholars put a lot of their research on hold during the pandemic because of the inability to collect data; however, infrastructure such as social media, online meeting platforms, and access to online participation has increased during the pandemic and is not likely to decrease post-pandemic.

NOTES

1. John Storey, *Cultural Theory and Popular Culture: An Introduction*, 5th ed. (Routledge, 2009).
2. Tony Bennett, "Popular Culture: A Teaching Object," *Screen Education* 34 (1980): 18.
3. Marcel Danesi, *Popular Culture: Introductory Perspectives* (Rowman & Littlefield, 2018).
4. Ray Browne, "Popular Culture: Notes toward a Definition," in *Popular Culture and Curricula*, by Ray Browne and Ronald Ambrosetti (Bowling Green University Press, 1972), 3–11.
5. John Fiske, *Understanding Popular Culture* (Boston: Unwin Hyman, 1989a), 23.
6. Storey, *Cultural Theory and Popular Culture: An Introduction*, 1.
7. Fred Niederman and Salvatore March, "The 'Theoretical Lens' Concept: We All Know What It Means, but Do We All Know the Same Thing?," *Communications of the Association for Information Systems* 44 (January 2019): 1–33, https://doi.org/10.17705/1CAIS.04401.
8. Ward H. Goodenough, *Culture, Language, and Society* (London: The Benjamin Cummings Publishing Company, 1981).
9. Paul DiMaggio, "Market Structure, the Creative Process, and Popular Culture: Toward an Organizational Reinterpretation of Mass Culture Theory," *Journal of Popular Culture* 11 (1977).
10. John Fiske, *Reading the Popular* (Boston: Unwin Hyman, 1989b), 2.
11. "53% of Americans Say the Internet Has Been Essential During the COVID-19 Outbreak," *Pew Research Center: Internet, Science & Tech* (blog), April 30, 2020, https://www.pewresearch.org/internet/2020/04/30/53-of-americans-say-the-internet-has-been-essential-during-the-covid-19-outbreak/.
12. "The Virus Changed the Way We Internet," *The New York Times,* April 7, 2020, https://www.nytimes.com/interactive/2020/04/07/technology/coronavirus-internet-use.html.
13. Robert L. Heath and H. Dan O'Hair, *Handbook of Risk and Crisis Communication*, 1st ed. (Taylor & Francis Group, 2008), http://search.ebscohost.com/login.aspx?direct=true&AuthType=ip,shib&db=cat06556a&AN=val.9922312981802931&site=eds-live&scope=site&custid=val1.
14. Mark Chong, "A Crisis of Epidemic Proportions: What Communication Lessons Can Practitioners Learn from the Singapore SARS Crisis?," *Public Relations Quarterly* 51, no. 1 (Spring 2006): 6–11.
15. Heidi Macdonald, "The Year Without Comic-Con," in *Publishers Weekly*, vol. 267 (Publishers Weekly, PWxyz LLC, 2020), 33–40,
16. "The Virus Changed the Way We Internet," *The New York Times*.

17. Heath and O'Hair, *Handbook of Risk and Crisis Communication.*

18. Derek Prall, "Connection Matters: Technology, Communication and Connection," *American City & County Exclusive Insight*, May 20, 2020, N.PAG-N.PAG.

19. Kim Kelly, "No New Normal: Who Will We Be When This Nightmare Is Over?," *Bitch Magazine: Feminist Response to Pop Culture*, no. 88 (Fall 2020): 24–31.

20. "Global Pc Gaming Hardware Market Forecast Expects Surge in 2020 Due to Covid," *Computer Graphics World* 43, no. 2 (March 2020): 6–6.

21. Smith, Michelle & Garrett, Stacie. "High leverage practices create transformative learning amid COVID-19" *The Delta Kappa Gamma Bulletin: International Journal for Professional Educators.*

22. William Visco, "Popping pedagogy: Making your classroom (traditional and virtual) pop with pop culture."

Index

ABC News, on hydroxychloroquine, 29, 35
Abdul-Jabbar, Kareem, 122, 128
accuracy, in journalism, 42–43
ACLU, 58
advocacy journalism, 26
Aggeler, Madeleine, 10
alcohol, 169
Ali, Muhammad, 128
Alito, Samuel, 64
Allsop, Joe, 46
Alsdurf, Phillis E., 194
Amazon, 96, 192, 215
ambient digital rhetoric, 2–6
Ambient Rhetoric (Rickert), 2
American Society of Newspaper Editors, 26
Anderson, C. W., 27
Anderson, Eric, 62
Angel Studios, 192
anti-Asian discrimination: health communication research on, 170–73; interpersonal communication and, 176–77
Antifa, 149
anti-vaccination groups, 148
anxiety: of athletes, 121; communitas and, 202; crisis communication and, 95; public relations and, 82; from social isolation, 169; sport communication and, 119, 120
"Applying Catholic Social Teachings to Ethical Issues in Marketing" (Klein and Laczniak), 196
Asians: discrimination against, 170–73, 176–77; as model minority, 171–72
Associated Press Managing Editors, Code of Ethics of, 26
Association of Tennis Professionals, *115*
Athletes for Hope, 121

Baker, Bradley J., 128
The Baker and the Beauty, 192
Bank of America, 94
Barreto, Matt, 172
Barth, Karl, 194
Baylor, Elgin, 124
Beehler, Donald Gene, 193
Bell, Emily, 27
Bennett, Tony, 213
Berg, David, 12
Berke, Andy, 63
Beshear, Andy, 63–64, 68
Bhardwaj, Anand, 4
bias: in journalism, 42; in MSM, 46; by omission, 52n61
Biden, Hunter, 44

Biden, Joe, 44; masks and, 69; on vaccinations, 122
Biles, Simone, 120
Billings, Andrew, 113
Bill of Rights, 141
Birx, Deborah, 34
Bitcoin, 13
Bitzer, Lloyd, 12
Black, Edwin, 12
Blackboard, 5
Black Lives Matter (BLM), 126; journalism on, 43; protests of, 67, 69; sport communication and, 123–24; Trump and, 149–54
Blake, Jacob, *116,* 126–28
Blasio, Bill de, 67
bleach injections, Trump and, 143–48, 161n45
BLM. *See* Black Lives Matter
Boyle, Casey, 2, 5
Brandeis, Louis, 74
Brands of Faith (Einstein), 193
Braun, Mike, 147
Breitbart News: on Floyd protests, 66; on hydroxychloroquine, 29, 30, 35, 36
Brock, Brian, 196
Broder, David, 26
Broom, Glen, 81
Brown, James J., Jr., 2
Browne, Ray, 213
Bruning, Stephen, 85–86
Bryan, Bill, 145
bubble: of NBA, 117, 121; of popular culture, 215, 217, 219–20; of WNBA, 117
Buice, Chris, 62
Burke, Kenneth, 12, 140
Bush, George W., 205
business impact of pandemic, 82

Calvary Chapel Dayton Valley v. Sisolak, 64
Campbell, Joseph, 200
Campbell Soup Company, 95

Canvas, 5
Carlos, John, 124, 126–27, 128
Carlson, Tucker, 66
Cassling, 88
CBS News: on hydroxychloroquine, 29, 30, 32; on police killings of Black people, 125
CDC. *See* Centers for Disease Control and Prevention
Center, Allen, 81
Centers for Disease Control and Prevention (CDC), 65, 69, 143; on bleach injections, 147, 148; on interpersonal communication, 176; on masks, 144; myths on, 200; religion and, 193; trust in, 90
Ceraso, Steph, 2
Chauvin, Derek, 125, 149
child abuse, 169
China, 9, 167
Choi, Mina, 175
The Chosen, 192
Choung, Hyesun, 175
Christian Ethics in a Technological Age (Brock), 196
Christianity Today Magazine, 194
"Christian Public Relations Strategies and 'The Last Temptation of Christ'" (Beehler), 193
circulation studies, 14
climate change, journalism on, 43
cloffice, 4
Clorox, 97
Cloud, Dana, 14, 15
CNN: on bleach injections, 146; on hydroxychloroquine, 29, 33
Code of Ethics: of Associated Press Managing Editors, 26; of RTDNA, 41; of Society of Professional Journalists, 30
Coinbase, 91
Colaner, Colleen Warner, 192
communitas, religious communication and, 198, 201–2, 206–7

comorbidities: framing and, 34; with hydroxychloroquine, 51n57
compelling state interest, First Amendment and, 58
contact tracing apps, 4
content neutrality: First Amendment and, 58–59; masks and, 74
contexualization, of science, 37
Coombs, Timothy, 81, 84, 88, 90, 92, 97–98
Cornell School, of rhetoric, 12
corporate social responsibility (CSR): crisis communication and, 93–97; in precrisis, 91; public relations and, 83–85
cosmology episodes, 87
Costantini, Rebecca, 90
Couric, Katie, 2
Couture, Barbara, 10
COVID-19 pandemic. *See specific topics*
Crane, Andrew, 84, 96–97
crisis: popular culture in, 213–23; public relations in, 87–89; self-efficacy in, 173–74
crisis communication, 92–97; for employees, 95–97
crisis event, public relations in, 92–97
Crisis Text Line, 171
Crowley, John P., 177
cryptocurrency, 13; in precrisis, 91
CSR. *See* corporate social responsibility
Cuomo, Andrew, 66, 67
Cuomo, Chris, 146
Curran, James, 26
Curry, Alexander L., 129
Curry, Stephen, 144
Cutlip, Scott, 81
CVS Health, 96

Danesi, Marcel, 213
Declaration of Independence, 141
deep mediatization, 14
deferential standard, in *Jacobson v. Massachusetts*, 58

Delta variant, 43, 116
democracy. *See* public address
Democrats, in journalism, 45
Department of Homeland Security (DHS), 145
Department of the Interior, 151–52
depression: of athletes, 121; interpersonal communication and, 175, 176–77; from social isolation, 169
DHS. *See* Department of Homeland Security
diffractive wearing, 3, 4
"The Digital" (Boyle), 5
digital rhetoric, 1–16; ambient, 2–6; hyperpublicity, 7, 9–11; postpandemic research and teaching on, 15–16; publics and privacy, 6–8; of reality, 12–14
Dilanian, Ken, 43
DiMaggio, Paul, 216
disinformation/misinformation: religion and, 197; on science, 143; on social media, 46
distance learning, sport communication and, 119
Dodd, Melissa, 84
Domestic Violence Helpline, 169–70
doomscrolling, 14
double standard, 66, 74–75
Doyle, Jason P., 128
Duarte, Jose, 45
Dunwoody, Sharon, 41
Duvivier-Dodds, Eleonora, 195

Edelman, Adam, 146
education, 3, 4; health communication research for, 178; for journalism, 25–29; popular culture and, 218–19, 221–22; sport communication and, 119, 130–31; on Zoom, 6–7, 10, 15–16, 130
Edwards, Harry, 127
Einstein, Mara, 193
elder abuse, 169

elderly, 168
Elements of Journalism (Kovach and Rosenstiel), 38
Emergency Broadband Benefit, 5
employees, crisis communication for, 95–97
ESPN, 112, 129
essential workers, 94, 97–98
ethics: in journalism, 26. *See also* Code of Ethics
Eyman, Douglas, 3
Ezike, Ngozi, 147

Facebook: family communication on, 174; interpersonal communication on, 175, 176; religion and, 196
Facebook Live, 5, 144
FaceTime, 11
fake Instagram (finsta), 8
fake news, media as, 146, 147
Faraj, Samar, 4
Fauci, Anthony, 69, 144; myths on, 200
FCC, 4–5
Feder, Lillian, 128
Federalist 10 (Madison), 137
Federalist 37 (Madison), 137
Federalist 41 (Madison), 137
Filo, Kevin, 129
finsta (fake Instagram), 8
First Amendment, 55–76; freedom of speech and, 55–56, 65–74; lockdowns and, 56; masks and, 56–57; religion in, 58–60, 61–65, 193; teaching and research implications of, 74–75
Fiske, John, 213, 216
flattening the curve, 23
Floyd, George, 56, 65–68, 124–25, 149, 152, 154; sport communication and, 114
Forbes, Bruce David, 191, 192–97
Forbes v. County of San Diego, 61
four-factor test, of *Jacobson v. Massachusetts*, 58

Fox News: on Floyd protests, 66; on hydroxychloroquine, 29, 35, 36; on sport communication, 120
framing: of hydroxychloroquine, 29–42; in journalism, 28–29; in MSM, 28–29, 34; of science, 36–37
Francis (Pope), 62, 197
Fraser, Nancy, 6
Frazier, Darnella, 125
Frederic, Katherine J., 194
freedom of speech: First Amendment and, 55–56, 65–74; masks and, 69–74
Free Exercise Clause, 61, 65
Friedberg, Anne, 10
Friesen, Norm, 10
Frith, Jordan, 13–14
frontline workers, 96–97

gathering restrictions. *See* First Amendment
Gavison, Ruth, 7–8
Geertz, Clifford, 189
Geller, Pamela, 66–68
General Motors, 94
George, Kurivilla, 194
George, Paul, 121
Givens v. Newsom, 59
Gobert, Rudy, 112
Good, Tiara, 129
Goodenough, Ward, 215
Google Meet, religious communication on, 206
Gorsuch, Neil, 60, 64, 65
The Gospel According to Peanuts (Short), 190
Gostin, Lawrence, 57
Gottlieb, Scott, 161n45
Gouge, Catherine, 3
GPS, reality and, 12
Graham, Gordon, 194
Greenwald, Glen, 44
Gries, Laurie, 14
grocery store apps, 5
groupthink, 45

Grunig, James, 86
Guardian, on social media misinformation, 46
Gumbel, Bryant, 2
Guttman, Nurit, 178

Habermas, Jürgen, 6–7, 140
Han, Byung-Chul, 208
Han, Yoon Kyoung, 196
handwashing, interpersonal communication on, 176
Hansen, Anders, 42
Hawk, Byron, 3
health communication research, 167–80; on anti-Asian discrimination, 170–73; on current pandemic situation, 167–70; family communication and, 172–73; interpersonal communication and, 174–77; on lockdowns, 168–70; practical implications of, 178; suggestions for, 179–80
Hearst, William Randolph, 24
Heath, Robert, 81, 84
hierophany, religious communication and, 199–200, 203–4, 207–8
Highway to Heaven, 192
Hilton, 94
Hitler, Adolf, 141
HIV/AIDS, 122–1223
Holladay, Sherry, 84
Hon, Linda, 86
Hoover, Stewart, 191, 210n9
Huffington Post, on hydroxychloroquine, 29
Hur, Won-Moo, 85
hydroxychloroquine: comorbidities with, 51n57; framing of, 29–42; MSM on, 25, 42; sandwiching of, 21–34; Trump and, 30, 31–34, 36, 42, 46; with zinc, 35, 52n65
hyperpublicity, 7, 9–11

identity: meatspace and, 10–11; privacy and, 8

"I Have a Dream" (King, M.), 141
Ihm, Jennifer, 175
Industrial Revolution, sport communication and, 117, 118
infrastructure, 4–5; of education, 15; reality and, 14
Inside Higher Ed, 6, 7
Instagram: finsta, 8; interpersonal communication on, 175
Intercept, 44
intermediate scrutiny, First Amendment and, 58, 60
International Journal of Sport Communication, 128
intimate partner violence, 169

Jacobson v. Massachusetts, 56, 57–61
James, LeBron, 120, 122
Johnson, Earvin "Magic," 122–23
Jones, John, 3
Jordan, Michael, 112, 126
journalism, 23–47; accuracy in, 42–43; biases in, 42; education for, 25–29; ethics in, 26; framing in, 28–29; future research in, 42–44; history of, 24–25; as knowledge brokers, 39; masks in, 23; pandemic impact on, 41–42; point of view in, 45–46; public relations and, 25–26; sandwiching in, 21–34; science in, 23–24, 27–28, 41–42; social media in, 43; truth in, 26–27. *See also* mainstream news media
Journal of Media and Religion, 192
The Journal of Religion and Popular Culture, 191
The Journal of Religion in Film, 191
The Journal of Religious Communication, 191
Jun, Jungmi, 176

Kaepernick, Colin, 124, 126
Kennedy, John F., 205
Kentucky Derby, *115*
keywords, in framing, 28–29

Kim, Hanna, 85
Kim, Heejung S., 193
King, Billie Jean, 124, 128
King, Martin Luther, Jr., 141
Kirkpatrick, David, 8
KKK. *See* Ku Klux Klan
Klein, Thomas A., 196
Kleinmann, Christie M., 129
Klinenberg, Eric, 205
knowledge brokers, journalism as, 39
Kovach, Bill, 38
Krizek, Robert L., 113
Ku Klux Klan (KKK), 71–72
Kushner, Jared, 127
Kuypers, Jim A., 28, 31–32

Laczniak, Gene R., 196
Ladies Professional Golf Association, *115*
Lancet, on hydroxychloroquine, 29–43, 46, 51n57
Lanham, Richard, 2, 16
Le, Thomas, 172
Ledingham, John, 85–86
Lee, Chul-Joo, 175
Lee, Suyeon, 177
Lerbinger, Otto, 88
Let Them Play v. Walz, 60
Lev, Eimi, 178
Levin, David, 29
liberal public sphere, 140–48; Trump and, 143–48
Liguori, Eric, 87
liminality, religious communication and, 198–99, 202–3, 207
Lincoln, Abraham, 138, 141
Lippmann, Walter, 27, 46–47
Litt, David, 139
Little Mosque on the Prairie, 192
Lloyd-Smith, Jamie, 63
lockdowns (stay-at-home orders): communitas and, 202; First Amendment and, 56; health communication research on, 168–70; journalism on, 43; MSM on, 24; public relations on, 82; religious communication in, 206; Zoom in, 9
Logan, Lara, 44–45
Logan, Robert K., 189
loneliness: communitas and, 202; interpersonal communication and, 175; from quarantine, 118; from social isolation, 169; sport communication and, 117
Los Angeles Times, 112
Love, Kevin, 121
Lyden, John C., 190–91
Lysol, 147

MacDougall, Robert, 189
Madison, James, 137, 139, 141, 153
Mahan, Jeffrey H., 190, 191, 192–97
mainstream news media (MSM): bias in, 46; framing in, 28–29; future research in, 42–44; on hydroxychloroquine, 25, 42; on lockdowns, 24
Major League Baseball (MLB), 90, 94, 114, 118; Blake and, 126; BLM and, 126; on racial injustice, 125; timeline of, *115–16*; on vaccinations, 122
Major League Soccer (MLS): BLM and, 126; timeline of, *115–16*; on vaccinations, 122
March, Salvatore, 215
Marist Center for Sports Communication, 119
Marriott, 94
masks: anti-Asian discrimination and, 172; case law on, 72–73; CDC on, 144; First Amendment and, 56–57; freedom of speech and, 69–74; health communication research on, 178; in journalism, 23; in precrisis, 90; public relations on, 82; religion and, 62, 65
Massie, Thomas, 64
Matten, Dirk, 84, 96–97
Mazur, Eric Michael, 190–91
McDonaldization of Church, 193

McEnany, Kayleigh, 146
McKinsey Group, 1–2
McManus, Jane, 119
meatspace, 10–11
media: on bleach injections, 146–48; as fake news, 146, 147; future research in, 42–44; reality from, 12; Trump in, 150–53. *See also* journalism; mainstream news media; popular culture; social media; *specific types*
mediations, 14, 15
memes, 217
mental health, sport communication and, 120–21
Michael Scott (fictional character), 12
Microsoft Teams, 5
MiLB. *See* Minor League Baseball
Millard, Egan, 149
Minor League Baseball (MiLB), *115*
misinformation. *See* disinformation/misinformation
MLB. *See* Major League Baseball
MLS. *See* Major League Soccer
monomyth, 200
Moore, Russell, 197
Mountifield, Charles, 129
MSM. *See* mainstream news media
MSNBC, on hydroxychloroquine, 29
Mulvihill, Mike, 120
Musk, Elon, 35
myth, religious communication and, 200, 204–5, 208

N95 masks, 94
National Association for Stock Car Racing (NASCAR), 111, 118; timeline of, *115*
National Basketball Association (NBA), 90, 112, 114, 118; Blake and, 126–27; BLM and, 123–24; bubble of, 117, 121; on racial injustice, 125; timeline of, *115–16*
National Football League (NFL), 111; on racial injustice, 125; on vaccinations, 122

National Hockey League (NHL), 90, *116,* 118; Blake and, 126; BLM and, 126; on vaccinations, 122
National Women's Soccer League (NWS), *115–16*; on vaccinations, 122
Nature, 148
Nazione, Samantha, 175–76
NBA. *See* National Basketball Association
NBC News: on bleach injections, 145; on hydroxychloroquine, 29, 30, 35
Netflix, 3, 215
new normal, 97–98
New York Times, 26; on Blake protests, 127; on hydroxychloroquine, 29, 32–33, 34, 36, 37, 40; Spayd and, 44; on Trump photo-op, 151
NFL. *See* National Football League
Nguyen, Thu, 170, 176
NHL. *See* National Hockey League
Niderman, Fred, 215
9/11: myths of, 205; sport communication and, 118
Nissenbaum, Helen, 8
Noah, Trevor, 144
NPR, on Trump photo-op, 151
nudists, on Zoom, 11
NWS. *See* National Women's Soccer League

Obama, Barack, 127, 140, 141
Occupational Safety and Health Administration, 193
Ochs, Adolph, 26
The Office, 12
Olympic Project for Human Rights, 127
Olympics, *115*; cancellation of, 203; protest at, 124
omission: bias by, 52n61; errors of, 26; framing and, 34
Osaka, Naomi, 121
Oshin-Martin, Moronke, 87
Osteen, Joel, 193
Ovide, Shira, 9
Oxford Internet Institute, 46

Pace, Kristin, 175–76
Paralympics Games, *115*
parent-child relationships, 174
Park, Young, 84
patient-provider communication, 177
Patterson, Orlando, 140
Patterson, Thomas E., 26, 27, 28, 39, 46–47
Paul, Rand, 63
pedagogy: of digital rhetoric, 6; of liberal public sphere, 140; of sport communication, 112, 128–31
Pedersen, Paul M., 113
peer review, lack of, 40
Perrault, Evan, 175–76
Perry, Ronald, 88
Pfister, Damien, 7
Pfizer-BioNTech vaccine, 114
PGA. *See* Professional Golfers' Association
Phelps, Michael, 121
Pinterest, 4
Pittz, Stephen, 87
point of view, in journalism, 45–46
politicization: of protests, 55–76. *See also* Black Lives Matter; First Amendment
Politico, on Trump photo-op, 151
PolitiFact, 146
Poppovich, Gregg, 122
popular culture: bubble of, 215, 217; in crisis, 213–23; defined, 213–14; education and, 218–19, 221–22; future research on, 222–23; religion and, 190–205; research on, 220–21; theoretical views of, 214–19
postcrisis, public relations in, 97–98
precrisis, public relations in, 89–91
prevention/mitigation stage, of precrisis, 89
Prinzivalli, Leah, 11
Pritzker, J. B., 63
privacy: in education, 15–16; publics and, 6–8

Professional Golfers' Association (PGA): on racial injustice, 125; timeline of, *115*; on vaccinations, 122
propaganda, of public relations, 25–26
Protagoras, 12
protests: of BLM, 67, 69; of Floyd murder, 56, 65–68, 125; of lockdowns, 56; politicization of, 55–76; sport communication and, 123–28; Trump and, 139–40, 164n90
PR Relationship Measurement Scale (Hon and Grunig), 86
PRSA. *See* Public Relations Society of America
public address, 137–57; implications for teaching and research, 153–55; liberal public sphere and, 140–48; of Trump, 139–40, 143–55
public concern: with masks, 72; in precrisis, 89
Public Health Emergency of International Concern, by World Health Organization, 167
public relations, 81–99; in crisis, 87–89; in crisis event, 92–97; CSR and, 83–85; defined, 81; journalism and, 25–26; on lockdowns, 82; on masks, 82; in postcrisis, 97–98; in precrisis, 89–91; RMT and, 85–87; on social distancing, 82; on sport communication, 129; on vaccinations, 82
Public Relations Society of America (PRSA), 81
publics, privacy and, 6–8
Pulitzer, Joseph, 24
"Pushing Back on the Rhetoric of 'Real' Life" (Frith), 13–14
Putin, Vladimir, 141

quarantine, 1; loneliness from, 118; religion and, 63; religious communication and, 205; remote work in, 95

racial injustice: sport communication and, 123–28. *See also* Black Lives Matter; Floyd, George
Racine, Karl, 151
Radio Television Digital News Association (RTDNA), 40; Code of Ethics of, 41
Ramsek v. Beshear, 68
Raoult, Didier, 35
Rapinoe, Megan, 120
Reagan, Ronald, 140, 141, 205
Real/ClearPolitics, 44–45
reality: digital rhetoric of, 12–14; virtual, 12
Redfield, Robert, 143
Redlener, Irwin, 148
"Reflections on the Past and Future of the Study of Religion and Popular Culture" (Mahan), 190
relationship management theory (RMT), public relations and, 85–87
religion: defined, 189; in First Amendment, 58–60, 61–65, 193; masks and, 62, 65; popular culture and, 190–205; vaccinations and, 197
Religion and Popular Culture in America (Mahan and Forbes), 191, 192–97
religious communication, 189–209; communitas and, 198, 201–2, 206–7; future research on, 205–9; hierophany and, 199–200, 203–4, 207–8; key principles of, 197–200; liminality and, 198–99, 202–3, 207; myth and, 200, 204–5, 208; pioneers of, 190–92
remote work, 95; liminality and, 202–3
Renno, Wadih, 4
Reny, Tyler, 172
republican remedy, 137, 139, 141
Republicans, in journalism, 45
Rethinking Media, Religion and Culture (Hoover), 191
retractions: journalistic ethics in, 42; journalistic failures in, 40–41;

of *Lancet* hydrochloroquine study, 29–43
rhetoric. *See* public address
The Rhetorical Presidency (Tulis), 138
Rickert, Thomas, 2
RMT. *See* relationship management theory
Roberts, John, 58, 64, 73
Roman Catholic Diocese of Brooklyn v. Cuomo, 60, 61, 64
Romney, Mitt, 154
Roosevelt, Franklin D., 140, 141
Roosevelt, Theodore, 138, 141
Rosenstiel, Tom, 38
Roth, Bill, 130
The Routledge Companion to Religion and Popular Culture (Lyden and Mazur), 190–91
Rowland, Robert, 140, 142
RTDNA. *See* Radio Television Digital News Association
Rubio, Katia, 203
Rucker, Phillip, 146
Russell, Bill, 122, 124

safety protocols: crisis communication on, 91; in NBA bubble, 121; public relations on, 82; in sport communication, 130. *See also* lockdowns; masks; social distancing
safety valve, in free speech, 74
sandwiching: of hydroxychloroquine, 21–34; in journalism, 21–34
Sasaki, Joni Y., 193
Schudson, Michael, 25–26
Schulz, Charles M., 190
science: contextualization of, 37; disinformation on, 143; failure to understand good practices in, 38–41; framing of, 36–37; in journalism, 23–24, 27–28, 41–42
Scripps National Spelling Bee, *115*
self-efficacy, in crisis, 173–74
Seton, Elizabeth Ann, 201
Sharpe, Stirling, 129

shelter-in-place. *See* stay-at-home orders
Shirky, Clay, 27
shopping: online, 5; safety protocols for, 91
Short, Robert L., 190
signal detection phase, of precrisis, 89
Silver, Adam, 90
Skype: interpersonal communication on, 175; religious communication on, 206
Slack, 93
Smith, Tommie, 124, 128
Smithfield Foods, 93
Snaza, Rob, 62
social compact theory, 57
social distancing: health communication research on, 178; interpersonal communication on, 176; public relations on, 82; religious communication and, 205; well-being and, 120
social isolation. *See* lockdowns; quarantine
social media, 1, 3; family communication on, 174; interpersonal communication on, 175, 176; in journalism, 43; masks on, 69–70; misinformation on, 46; religion and, 195–96; Trump and, 46. *See also specific platforms*
Society of Professional Journalists, 26, 39; Code of Ethics of, 30
South Bay Pentecostal Church v. Newsom, 58–60, 64–65
Souza e Silava, Adria de, 13
Spayd, Liz, 44
Spencer, Craig, 148
Spicer, Sean, 66
sport communication, 111–31; declining television ratings for, 118–20; defined, 112–14; education and, 119, 130–31; Industrial Revolution and, 117, 118; mental health and, 120–21; 9/11 and, 118; pedagogy of, 112, 128–31; protests and, 123–28; public relations on, 129; racial injustice and, 123–28; religion and, 194; timeline for, *115–16*; vaccinations and, 114, 122–23; well-being and, 120–21; on Zoom, 130
Stahl, Lesley, 147
Stalin, Joseph, 141
Starbucks, 93–94, 96; religion and, 193
stay-at-home orders. *See* lockdowns
Stop AAPI Hate, 171
"Stop the Spread" campaign, 94
Storey, John, 213, 214
Streeter, Kurt, 127
strict scrutiny, First Amendment and, 58, 65
Su, Yiran, 128
suicides/suicidal ideation, 169, 173
super-spreader events, with religion, 63
surround systems, 4
symbolic speech, masks as, 56, 73
systems theory, 117

Tandon v. Newsom, 65
Tavani, Herman, 8
Taylor, Breonna, 125
Telegram, interpersonal communication on, 176
Texas Tech University (TTU), 72
3M, 94
TikTok, 128–29
Time magazine, on public address, 139
Today Show, 2
Touched by an Angel, 192
Trump, Donald J., 6; on Blake protests, 127; bleach injections and, 143–48, 161n45; BLM and, 149–54; fake news and, 146, 147; Fauci and, 144; on Floyd protests, 66; hydroxychloroquine and, 30, 31–34, 36, 42, 46; liberal public sphere and, 143–48; on masks, 69, 73, 90; in media, 150–53; photo-op at church by, 149–53; protests and, 139–40, 164n90; public address of, 139–40,

143–55; on religion, 61; social media and, 46; on Twitter, 144
trust: in CDC, 90; crisis communication for, 92, 93; of employees, 95; RMT and, 86–87
truth, in journalism, 26–27
TTU. *See* Texas Tech University
Tulis, Jeffrey K., 138
Turner, Edith, 198
Turner, Victor, 198
Twitter, 4; anti-Asian discrimination on, 170; family communication on, 174; interpersonal communication on, 176; sport communication on, 112; Trump on, 144

Ultimate Fighting Championship (UFC), *115*
underlying medical conditions, 168
unemployment, 143
University of Iowa, 24
University of Wisconsin, 24
Urs von Balthasar, Hans, 194
U.S. Open Tennis, on racial injustice, 125

vaccinations: hesitancy for, 98; myths on, 200; public relations on, 82; religion and, 197; sport communications and, 114, 122–23
Vargas, Elizabeth, 2
Varnelis, Kazys, 10

video games, 3, 172, 208, 214
virtual reality, 12
Volokh, Eugene, 63
vulnerable populations, 168

Wall Street Journal, on hydroxychloroquine, 29, 30
Walmart, 92, 95
Warren, Rick, 193
Washington, George, 138
Washington Free Beacon, on social media misinformation, 46

Washington Post: on bleach injections, 146; on hydroxychloroquine, 29, 36, 37; on hydroxychloroquine with zinc, 52n65; on social media misinformation, 46; on sport communication, 119–20; on Trump photo-op, 151
Waters, Sara, 177
Waymer, Damion, 83–84
"We Can Do This," 122
WeChat, 176
Weick, Karl, 87
well-being: in crisis, 82, 93; interpersonal communication for, 175; sport communication and, 120–21
WestWind Pictures, 192
WhatsApp, interpersonal communication on, 175, 176
Whitehead, John, 62
Whitney v. California, 74
Will, George, 146
Williams, Serena, 120
Wilson, Woodrow, 138
Winfrey, Oprah, 193
Women's National Basketball Association (WNBA), *115–16,* 118; Blake and, 126; BLM and, 123–24; bubble of, 117; protests of, 124; on racial injustice, 125; on vaccinations, 122
Woo, Bongki, 176
work. *See* remote work
World Health Organization, 114; on hydroxychloroquine, 37; Public Health Emergency of International Concern by, 167
World Wrestling Entertainment, 122
Wu, Cary, 170

Yan, Meimi, 128
yellow journalism, 24
Yeo, Junsang, 85
yoga, on Zoom, 11
YouTube, 13

Yuan, Eric, 9

Zarefsky, David, 138
Zhang, Peter, 189
zinc, hydroxychloroquine
    with, 35, 52n65

Zoom, 3, 5; education on, 6–7, 10,
    15–16, 130; hyperpublicity of, 9–11;
    interpersonal communication on,
    175; in lockdowns, 9; reality and,
    13–14; religious communication on,
    206; sport communication on, 130
Zuckerberg, Mark, 8, 144

About the Editor and Contributors

Jim A. Kuypers (Ph.D. Louisiana State University) is a professor of rhetoric and political communication at Virginia Tech. He is the author, editor, or co-author of 15 books, including *Purpose, Practice, and Pedagogy in Rhetorical Criticism* (winner of the Everett Lee Hunt Award for Outstanding Scholarship) and *Partisan Journalism: A History of Media Bias in the United States* (a *Choice* Outstanding Academic Title for 2014). He is a former co-editor for the *American Communication Journal*. He is the recipient of the American Communication Association's Outstanding Contribution to Communication Scholarship Award, the Southern States Communication Association's Early Career Research award, and Dartmouth College's Distinguished Lecturer Award. His research interests include political communication, news media framing of political events, metacriticism, and the moral/poetic use of language.

* * *

Shristi Bhochhibhoya (Ph.D. University of Oklahoma) is a post-doctoral research associate at the Center for Research on Interpersonal Violence at Georgia State University. She research interests include adolescent & sexual health, adolescent risk behaviors, and adolescent pregnancy among the diversified population.

Ann E. Burnette (Ph.D. Northwestern University) is a professor in the Department of Communication Studies at Texas State University. She publishes scholarship on political communication and freedom of expression issues. Her work has been published in national and international journals and she has received the James Madison Prize for Outstanding Free Speech Scholarship from the Southern States Communication Association. She has also received numerous teaching awards, including the Southern States

Communication Association John I. Sisco Excellence in Teaching Award and the Minnie Stevens Piper Professor Award.

Dennis D. Cali (Ph.D. Louisiana State University) is a Distinguished Professor of Arts and Sciences at the University of Texas at Tyler. He is the recipient of the Louis Forsdale Award for Outstanding Educator in the Field of Media Ecology; the President's Scholarly Achievement Award at the University of Texas at Tyler; and the Media Ecology Association's Top Paper Award for his essay on "The Sacramental View of Marshall McLuhan, Walter Ong, and James Carey," which appears in the *Explorations in Media Ecology* journal. He is also the author of *Mapping Media Ecology: Introduction to the Field*, two other books, and numerous scholarly articles in communication journals. He teaches in the areas of media ecology, rhetorical criticism, political communication, and religious communication. His primary researchinterest areas are in media ecology and religious and sacramental communication.

Amber Davisson (Ph. D. Rensselaer Polytechnic Institute) is an associate professor of communication at Keene State College. She is the author of *Lady Gaga and the Remaking of Celebrity Culture* and co-author of *Poaching Politics: Online Communication during the 2016 US Presidential Election*. Her interdisciplinary scholarship on identity, politics, and digital technology has appeared in such journals as *Rhetoric & Public Affairs, Journal of Media & Digital Literacy, Journal of Visual Literacy*, and the *American Communication Journal*. Davisson has been interviewed on NPR's *1A* and quoted in the *New York Times, Forbes*, and *Wired*.

David R. Dewberry (Ph.D. University of Denver) is a professor in the Department of Communication and Journalism at Rider University. He primarily examines free speech and the First Amendment in public discourse. His work has been recognized with the Franklyn S. Haiman Award for Distinguished Scholarship in Freedom of Expression by the National Communication Association and the James Madison Prize for Outstanding Free Speech Scholarship by the Southern States Communication Association.

Michael Eisenstadt (Ph.D. The University of Kansas) is an assistant professor & Director of Forensics at California State University, Long Beach. His research has been published in *Argumentation & Advocacy, First Amendment Studies, Review of Communication*, and in several edited volumes. He is a two-time Cross-Examination Debate Association Critic of the Year and has won numerous awards for service to the competitive speech and debate community. Eisenstadt's research interests include public argument, public address, legal argument, and political communication.

Rebekah L. Fox (Ph.D. Purdue University) is a professor at Texas State University. Her research focuses on organizational rhetoric and resilience, as well as the rhetoric of environmental and political issues specifically related to the First Amendment. Her work has been published in a variety of journals, and she has been recognized by the Southern States Communication Association's Free Speech Division with the James Madison Prize.

Michelle Gibbons (Ph.D. University of Pittsburgh) is an associate professor in the Department of Communication at the University of New Hampshire, where she regularly teaches courses in Rhetorical Theory & Criticism and Digital Rhetoric. Her research includes studies of digital phenomena, such as search engine optimization, and medical technologies, including fMRI and x-rays. She also investigates the rhetorical deployment of commonsense psychological precepts in public culture. Her work has been published in *Rhetoric Society Quarterly*, *Technical Communication Quarterly*, *Philosophy of Science*, *Journalism History*, and *Argumentation and Advocacy*, among other places.

Michael Horning (Ph.D. Penn State University) is an associate professor of multimedia journalism at Virginia Tech where he is also an affiliate with Virginia Tech's Center for Human Computer Interaction. Before entering the academy, he was a general assignment news reporter for a community newspaper in Southwest Virginia where he regularly covered government and politics. His research interest includes how emerging media technologies influence audience experience and response to news, and how such technologies shape journalistic practices. His published research examines topics as varied as how audiences responded to the use of YouTube in the 2008 election debates, how mobile devices impact audience interest in news content, and how journalistic norms and value influence political cartoonist's coverage of sensitive political topics. Horning is also recipient of the Association in Journalism and Mass Communication's top research award in new media and politics.

Justin W. Kirk (Ph.D. The University of Kansas) is an assistant professor of practice at the University of Nebraska-Lincoln: He received top paper award in Argumentation and Forensics from the Central States Communication Association in 2019 and the National Communication Association in 2020. He is the director of debate at the University of Nebraska-Lincoln and his research interests include competitive and public debate, presidential communication, public policy, gun control discourse, and argumentation theory.

Kimberly Kulovitz (Ph.D. University of Wisconsin Milwaukee) is an assistant professor of communication at Valdosta State University. Teaching and research areas focus on game theory and culture, organizational communication, and gamification.

Nneka Logan (Ph.D. Georgia State University) is an associate professor of public relations at Virginia Tech, where she is also a research associate with Virginia Tech's Center for Humanities. Prior to joining the academy, she worked in a variety of corporate communications management roles for a multibillion corporation and its subsidiaries. She has also worked as a freelance music and entertainment writer. Her research interests include public relations, organizational communication, corporate social responsibility, race, and rhetoric. Her published research explores how corporations can communicate in ways that improve society. Her industry work has won several awards from organizations such as the International Association of Business Communications and Public Relations Society of America. Her academic work has also earned awards from the public relations divisions of the National Association of Communication and the Association for Education in Journalism and Mass Communication.

Yu Lu (Ph.D. Pennsylvania State University) is an assistant professor in the Department of Health and Exercise Science at the University of Oklahoma. Her primary research interests are in health disparities and global health in the context of substance use and interpersonal violence. She also is interested in research methods particularly working with diverse cultural groups, such as accessing and gaining trust with minority populations and cross-cultural theory/measure adaptation. Her publications appear in *Health Communication, Preventive Medicine,* A*ddictive Behaviors, Journal of Research on Adolescents, Health Education Research,* among other places.

Benjamin Medeiros (Ph.D. University of California, San Diego) is an assistant professor in the Department of Communication Studies at the State University of New York at Plattsburgh. His research concerns digital media policy, internet culture, and the political history of communications regulation. He is a past recipient of the Robert O'Neill top paper award from the National Communication Association's Freedom of Expression Division and serves on the editorial board of the journal *First Amendment Studies*.

David Nelson (Ph.D. University of Southern Mississippi) is associate professor of communication at Valdosta State University. Teaching and research areas focus on social media, humor, and rhetoric.

Robert C. Rowland (Ph.D. The University of Kansas) is a professor at the University of Kansas. His many publications include *Shared Land/ Conflicting Identity: Trajectories of Israeli & Palestinian Symbol Use* (with David Frank), which won the inaugural Kohrs-Campbell Book Award; *Analyzing Rhetoric*; and more than eighty essays on rhetorical criticism, argumentation, and narrative. He received the Douglas W. Ehninger Distinguished Rhetorical Scholar Award from the National Communication Association in 2011. Rowland's research interests include critical methodologies, public argument, argumentation theory, and political communication.

YoungJu Shin (Ph.D. Pennsylvania State University) is an associate professor of health communication in the Hugh Downs School of Human Communication at Arizona State University. She has been dedicated to extending the scope of health communication and prevention intervention with the focus of culture. Her research intersects with four main areas: (1) substance use and other risky behavior prevention, (2) implementation quality and effect of prevention interventions, (3) media effect and narrative persuasion, and (4) immigrant health and communication. Her research appears in journals such as *Communication Monographs*, *Health Communication*, *Health Education Research*, *Journal of Adolescence*, *Journal of Applied Communication Research*, *Journal of Health Communication*, *Journal of Immigrant and Minority Health*, *Journal of International and Intercultural Communication*, and *Prevention Science*.

Brandi Watkins (Ph.D. The University of Alabama) is an associate professor of Communication at Virginia Tech where she teaches courses in social media and public relations. Her research examines the role of social media in brand communication and as a way to build, enhance, and maintain organization-public relationships. She is the author of the book *Sports Teams, Fans, and Twitter: The Influence of Social Media on Relationships and Branding.*" Her work has been published in *Public Relations Review*, *Journal of Brand Management*, and *International Journal of Sport Communication*.

Chelsea Woods (Ph.D. University of Kentucky) is an assistant professor of public relations at Virginia Tech. Her research interests include crisis communication, reputation management, and activism. Her published research examines topics including effective communication practices amid crises and disasters, how governing sport bodies employ corporate social responsibility, and activist groups' efforts to erode corporate reputations. Her research appears in journals such as *Public Relations Review* and *Public Relations Inquiry*, and has earned awards from the public relations divisions of the

National Association of Communication and the Association for Education in Journalism and Mass Communication. Before pursuing her Ph.D., Woods practiced public relations in the nonprofit and hospitality sectors.

www.ingramcontent.com/pod-product-compliance
Lightning Source LLC
Chambersburg PA
CBHW020114010526
44115CB00008B/827